Sickle Cell Disease in Sub-Saharan Africa

This important collection provides an epidemiological perspective on the continuing scope of sickle cell disease (SCD) in sub-Saharan Africa, alongside the clinical attempts to provide comprehensive care in a resource-limited setting.

The book moves from a clinical profile of SCD to screening for the disease and ongoing patient care. There are chapters on pain management, organ failure, infections and transfusions, as well as nutrition and neurocognitive complications. The book concludes with chapters on anti-sickness medication, cell transplantation and nursing care.

The first in a two-volume set offering a multi-disciplinary perspective on SCD, this is a comprehensive resource that applies clinical knowledge to the practical challenges faced in sub-Saharan Africa. It will be an important reading for medical students taking courses in haematology as well as those studying Public Health in sub-Saharan Africa. Practitioners in the region will also find it invaluable in developing their understanding of this pervasive disease.

Baba Inusa, MBBS (ABU 1984), FMCPaed (Nigeria, 1992), FRCPCH (UK, 1997), is Professor of paediatric haematology, Evelina London Children's Hospital, Guy's and St Thomas NHS Foundation Trust.

Kanayo Nwankwo, MD, is the Chief Resident and a lifespan sickle cell advocate, currently serving at Brookdale University Hospital in Brooklyn, NY.

Nkechikwu Azinge-Egbiri, LLB (Hons), BL, LLM, PhD (Warwick), is a Lecturer at the School of Law, Lancaster University and Founder of the Sickle Cell Aid Foundation (SCAF), a youth-led NGO she established to raise awareness of Sickle Cell Disease (SCD) and support those living with it.

Bukola Bolarinwa is a qualified legal practitioner with an LLM in International Economic Law from the University of Warwick and LLB from the University of Leicester.

'This edited book is a timely and significant contribution to the otherwise scarce literature on sickle cell disorder (SCD) from the global south. In many ways, the book unravels the intricacies of SCD by blending cutting-edge multidisciplinary research with poignant personal narratives. Packed with recognised SCD experts, this book tells a coherent story that commences by examining the micro-level cellular battles associated with SCD and then investigates relevant macro-level societal challenges. As such, the book gives its readers a holistic outlook on SCD. This is a must-read publication that I heartily recommend. It should be read by anyone seeking to appreciate the full spectrum of SCD in Africa.'

Professor Dame Elizabeth Nneka Anionwu,
OM DBE FRCN FQNI, Patron: UK Sickle Cell Society

Sickle Cell Disease in Sub-Saharan Africa

Biomedical Perspectives

Edited by Baba Inusa, Kanayo Nwankwo, Nkechikwu Azinge-Egbiri and Bukola Bolarinwa

Routledge
Taylor & Francis Group

LONDON AND NEW YORK

First published 2024
by Routledge
4 Park Square, Milton Park, Abingdon, Oxon OX14 4RN

and by Routledge
605 Third Avenue, New York, NY 10158

Routledge is an imprint of the Taylor & Francis Group, an informa business

© 2024 selection and editorial matter, Baba Inusa, Kanayo Nwankwo, Nkechikwu Azinge-Egbiri and Bukola Bolarinwa; individual chapters, the contributors

British Library Cataloguing-in-Publication Data
A catalogue record for this book is available from the British Library

Library of Congress Cataloging-in-Publication Data
Names: Inusa, Baba, editor, author. | Nwankwo, Kanayo, editor, author. | Azinge-Egbiri, Nkechikwu Valerie, editor, author. | Bolarinwa, Bukola, editor, author.
Title: Sickle cell disease in Sub-Saharan Africa, biomedical perspectives / edited by Baba Inusa, Kanayo Nwankwo, Nkechikwu Azinge-Egbiri and Bukola Bolarinwa.
Description: New York : Routledge, 2024. | Includes bibliographical references and index. |
Identifiers: LCCN 2023050297 (print) | LCCN 2023050298 (ebook) | ISBN 9781032183671 (hardback) | ISBN 9781032733852 (paperback) | ISBN 9781003463931 (ebook)
Classification: LCC RC641.7.S5 S543 2024 (print) | LCC RC641.7.S5 (ebook) | DDC 616.1/52700967--dc23/eng/20231026
LC record available at https://lccn.loc.gov/2023050297
LC ebook record available at https://lccn.loc.gov/2023050298

ISBN: 978-1-032-18367-1 (hbk)
ISBN: 978-1-032-73385-2 (pbk)
ISBN: 978-1-003-46393-1 (ebk)

DOI: 10.4324/9781003463931

Typeset in Times New Roman
by KnowledgeWorks Global Ltd.

Dear Sickle Cell Warrior,

This book is dedicated to you, with the sincere intention of positively impacting your life. Our ultimate goal is to empower doctors, nurses, caregivers, researchers, and policymakers to enhance their knowledge, practices, and policies, all for the betterment of your well-being.

We would like to honor the memory of *Awele Nwosu Akeh (1989–2015)*, a courageous advocate for sickle cell who fearlessly spoke out when stigma silenced so many warriors. Your unwavering voice has served as an inspiration for us, compelling us to pen these pages.

For you, we wrote this book.

Your Advocates

Dr. Baba Inusa, Dr. Kanayo Nwankwo,
Dr. Nkechikwu Azinge-Egbiri, Dr. Bukola Balarinwa

Contents

Figures

Tables

Contributors

Editors

Baba Inusa, MBBS (ABU 1984), FMCPaed (Nigeria, 1992), FRCPCH (UK, 1997)
  Professor of Paediatric Haematology, Evelina London Children's Hospital, Guy's and St Thomas NHS Foundation Trust
  Main research in sickle cell disease includes stroke, newborn screening, renal complications and clinical trials leadership with over 130 publications and book chapters.
  Chair, National Haemoglobinopathy Panel (NHP), www.nationalhaempanel-nhs.net, and co-lead South East/South London Haemoglobinopathy centre from 2020
  Chair, Steering Committee, Sickle Cell Improvement Project, England from April 2022 to institute changes in response to "No one's listening" report, England from April 2022
  Chief investigator for African Research and Innovative Initiative for Sickle Cell Education (ARISE) Horizon 2020 funded project 2019–2024
  Founder, Academy for sickle cell and thalassaemia (ASCAT), a leading world scientific conference in sickle cell disease and thalassaemia from 2006
  Co-chair of the treatment subcommittee for consortium for newborn screening for Africa (CONSA), an international network that seeks to demonstrate benefit of newborn and early diagnosis of sickle cell disease from 2019
  Member WHO expert group for African sickle cell centre of excellence from 2022
  Chair, grants and publication subcommittee, British Society of Haematology from June 2023

Kanayo Nwankwo, MD, is a life-span sickle cell advocate who is currently a resident physician at Brookdale University Hospital, Brooklyn, NY, where he is serving the position of the chief resident. He was elected president of the Sickle cell Aid Foundation Nigeria where he served for a period of time. During his tenure he led and energized a growing team of volunteers towards medical outreaches aimed at breaking the sickle cycle and increasing genotype awareness in very remote villages. He also advocated for the first sickle cell neonatal screening bill in the Nigerian legislative system. His research interests include gene therapy, stem cell transplant and other novel disease-modifying therapies for sickle cell disease.

Nkechikwu Azinge-Egbiri, LLB (Hons), BL, LLM & PhD (Warwick), is a Lecturer at the School of Law, Lancaster University. She is the Founder of the Sickle Cell Aid Foundation (SCAF), a youth-led NGO she established to raise awareness of Sickle Cell Disorder (SCD) and support those living with it. She is also the Co-Founder of Haima Health Initiative (HHI), established to provide blood products in real time within Nigeria. Nkechikwu has worked in numerous capacities to amplify youth involvement in non-communicable diseases (NCDs), for instance she served as a team lead with the Commonwealth Youth Health Network (CYHN) and currently volunteers for the Sickle Cell Society, UK. Nkechi's interest spans beyond sickle cell. She researches on financial crime, specifically anti-money laundering and terrorist financing regulation. She is the Founder of the Global South Dialogue on Economic Crime, a multi-disciplinary platform for advancing dialogue and combatting matters of economic crime in global south countries. Nkechi has presented and authored many articles, papers, chapters and books on her research areas.

Bukola Bolarinwa is a qualified legal practitioner with an LLM in International Economic Law from the University of Warwick and LLB from the University of Leicester. Bukola is a sickle cell advocate and founder of Haima Health Initiative, a West African NGO established to improve blood supply for patients. Bukola has received several awards for her work including the Queen's Young Leaders award and was selected as an Obama Foundation Africa Leader for her work to raise awareness about the importance of giving blood.

Contributors

Miguel Abboud, MD, MHA Professor and Chairman Department of Pediatrics and Adolescent Medicine, American University of Beirut, Beirut Lebanon, is a Pediatric Hematologist-Oncologist and sickle cell expert who has participated in many pivotal clinical trials in SCD such the STOP and STOP II studies, and the preop transfusion study. Recently he is a major contributor to developing clinical trials with new agents for the disease. He also is a member of the Medical and Research Advisory Committee of the SCDAA, the National Committee for SCD in Lebanon and contributed to the Lancet Hematology Commission on SCD.

Ademola Samson Adewoyin, MBBS, MSc, FMCPath(Haem), FWACP (Lab Med), Cert-Cellular Therapies (Wash), EMBA, is a Clinical Lecturer at the Department of Haematology and Blood Transfusion, University of Lagos. Dr. Ademola Adewoyin has been involved in academic and clinical management of persons living with SCD for over a decade. His practice also covers other anaemias, transfusion medicine, haemopoietic stem cell transplantation, blood cancers, bleeding disorders and thrombosis, cellular therapies, laboratory quality systems, business administration, operations management, public health including informatics, electronic medical records and telemedicine. He has been active in clinical research and collaborations with over 30 well-cited publications in peer-reviewed journals, alongside abstract presentations at local and international conferences.

Bosede Bukola Afolabi, MBChB (Ife), DM (Notts), FRCOG, FWACS, FMCOG, is a Professor of Obstetrics and Gynaecology, with a confirmed faculty position at the College of Medicine, University of Lagos (CMUL), Lagos, Nigeria. She is the current Head of Department, has interests in maternal and fetal medicine, and medical education, and is internationally recognized for her research and clinical care in sickle-cell pregnancy. She is a fellow of Academy of Medicine Specialties of Nigeria and lead investigator of several research projects including clinical trials and implementation science with grants from TETFund Nigeria, NIH, USA and Bill & Melinda Gates Foundation, among others. She has supervised over 20 postgraduate theses and PhDs and has over 102 peer-reviewed publications. She is Director of the Centre for Clinical Trials, Research and Implementation Science (CCTRIS) of the University of Lagos.

Annette Akinsete, MBBS, DTM&H, MPH, FMCPH, Dipl Broadcasting, is an Associate Lecturer at the Eko University of Medicine. She was Director in the Public Health Department of the Federal Ministry of Health for many years and has represented the Federal Government of Nigeria on various platforms all over the world. At a global level, she has contributed to World Health Organisation (WHO) publications on NCDs, served as WHO Fellow in Geneva and as UN Cares Facilitator at the United Nations Headquarters in New York. She is on the board of University of Ibadan Research Foundation. She is a key resource person for the West African Health Organisation and represents the Women's Board at the United Nations. She has been the CEO/National Director of Sickle Cell Foundation Nigeria since 2013.

Mary Ampomah, PhD, is a Lecturer at the University of Health and Allied Sciences, Ho, Volta, Ghana. She was previously a Clinical Psychologist at the Ghana Institute of Clinical Genetics where the adolescent and adult SCD clinic is located. She was a part-time lecturer at the Department of Psychology of the University of Ghana, Legon and taught at the Regent University of Science and Technology. She obtained her PhD in Clinical Psychology at the University of Ghana, Legon. Her career objective is to seek a challenging opportunity to utilize her professional and educational experiences in academia and participate in innovative teaching, clinical and community-based research. Mary is particularly interested in the psychological well-being and quality of life of SCD patients. She is also interested in the neuropsychology of SCD patients in Ghana. She is currently collaborating with Sickle Cell Foundation Ghana on their GENECIS tour which aims at implementing a culturally sensitive and evidence-based SCD counselling in Ghana.

Nwabundo I. Anusim, MD, MPH, is an Assistant Professor of Hematology and Oncology at The University of Texas at Austin and courtesy Assistant Professor at the Department of Pediatrics. Her areas of interest are classical and malignant haematology. Anusim is a medical educator providing haematology training to medical professionals. Anusim is the recipient of the American Society of Hematology Medical Educator Institute award where she developed a curriculum for management of acute complications of SCD. Anusim is collaborating with the paediatric haematologists at The University of Texas at Austin to develop a transition programme for the paediatric sickle cell patients to the adult clinic and is spearheading the establishment of a Comprehensive Sickle Cell Disease centre focused on the care of adults with SCD in Austin, Texas. Anusim is the Principal Investigator on a grant involving sickle cell research and has published several manuscripts in leading international journals and presented papers in international conferences. Anusim is a member of the American Society of Hematology Leadership Institute where she advocates for patients with SCD.

Nnenna Ukachi Badamosi, MD, MPH, is an Assistant Professor in the Department of Pediatric Hematology and Oncology, Augusta University Medical Center, Georgia, USA. Her clinical focus is benign haematology and SCD. Her research interests include lung function of young children with SCD, transition of care in adolescents and young adults, and optimizing outcomes of children with SCD.

Sabrina Bakeera-Kitaka is a Senior Lecturer at the Department of Paediatrics and Child health at the Makerere University, College of Health Sciences. She completed her MBChB in1995; Masters of Paediatrics and Child Health in July 2002, both at Makerere University. She was a Gilead Fellow, and then Research Scholar at the Infectious Diseases Institute from 2003 to 2011 where she undertook a Fellowship in Paediatric Infectious Diseases and did research on HIV-infected adolescents. She has a PhD from the School of Medical Sciences at the University of Antwerp, Belgium. She is involved in conducting basic research in various Paediatrics Infectious Diseases and offers clinical care to HIV-infected children and adolescents, most of whom are perinatally infected. She directs the Adolescent Health training programme at the Makerere University College of Health Sciences and is the Founder President of the Society of Adolescent Health in Uganda (www.sahu.ug). Dr. Kitaka is also an active member of the African Paediatric Society of Infectious Diseases (AFSPID).

Suparno Chakrabarti, MD (PGIMER, Chandigarh), Doctor of Med (Univ of B'ham, UK), FRCPATH (London), is the Director, Institute of Cellular Therapy and Transplantation Research Centre, Manashi Chakrabarti Foundation and Head, Dept of BMT & Hematology, Dharamshila Narayana Hospital, New Delhi, India. Dr. Chakrabarti trained in Internal Medicine at PGIMER, Chandigarh in India. Subsequently, he spent 13 years in the UK, initially as a research fellow and subsequently as a consultant in the field of Bone Marrow Transplant (BMT). During this period, he played a substantial role in developing Campath-1H-based T-cell depletion and reduced intensity conditioning. The bulk of his research also focused on post-transplant virus infections and immune reconstitution. Dr. Chakrabarti received FRCPATH based on his published work. He is credited to have initiated the first haploidentical BMT programme in India and along with Dr. Sarita Jaiswal has developed this as a sustained alternate donor programme with over 180 haploidentical transplants in the past eight years. They have innovated newer methods of carrying out haploidentical BMT in patients with advanced leukaemia as well as haemoglobinopathies and aplastic anaemia incorporating T-cell costimulation blockade, with excellent results. His key area of research is transplant immunology in relation to haploidentical BMT. Dr. Chakrabarti's lab actively investigates the role of adaptive NK cells in transplantation and viral infections. Their novel approach to NK-cell-based immunotherapy using T-cell costimulation blockade has been considered path-breaking. He has over 100 publications to his credit and is peer-reviewer and Editorial Board member for several reputed journals.

Ekaete David, MBBS, MSc Medical Genetics, FMCPath, is currently a Consultant Haematologist at the National Hospital Abuja, Nigeria. Dr. David has been involved in clinical practice and has been involved in teaching at the postgraduate level. She has supervised four postgraduate dissertations. She is currently involved in clinical trials for emerging treatments for sickle cell anaemia. Her areas of interest are sickle cell anaemia and haemato-oncology. Dr. David has co-authored several articles in peer-reviewed journals.

Livingstone Dogara, MBBS (ABU), FMCPath (Haematology), Nigeria, is a Senior Lecturer of Haematology at the Kaduna State University (KASU) and a Consultant Haematologist at its academic hospital, Barau Dikko Teaching Hospital (BDTH) all in Kaduna. He has been a regional leader in haematology and an active member of some of the largest SCD cohort study teams in Nigeria. He has an established reputation as a leading clinician and a capacity-builder and has provided leadership and guidance for trainees and senior physicians interested in health system haematology research. Dr. Dogara has been leading research programmes in sickle cell and in bleeding disorders as one of the few academics in classical haematology. A major accomplishment of his career is the launch of pilot programmes for sickle cell screening in Kaduna, Nigeria. He provides training support for the community health workers, community nursing preceptorship programmes in Kaduna. In the over ten years' experience in SCD care, he has contributed in major publications, conferences, workshops and sickle community engagements. As a dedicated innovator and programme-builder, he is attracting others into implementation research and health services research for haematologists who want to do more than clinical care.

Dunia Hatabah is a Postdoctoral Fellow in the Department of Pediatrics, Division of Pediatric Emergency Medicine at Emory University School of Medicine under the mentorship of Dr. Claudia Morris. She received her Medical Doctorate from the American University of Beirut (AUB) in 2022. She was mentored by Dr. Miguel Abboud, a Professor of Pediatrics, Hematology-Oncology, Head of Sickle Cell Disease Program and Chairman of the Department of Pediatrics and

Adolescent Medicine in AUB. She worked with Dr. Abboud for two years on patient diagnosis, physical exams and history taking. She has been actively involved in clinical research for the past three years. Her research area of interest is paediatric benign haematology with an emphasis on SCD.

Lewis Hsu, BS (Cornell), MD, PhD (University of Rochester), is a Professor of Pediatric Hematology and Director of Pediatric Sickle Cell at University of Illinois Chicago. His career is devoted to SCD. Hsu has 29 years of experience in leadership of some of the largest sickle cell programmes in the USA. His over 100 publications include landmark studies in SCD on stroke prevention and on matched-sibling haematopoietic stem cell transplant. Current research includes improving delivery of SCD therapies using dissemination and implementation science, health education and global community engagement. He trains community health workers in the USA and Nigeria. Hsu has global experience in community engagement in Nigeria plus Brazil, developing health education (books, websites, videos, conferences, and health fairs) to empower families to overcome the complex problems of SCD.

Richard Idro is an Associate Professor at Makerere University School of Medicine and Consultant Paediatrician/Paediatric Neurologist at Mulago, the teaching hospital for Makerere University. He is also the Immediate Past President, Uganda Medical Association. Dr. Idro leads a paediatric neuroscience group in Uganda. His group is studying the pathogenesis and interventions to improve the outcomes of children exposed to central nervous system infections, childhood epilepsy, and malaria chemoprophylaxis and prevention of stroke in children sickle cell anaemia. He is a Medical Research Council (UK) 2015 African Research Leadership Awardee (through which he is studying the pathogenesis and treatment of nodding syndrome) and the Inaugural Greenwood Africa (2019) Awardee. He sits on Boards of the International League against Epilepsy and the International Child Neurology Association.

Mboka Jacob, PhD, is a Senior Lecturer at Muhimbili University of Health and Allied Sciences, school of medicine and a Consultant Radiologist and head of Department at Muhimbili National Hospital in Dar es Salaam, Tanzania. She obtained her PhD by publishing manuscripts exploring brain injury in children with sickle cell disease (SCD) by using conventional and advanced neuroimaging techniques. Her main area of interest is clinical neuroradiology consultancy and Research. She teaches Radiology for both undergraduate and postgraduate students, conducts and supervises students' research. Dr. Jacob also arranges international live lectures for radiology residents at Muhimbili.

Sarita Rani Jaiswal, BSc, MD, is the lead consultant for haploidentical BMT and Program Director, BMT at Dharamshila Hospital and Research Centre, New Delhi. Dr. Jaiswal trained in Internal Medicine, Critical Care Medicine and Pathology before initiating her career in Hematology and BMT. She did her fellowships in BMT under Dr. Suparno Chakrabarti in India, in Italy at University of Parma under Professor Franco Aversa and San Martino Hospital at Genova under

Professor Andrea Bacigalupo. Subsequently, she trained at Fred Hutch Cancer Centre, Seattle, Washington as Vising Physician Fellow. Since her return from the USA, she has been instrumental in setting up a comprehensive haploidentical BMT programme at Dharamshila Hospital, New Delhi, along with Dr. Chakrabarti. The programme is one of its kind in India with a dedicated patient-care wing as well as basic research facilities. Dr. Jaiswal and team has carried out over 180 haploidentical HCT during this period, with innovative and novel approaches for both malignant and non-malignant diseases. The use of Abatacept in haploidentical HCT as conceptualized and protocolized by her group has literally changed the landscape of haploidentical HCT for non-malignant diseases. Her work on haploidentical BMT for SCD and thalassaemia with emphasis on understanding the phenomenon of post-transplant macrophage activation deserves special mention. The wor\k of her team has been selected for oral presentation at the BMT Tandem Meetings in the USA for seven consecutive years from 2015 onwards. The other major area of research has been post-transplant NK-cell-based immunotherapy and simultaneous prevention of GVHD following haploidentical BMT. This has led to some novel developments in this field. Dr. Jaiswal has had over 50 international publications and presentations in the last three years.

Philip Kasirye, MBChB, MMed, Cert. PHO, is a Paediatric Haematologist working at the Mulago National Referral Hospital. He is the Head of the Sickle Cell Clinic and Day Care Centre and leads the care and treatment of people living with SCD. He is very passionate about improving care and treatment of children with SCD. He is a member of the National Task force for SCD. He has participated in numerous research initiatives to improve care in SCD.

Fenella Kirkham is a Professor of Paediatric Neurology, Developmental Neurosciences Unit, UCL Great Ormond Street Institute of Child Health and Clinical and Experimental Sciences, University of Southampton; Consultant Paediatric Neurologist, University Hospital Southampton. She obtained her MD from the University of Cambridge for a thesis entitled 'Cerebral haemodynamics in Children in Coma'. She now focuses on neurocognitive complications of SCD, collaborating with haematologists in England, Europe, the USA, the Middle East, India and Africa. Her UK, European, Middle Eastern, Indian, Ghanaian and Tanzanian students and post-docs have successfully defended MSc/PhD theses and published on neuroimaging and cognition. She was a member of the American Society for Hematology Guidelines and Endpoints working groups looking at the Neurology of Sickle Cell Disease. She ran a randomized controlled trial (RCT) of auto-adjusting CPAP with cognitive and MRI endpoints and collaborated with the Kano/Kaduna team in Nigeria on an RCT of low/moderate hydroxurea doses for primary stroke prevention. In 2023, she will commence an RCT of Montelukast in young children (primary endpoint processing speed).

IkeOluwa Lagunju is a Professor of Paediatrics at the College of Medicine, University of Ibadan and a Consultant Paediatric Neurologist at the University College Hospital, Ibadan, Nigeria. She holds the Fellowship and the Doctor of Medicine (MD) degree of the National Postgraduate Medical College of Nigeria and the Fellowship of the West African Postgraduate Medical College. In recognition of her outstanding contributions to Child Health in Nigeria, she was awarded the Fellowship of the Royal College of Paediatrics and Child Health, UK, in 2012. Her research work focuses on childhood epilepsy, neurodisability and stroke prevention in SCD. She established the first service for routine transcranial Doppler ultrasonography for primary stroke prevention in SCD in Nigeria and her work has significantly reduced the burden of stroke in Nigerian children. She served as the Head of Department of Paediatrics, University of Ibadan from October 2015 to July 2022. She is the current AHA International Training Centre Coordinator for the College of Medicine ITC and the immediate past President of the Child Neurology Society of Nigeria. Professor Lagunju's research interests focus on early child development, childhood epilepsies, developmental disabilities and stroke in SCD. She has over 100 publications in peer-reviewed journals and has made presentations at a number of international conferences. She is a well sought-after speaker at local and international meetings. Professor Ike Lagunju is the current Head of the Paediatric Neurology Unit, University College Hospital, Ibadan.

Juliana Olufunke Lawson, MBBCh, FWACP, MSc (Public Health), is a Consultant Paediatrician/Vice Chairman of Zankli Medical Centre, Abuja, Nigeria. She is a member of the Paediatrics Association of Nigeria, Nigeria Medical Association, Nigeria Society of Neonatal Medicine, American Academy of Paediatrics, Fellow of the West African College of Physicians, member of the American Academy of Paediatrics and a Past National Secretary, Medical Women's research work mainly in Rickets and SCD in the community and has 19 published papers in peer-reviewed journals.

Deogratais Munube, MBChB, MMed, Cert. PHO, is a Paediatric Haematologist-Oncologist working at the Directorate of Paediatrics and Child Health, Mulago National Referral Hospital, Kampala, Uganda. His goal is to improve the care and treatment of children with paediatric haematological and oncological diagnosis. He has a key interest in the neurological outcomes of children with SCD in particular stroke incidence, risk factors and outcomes. In addition, he is faculty at the College of Health Sciences, Makerere University.

Catherine Nabaggala is a Pediatric Haematologist-Oncologist currently based at Mulago National Referral Hospital in Uganda. She attained her Master of Medicine in Paediatrics and Child health from Makerere University and recently completed her fellowship training through the Makerere College of Health Sciences – Global Hope Program in Uganda. She has been involved in some of the research at the Mulago Hospital Sickle Cell Clinic including the NOHARM MTD "Optimizing Hydroxyurea Therapy in Children with Sickle cell Anemia in Malaria Endemic Areas" (*New England Journal of Medicine*, 2020), a pivotal study in advocacy and providing guidance for hydroxyurea use in SCD in Uganda. She also continues to be involved in the management of children with SCD in Uganda.

Annet Nakirulu, MBChB (Kampala International University), PPC (Mildmay), MMED Paed (Uganda Martyrs University), PHO (Makerere University), is a Paediatrician/Paediatric Haemato-Oncologist/Lecturer Haematology/Oncology Wards/Sickle Cell and Day Care Centre, Directorate of Paediatrics and Child Health Mulago National Referral Hospital. In her current position, she is involved in patient care with teaching and supervision of undergraduate and postgraduate students. She is engaged in paediatric palliative care activities including research that are key in facilitating improved quality of lives and thus outcomes in affected children and families.

Ruth Namazzi, MBChB, MMED, Cert. PHO, is a paediatrician and paediatric haematologist, and faculty at Makerere University College of Health Sciences, Kampala Uganda. Her goal is to improve outcomes of children SCD through improved clinical care, research and training. She conducts research, clinical care and medical education at Makerere University College of Health Sciences and Mulago National Referral Hospital, Kampala, Uganda.

Eunice Ndirangu-Mugo, BSc, Nursing summa cum laude (University of Eastern Africa, Baraton), MSc, Advanced Nursing Practice & PhD Nursing Studies (University of Nottingham, UK), is a Professor and Dean at the Aga Khan University, School of Nursing & Midwifery, East Africa and an Associate Faculty with the Brain and Mind Institute (BMI) at Aga Khan University. She is also the Char of Nursing Council of Kenya, the body that regulates Nursing & Midwifery education and practice in Kenya. Eunice has attended and presented in a number of national and international conferences and published throughout the span of her academic career on a wide variety of topics. She is also an Associate Fellow of the Higher Education Academy in the UK and holds a Postgraduate Certificate of Teaching in Higher Education from Oxford Brookes University in the UK. Eunice is a graduate of the Adaptive Leadership for Africa: Chaos, Complexity and Courage course from the Harvard Kennedy School, Executive Education. She has served in a number of Technical Working Groups such as Kenya Nursing & Midwifery Policy (Chair), Kenya Nurses & Midwives Strategic Plan (Member) and QUAD (Member). Eunice is interested in the intersection between education and implementation science, generating cultural and social responsive evidence, and linking this to education, practice, research and policy.

Lilian Nuwabaine obtained a Master of Nursing (Midwifery and Women's Health) and a Bachelor of Science in Nursing, all from Makerere University. She is a certified trainer in Advanced Life Support, Basic Emergency and Obstetric Newborn Care, Leadership and Management. She is currently working as the Continuous Professional Development Coordinator with Aga Khan University. Lilian also emerged as the Midwife of the year 2021 in the Heroes in Health Awards Uganda, an award by the Ministry of Health Uganda. She was also one of the staff that received an award of excellence in research scholarly outputs in June 2023 by The Aga Khan University School of Nursing and Midwifery, East Africa. Since 2022, Lilian has published over ten manuscripts in reproductive maternal newborn child and adolescent health (RMNCAH). From September 2019, with Aga Khan University, Lilian has conducted over 90 trainings to over 3,000 nurses and midwives from different health facilities across Uganda in areas such as RMNCAH, Basic Emergency Care, SRHR, Gender Based Violence and leadership and management among others.

Ugochi O. Ogu, MD, is an Associate Professor of Medicine at the University of Tennessee Health Science Center (UTHSC) and the Medical Director of the Diggs-Kraus Comprehensive Sickle Cell Center. Her clinical and research interests focus on SCD and transition of care from paediatrics to adult. Dr. Ugochi O. Ogu is renowned for discovering a novel variant of SCD, Hb S/Haringey, published in 2021. She provides care for people living with SCD, across their lifespan, and is heavily invested in the education of the next generation of physicians who will continue to provide excellent care for people living with SCD.

Vivian Omuemu, MBBS (Benin), MPH, MD, FRSPH, FMCPH, FWACP, is a Professor of Public Health and Community Medicine and a Consultant Public Health Physician at the University of Benin and University of Benin Teaching Hospital, Benin-City Nigeria. Her areas of special interests include Epidemiology, Public Health Nutrition, Reproductive & Family Health and Rehabilitative Medicine. She was Editor-in-Chief of the *Journal of Community Medicine & Primary Health Care* from 2017 to 2023 and currently the Editor of the *Journal of Medicine & Biomedical Research*. She is the Deputy Provost of the College of Medical Sciences, University of Benin. She has published several papers in peer-reviewed local and international journals and also presented several papers at local and international conferences.

Oluseyi Oniyangi, MBBS (Nigeria), FWACP (Paeds) Fellow, West African College of Physicians – specialty Paediatrics, is a Chief Consultant Paediatrician with many years of clinical practice at the National Hospital Abuja Nigeria. Her clinical and research interests focus on SCD and care of children with the disorder. She was a part of the editorial team that produced the guidelines of care for SCD for Nigeria and has written and co-authored multiple academic papers on SCD, including a Cochrane systematic review on phytomedicines in SCD. She provides care for children and adolescents with SCD.

Adaeze Oreh, MBBS (University of Nigeria); MSc (Imperial College London); MSc Public Health (London School of Hygiene & Tropical Medicine); FWACP (Family Medicine) is a Senior New Voices Fellow in Global Health with the Aspen Institute, Washington D.C, PhD candidate at University of Groningen, the Netherlands, and Adjunct Senior Lecturer College of Medicine and Health Sciences, Baze University, Abuja. She is currently the Honorable Commissioner for Health in Rivers State, and was previously the Country Director of Planning, Research and Statistics at Nigeria's National Blood Service Commission where she was involved in the process leading up to the enactment of the National Blood Service Commission Act 2021. Adaeze is a member of the International Society of Blood Transfusion (ISBT) COVID-19 Working Group and has presented and authored several papers and book chapters locally and internationally on blood transfusion services, primary healthcare, infectious diseases such as COVID-19, and health systems.

Ahmed Mohammed Sarki, BSc (Hons) (Bayero University Kano), MPH (Oxford Brookes), PhD (Warwick), is an Assistant Professor at the School of Nursing and Midwifery, Aga Khan University, Uganda Campus. He is also the Chair for Research at the School of Nursing and Midwifery East Africa (Kenya, Tanzania, and Uganda). Dr. Sarki is a Fellow of the Royal Society for Public Health, UK, an Associate Fellow of Advanced HE, UK and a Member of the International Epidemiological Association. Dr. Sarki has held different research roles at Oxford Brookes University, Population Council Kenya, and a Joint Project with Massachusetts Institute of Technology and Planned Parenthood Federation of Nigeria. He has written and published several articles on topics ranging from chronic diseases, mental health and adolescent health.

Dawn E. Saunders has had a long-standing interest in the neuroradiology of SCD, is currently an Associate Professor at UCL Institute of Child Health in London, UK and a Consultant Neuroradiologist at Epsom hospital. She trained at King's College hospital, Boston Children's Hospital, Imperial College Healthcare, St George's Hospital and the National hospital for Neurology and Neurosurgery and obtained her MD from St George's Hospital Medical school.

Maryam Shehu is a Consultant Paediatrician and Lecturer in Paediatrics at Bingham University in Jos, Nigeria. She has been an ARISE (African Research and Innovative Initiative for Sickle Cell Education) scholar funded by the European Union. She is focusing on the comparison of Imaging and Non-Imaging transcranial Doppler and on long-term outcomes for neonatally screened children with SCD.

Léon Tshilolo, MD, PhD, is a Professor of Pediatrics and Haematology at Ufficial University of Mbujimayi (UOM) and Visitor at University of Kinshasa and University of Lubumbashi, DRC. He is also the Director of Research in the Institut de Recherche Biomédicale (IRB) associated to Monkole Hospital in Kinshasa, DRC. He is a WHO Temporary Consultant concerning the Sickle Cell Disease and President, co-founder of the African network of SCD in Africa "REDAC." Member of the Académie de Médecine de France and the Académie Congolaise des Sciences (ACCOS), Léon is also the DRC leader Investigator of REACH-Realizing Effectiveness Across Continents with Hydroxyurea and Co-Chair in Sickle in Africa Consortium. He has written more than 100 papers mostly dedicated on SCD and malaria.

Sophie Uyoga, BSc (Hons), MSc, Phd (Heidelberg), is a research scientist at the Kenya Medical Research Institute Wellcome Trust Research Programme Kilifi, Kenya. She leads research on the impact of transfusion in SCD. She has contributed to 72 publications in the area of transfusion in African children and the epidemiology malaria and red blood cell genetic polymorphisms.

Tamunomieibi Wakama, MBBS, FMCPath, is currently a Consultant Haematologist at the Babcock University Teaching Hospital and Associate Professor of Haematology at the Department of Haematology, Benjamin Carson (Snr) College of Health and Medical Sciences, University of Babcock, Ilisan Ogun State, Nigeria. He was previously at the National Hospital Abuja as Consultant Haematologist and Snr Lecturer at the Department of Haematology, University of Abuja, Nigeria. Dr. Wakama has taught and practised Haematology at both undergraduate and postgraduate levels having supervised and mentored over 11 postgraduate dissertations in Haematology. He was a 2014 recipient of the ASH VTP programme at the Roswell Park Cancer Institute Buffalo, USA and has co-authored a book chapter and several articles in peer-reviewed journals with special interest in sickle cell aneamia.

Thomas N. Williams, MBBS, FRCPCH, PhD, FMedSci, is the Professor of Haemoglobinopathy Research at Imperial College, London, and Chair of the Department of Epidemiology and Demography at the KEMRI-Wellcome Trust Research Programme, Kilifi, Kenya. A major focus of Professor Williams' research work is the positive and negative health consequences of a range of human genetic conditions among children in Africa, particularly those that affect the structure or function of red blood cells. He addresses these questions through a range of approaches that include large-scale epidemiological studies, laboratory-based studies and clinical trials. In recent years, Professor Williams has published some of the most influential and widely cited studies on the clinical epidemiology of SCD conducted in Africa to date.

Foreword

During medical school in Nigeria, I observed first-hand the devastating consequences of sickle cell disorders (SCD) on families in sub-Saharan Africa (SSA). The experiences were poignant: a two-year-old who died in my arms from severe anaemia and acute malaria, a neighbor who lost several infants over the years to what was colloquially called "ogbanje" or "spirit child." These early observations instilled in me a resolve to improve the healthcare conditions for this vulnerable population.

Now, as a 30-year veteran haematologist who has practiced across the globe, I find it exhilarating to see how modern medicine has improved the lives of SCD patients in high-income countries like the USA and Europe. However, it remains disheartening that individuals in SSA still face stigma, ignorance, and a severe lack of resources, contributing to an abysmally low life expectancy.

This urgent need for systemic change forms the basis for the two-part edited volumes *Sickle Cell Disorder in Sub-Saharan Africa: Biomedical Perspectives* and *Sickle Cell Disorder in Sub-Saharan Africa: Public Health Perspectives.* Designed to be read as companion pieces, these volumes provide a comprehensive overview that spans both biomedical and public health perspectives unique to SSA.

The works cover several key aspects of SCD relevant to SSA, such as updated epidemiological data, attention to vital clinical complications including nutrition and infectious diseases, and the role of traditional medical practices. These volumes are aimed to serve as reference texts for healthcare providers, researchers, and policymakers, ultimately guiding improvements in healthcare policy and delivery for SCD patients in SSA.

SCD in SSA can only be tackled through comprehensive approaches that involve advocacy, public-private partnerships, and a multi-disciplinary ethos. These twin volumes aim to fill the knowledge and advocacy gaps, providing a substantive resource for a resource-limited population.

In the words of Kofi Annan, "Knowledge is power. Information is liberating. Education is the premise of progress in every society and in every family." These volumes, I firmly attest, offer the power of knowledge, the liberation of information, and the promise of educational advancement, tailored specifically to the challenges and opportunities present in SSA.

I have every belief that they will make a significant contribution to improving the state of SCD healthcare in SSA.

Sincerely,

Ifeyinwa (Ify) Osunkwo MD, MPH
Lifespan Sickle Cell Expert and Hematologist
Chief Patient Officer, Novo Nordisk Rare Disease
Professor of Medicine and Pediatrics
Maya Angelou Center for Health Disparities, Wake Forest University

Acknowledgements

At the tail end of the COVID-19 pandemic, the book editors met to discuss the prospects of amplifying sickle cell research through expert voices from the global south where the disease is predominant. This book is a brainchild of that meeting. It took an immense amount of work, and it would not have been possible without the invaluable contributions of several supportive persons, including:

Baba Inusa, our foremost co-editor and a phenomenal person. Professor Baba supported this project every step of the way, from the point of conceptualization to publication – offering insights, resources, timely encouragement and administrative support.

Nkechikwu Azinge-Egbiri and Bukola Bolarinwa, my co-editors equally dedicated time to ensure the quality and standard of this book. Their involvement at the conceptualization stage meant that they wrote and ran with the vision of developing the foremost multi-disciplinary book on sickle cell disease targeted at pushing for a systemic shift in how sickle cell care is approached.

Our vision was shaped by our interactions with Simon Dyson and Stuart Edelstein, prominent researchers in the field, who provided critical feedback and invaluable guidance.

Adeola Adegbusi, our administrative lead, was the glue that held the project together. She understood what we were trying to accomplish, and she was meticulous in helping us achieve this. She meticulously organized and coordinated meetings, liaised with authors and ensured the accuracy of information, investing extraordinary hours of care into ensuring this finished product.

I acknowledge Dr. Matthew Nwankwo, our brilliant editor who read all early drafts and provided valuable feedback.

I acknowledge the Routledge Publishing Press, George Russell and Amy Thomson, for their patient correspondence and assistance throughout the publication process. Their expertise and professionalism have been instrumental in bringing this book to fruition.

Individually, I want to thank the Sickle Cell Aid Foundation (SCAF)'s team members: Dr. Victor Oyoyo, Scott Adamu-Oyegun, Elmer Aluge, Yejide Adewakun, Ayobami Bakare, Amina Jibrin, Bashira Hassan, Odidi Oluwaseun, Dr. Justice Igbiti, Nkemdilim Azinge, Olisa Azinge, Larry Jacob, Aisha Ali Ameh, Joshua Olatunde Adedamola, Nura Abdullahi (1988–2016), Awele Nwosu Akeh

(1989–2015), Jake Okechukwu Effoduh, Dr. Tochukwu Nnamoko, Harrison Oliver, Majekodunmi Olasumbo Opemipo, Grace Usman (1989–2021), Rukaiya Muhammed, Dozie Nwafor, Minta Yusuf, Hauwa Ibrahim, Ikechwuku Oleka, Oluwatobi Olusesi, Abimbola Ogunmekan, Oyesola Oni, Muhammed Nurudeen, Bolaji Alamu, Subulola Jiboye, Sheriffdeen Owokunle, Adebimpe Shenbote, Uche Okoye (1987–2019), Ridwan Adewale (1995–2019), and Tochukwu Nwonu. Their endless commitment to raising awareness and combatting SCD culminated in the embryonic ideas discussed at the initial meeting, which birthed this book.

My greatest acknowledgement is our authors, who have individually and collectively given SCD a voice of origin. Inspired by the words of Toni Morrison, a literature Noble Laurette, "If there's a book that you want to read, but it hasn't been written yet, then you must write it" – we took on the challenge of addressing sickle cell in Sub-Saharan Africa, aiming for the depth of knowledge required. Recognizing the complexity of the task, we drew on experts from Africa or with research interest on the continent who specialize in different aspects of the disease. With their involvement, we are positive that SCD will garner the attention it deserves, and sickle cell warriors will get improved holistic care.

I acknowledge my wife Rita Offor and amazing daughter Olanma Nwankwo, who offered love, silence, and the moral support needed to co-edit this book.

With profound gratitude,

Kanayo Nwankwo, MD
For, and on behalf of the Co-Editors.

Introduction

Sickle Cell Disease in Sub-Saharan Africa: A Multidisciplinary Approach

Baba Inusa, Kanayo Nwankwo,
Nkechikwu Azinge-Egbiri and Bukola Bolarinwa

Sickle cell disease (SCD) is a hereditary haemoglobin condition. In early infancy, it often presents with symptoms like anaemia, infections, and generalized pain. As individuals grow older, they frequently encounter chronic organ complications and may have a shortened life expectancy. The severity of SCD varies across patients (Lokanatha et al., 2016). While some patients have minimal poor-health interferences with their daily lives, many suffer in untold ways. Clinical findings show significantly affected quality of life (McClish et al., 2005; Osunkwo et al., 2020) impacting education outcomes, lifestyle choices, and career progression. Additionally, patients are exposed to stigma and disability or race discrimination, issues that culminate in poor mental health outcomes for them and their caregivers.

Discovered in 1910, SCD which was originally predominant in Sub-Saharan Africa now has an increasing burden in Western countries partly due to migration from high-prevalence countries. Studies estimate that 75% of live SCD births totalling 400,000 annually occur in Sub-Saharan Africa, although India has a significant prevalence level (Piel et al., 2013; Therrell et al., 2015). However, with rising migration attributable to endogenous factors such as civil wars, military coups and rising living cost or exogenous factors such as foreign intervention, economic recession, or the recent COVID-19 pandemic (Orozco, 2020), one can argue that the demographic of SCD has expanded beyond the global south. For instance, the United Kingdom records that at least 350 more babies are born with SCD each year (Meremikwu et al., 2015). Indeed, the SCD index case which concerned Walter Noel, a United States immigrant student from Grenada in the Caribbeans is testament to the impact of migration on disease demographic – demonstrating that SCD is now a global phenomenon.

SCD research and management has however yet to advance to align with its now globalized positioning. There is a dearth of research particularly from a global south or multidisciplinary perspective. Additionally, there is no affordable cure for SCD, neither are the therapies easily accessible. For instance, Western countries have adopted newborn screening, penicillin prophylaxis, and curative therapies (such as gene therapy and bone marrow transplants) to checkmate childhood mortality. Additionally, hydroxyurea therapy – the leading disease-modifying therapy – has been used for 30 years with increasing benefit globally (Frempong & Pearson, 2007). Yet, qualification standards for curative therapies are exclusionary and

DOI: 10.4324/9781003463931-1

insurance is necessary for treatment – a challenge for the under-deserved or the undocumented. The struggles faced by the global south are significantly different. As it stands, Sub-Saharan African countries and India are still struggling to achieve universal newborn screening. Particularly, SCD patients are unlikely to benefit from new therapies such as voxelotor or crizanlizumab, and curative therapies are out of reach for most patients (Robbins, R., & Nolen, S., 2023).

To address the scourge of SCD and the disparity in access to therapies, it became imperative to provide a resource that brings together recent development in disease pathology, genetics, and clinic pattern, psychosocial issues, and new therapies. The idea of editing this book on SCD *was* borne out of first-hand experience of living with family members affected by SCD which initially led to the establishment of a sickle cell foundation known as Sickle Cell Aid Foundation (SCAF) by Nkechikwu Azinge-Egbiri. Members of SCAF's leadership team, Dr Kanayo Nwankwo, have treated sickle cell warriors for over ten years, and Bukola Bolarinwa is a sickle cell warrior/advocate. The combined experience of watching family members/patients suffer and living with SCD motivated the search for holistic information to facilitate practical change.

This title of this edited book reflects the aspiration of the above trio to highlight the plight of people affected by SCD in Sub-Saharan Africa. However, the chapter authors have been deliberately drawn from leading experts in Africa, India, Europe, the United States, and the Middle East. The experts selection is aimed at providing up-to-date research on diagnosis, treatment strategies, psychosocial management, and epidemiology. We have been fortunate to attract leading experts to provide authoritative multidisciplinary perspectives while addressing the specific issues on newborn screening and transition from paediatrics to adults, amongst others.

This edited book has two volumes that should be read together. The first volume titled 'Sickle Cell Disorder in Sub-Saharan Africa: A Multi-Disciplinary Approach - Biomedical Perspectives' focuses on the epidemiology of SCD alongside the clinical attempts to provide comprehensive care in a resource-limited setting. It considers, for instance, the evolution of bone marrow transplants in Sub-Saharan Africa and the utilization of home-grown anti-sickling medications. The second volume is titled 'Sickle Cell Disorder in Sub-Saharan Africa: A Multi-Disciplinary Approach – Public Health Perspective'. The volume examines the socio-economic factors that impact patient well-being and the critical importance of patient advocacy. Collectively, these volumes are synchronized to advance patient well-being in Sub-Saharan Africa. Indeed, this nuanced approach of the two-part edited book is unique as it recognizes that the SCD management requires a holistic approach that spans beyond medical care and into patient advocacy, alongside socio-economic factors. Given the book's multidisciplinary approach, which bridges the typically separate realms of science and social sciences, its primary focus is on addressing tropical issues related to SCD in Sub-Saharan Africa. This focus fills an existing literature gap and would further spur continental strategies towards the prevention of, and improved management of, SCD in the region.

To all professionals, caregivers, and advocates in the realm of SCD research and care, this publication has been meticulously curated with you in mind. Our aim is to provide a comprehensive resource that bridges the gap between advanced scientific knowledge and practical applications, especially concerning the intricacies faced in Sub-Saharan Africa. Policymakers and philanthropists, this is an imperative read to understand the current landscape and the ways in which your support can be transformative. With insights from esteemed entities such as the Lancet Commission on Sickle Cell Disease 2023, this book stands as a beacon of current knowledge and innovative approaches in the field. We invite you to immerse yourself in this work, which promises to inform, challenge, and inspire.

References

Lokanatha, H., Rudramurthy, P., & Ramachandrappa, R. M. (2016). Spectrum of sickle cell diseases in patients diagnosed at a tertiary care centre in Karnataka with special emphasis on their clinicohaematological profile. *J Clin Diagn Res, 10*(2), EC09–EC11. https://doi.org/10.7860/JCDR/2016/18280.7221

McClish, D. K., Penberthy, L. T., Bovbjerg, V. E., Roberts, J. D., Aisiku, I. P., Levenson, J. L., Roseff, S. D., & Smith, W. R. (2005). Health related quality of life in sickle cell patients: The PiSCES project. *Health Qual Life Outcomes, 3*, 50. https://doi.org/10.1186/1477-7525-3-50

Osunkwo, I., Andemariam, B., Minniti, C. P., Inusa, B. P. D., El Rassi, F., Francis-Gibson, B., Nero, A., Trimnell, C., Abboud, M. R., et al. (2020). Impact of sickle cell disease on patients' daily lives, symptoms reported, and disease management strategies: Results from the international Sickle Cell World Assessment Survey (SWAY). *Am J Hematol*. https://doi.org/10.1002/ajh.26063

The sickle cell disease Commissioners. (2023). The Lancet Haematology Commission on sickle cell disease: Key recommendations. *Lancet Haematol, 10*(8), e564–e567. https://doi.org/10.1016/S2352-3026(23)00154-0

Piel, F. B., Hay, S. I., Gupta, S., Weatherall, D. J., & Williams, T. N. (2013). Global burden of sickle cell anaemia in children under five, 2010-2050: Modelling based on demographics, excess mortality, and interventions. *PLoS Med, 10*(7), e1001484. https://doi.org/10.1371/journal.pmed.1001484

Therrell, B. L., Padilla, C. D., Loeber, J. G., Kneisser, I., Saadallah, A., Borrajo, G. J., & Adams, J. (2015). Current status of newborn screening worldwide: 2015. *Semin Perinatol, 39*(3), 171–187. https://doi.org/10.1053/j.semperi.2015.03.002

Suárez-Orozco, M. M. (2020). Global migration, education, and the nation-state. *Intercult Educ, 31*(5), 506–518. https://doi.org/ 10.1080/14675986.2020.1795373

Meremikwu, M. M., & Okomo, U. (2016). Sickle cell disease. *BMJ Clinical Evidence, 2016*, 2402.

Frempong, T., & Pearson, H. A. (2007). Newborn screening coupled with comprehensive follow-up reduced early mortality of sickle cell disease in Connecticut. *Conn Med, 71*(1), 9–12.

Robbins, R., & Nolen, S. (2023, December 8). New sickle cell therapies will be out of reach where they are needed most. *The New York Times*. https://www.nytimes.com/2023/12/08/health/casgevy-lyfgenia-sickle-cell-africa.html

1 The Clinical Epidemiology of Sickle Cell Disease in Sub-Saharan Africa

Thomas N. Williams

Introduction

Normal adult haemoglobin, haemoglobin A (HbA), is predominantly composed of two α- and two β-globin polypeptide chains, encoded, respectively, by the *HBA* gene on chromosome 16 and *HBB* gene on chromosome 11. In persons with sickle cell disease (SCD), the majority of the haemoglobin produced is an abnormal variant of HbA known as haemoglobin S (sickle haemoglobin; HbS). HbS is identical in structure to HbA with the exception of a single amino acid: the glutamic acid residue normally found at position 6 of the β-globin chain is replaced by a valine residue (Ingram, 1957), the result of a single nucleotide polymorphism (rs334 c.20A>T [p.Glu7Val]) in *HBB*. HbS behaves very differently from HbA when subjected to low oxygen tensions. The altered amino acid sequence results in a hydrophobic motif that triggers the polymerization of HbS inside erythroycytes on de-oxygenation (Figure 1.1), disrupting their architecture to result in misshapen cells that frequently adopt the shape of a sickle (Figure 1.2), a process that is central to the pathophysiology of SCD.

Classification of Sickle Cell Disease

The most common form of SCD results from homozygosity for the rs334 mutation (HbSS), commonly known as sickle cell anaemia (SCA). SCA accounts for approximately 70% of all cases of SCD in sub-Saharan Africa, while most of the remaining cases are caused by the coinheritance of rs334 with another single nucleotide polymorphism in *HBB*, rs33930165 c.20G>A [p.Glu7Lyc], which encodes a different structural variant of β-globin known as haemoglobin C (HbC) (Modiano et al., 2008). The resulting condition, HbSC, is similar to but somewhat less severe than HbSS (Steinberg, Forget, Higgs, & Weatherall, 2009). Finally, SCD can also result from the coinheritance of rs334 and other *HBB* mutations including various β-thalassaemia mutations that result in the reduced or absent production of stable normal β-globin chains (HbS/β-thalassaemia) and mutations that result in other structural haemoglobin variants such as HbO^{Arab} (HbS/O^{Arab}). The main molecular forms of SCD are summarized in Table 1.1.

DOI: 10.4324/9781003463931-2

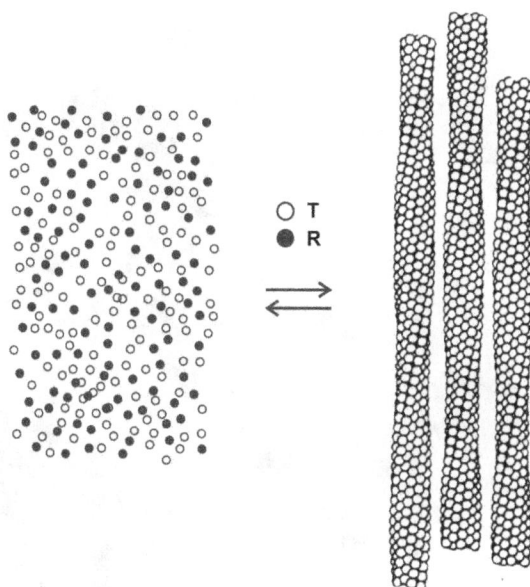

Figure 1.1 Intraerythrocytic polymerization of HbS.

Molecular Origins of the rs334 Mutation

Two main hypotheses have been put forward regarding the origin of the rs334 mutation. The first – the so-called single origin theory – is that it arose just once in an isolated population, increased in frequency within that population and then subsequently spread to other populations in which new haplotypes were formed by gene conversion (Flint, Harding, Clegg, & Boyce, 1993; Livingstone, 1989). A second hypothesis invokes independent occurrences of the same mutation in multiple different populations (Currat et al., 2002; Kurnit, 1979; Mears et al., 1981; Pagnier et al., 1984). This hypothesis was supported by the discovery of five main haplotypes in early studies based on restriction fragment length polymorphism analyses, which were named after their supposed origins – Benin, Cameroon, Central African Republic (CAR)/Bantu, Senegal, and Arab/Indian (Kan & Dozy, 1978a, 1978b). The latter hypothesis was widely favoured for much of the last few decades.

The clinical severity of SCA can vary substantially, from a mild condition with few complications at one extreme to a severe condition associated with frequent painful crises and early death at the other. Following the description of these various haplotypes, studies began to suggest that they may be relevant to disease phenotype, particularly given that some are associated with higher levels of haemoglobin F (HbF) which has been shown to be a powerful disease-modifying factor. In particular, it was suggested that the Arab/Indian haplotype might be less severe than the African haplotypes (Kulozik et al., 1986) and that within Africa, the CAR/Bantu haplotype is the most severe and

NORMAL RED BLOOD CELLS

Normal red blood cells flow
freely within blood vessel

Normal
hemoglobin

ABNORMAL, SICKLED RED BLOOD CELLS
(SICKLE CELLS)

Sickle cells blocking
blood flow

Abnormal
hemoglobin
form strands
that cause
sickle shape

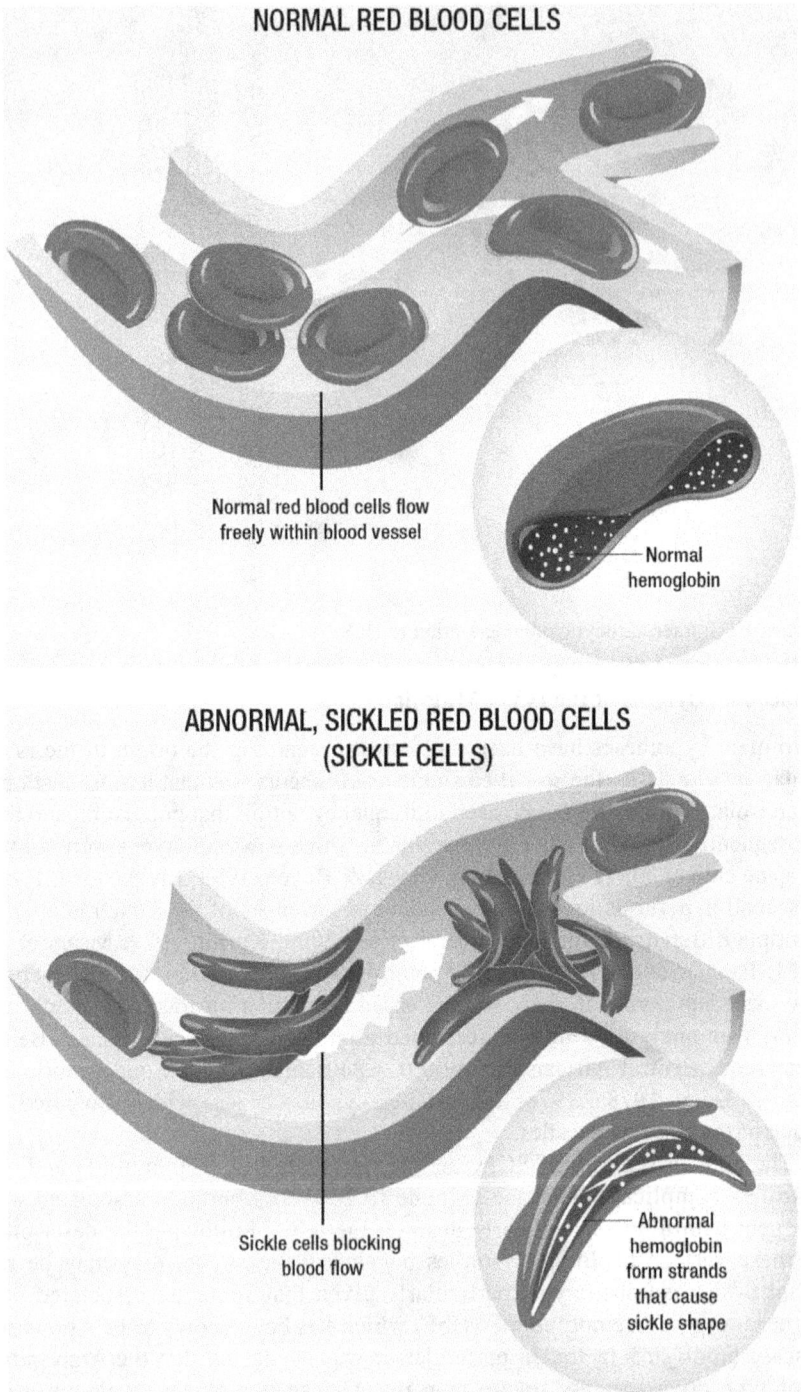

Figure 1.2 "Sickled" red cells due to intraerythrocytic HbS polymerization.

Table 1.1 Molecular classification of the main forms of sickle cell disease.

Molecular forms of SCD, listed by severity		Notes
Severe	HbS/S (β6Glu>Val/β6Glu>Val)	Homozygosity for the rs334c.204>T mutation. Commonly known as sickle cell anaemia. Approximately 70% of all cases of SCD.
	HbS/β⁰-thalassaemia	The most prevalent form of SCD in the Eastern Mediterranean region and India.
	HbS/β⁺-thalassaemia	Severe forms of β⁺-thalassaemia mean that only 1–5% of Hb produced is HbA. This form is most prevalent in India and in the Eastern Mediterranean.
	HbS/O Arab (β6Glu>Val/β121Glu>Lys)	A rare form of severe SCD is found most commonly in North Africa, the Middle East, and the Balkans.
	HbS/D Punjab (β6Glu>Val/β121Glu>Gln)	Through migration, this has been reported globally but is predominantly found in Northern India.
	HbS/C Harlem (β6Glu>Val/β6Glu>Val, β73Asp>Asn)	Electrophoretically, this rare form of SCD resembles HbSC, but is clinically more severe.
	HbC/Antilles (β6Glu>Lys/β6Glu>Val, β23Val-Ile)	HbS Antilles results from two separate single-point mutations in *HBB*. Results in a severe form of SCD when coinherited with HbC. Very rare.
Moderate	HbS/C (β6Glu>Val/β6Glu>Lys)	Twenty-five to thirty per cent of cases of SCD in populations of African origin.
	Moderate HbS/β⁺-thalassaemia	Less severe forms of β⁺-thalassaemia mean that 6–15% of Hb is HbA. Most commonly found in the Eastern Mediterranean.
	HbA/S Oman (βᴬ/β6Glu>Val, β121Glu>Lys)	HbS Oman results from a double mutation in *HBB*. Very rare.
Less severe	HbS/β⁺⁺-thalassaemia	Coinheritance of HbS with less severe forms of β⁺⁺-thalassaemia means that 16–30% of Hb is HbA. Most often seen in populations of African origin.
Mild	HbS/HPFH	HPFH – Hereditary Persistence of Fetal Haemoglobin – denotes a group of conditions caused by large deletions in the haemoglobin gene complex. Typically, 30% of total Hb is haemoglobin F (HbF).

the Benin haplotype the least (Steinberg, 2005). However, a lack of systematic studies makes it difficult to confirm such relationships, and more recent studies have suggested that severe disease is more common than previously recognized among patients with the Arab/Indian haplotype (Alsultan et al., 2014; Italia et al., 2015).

In a recent whole-genome-sequence-based analysis using data from the 1000 Genomes Project, the African Genome Variation Project and Qatar, Shriner and Rotimi presented data to suggest that the single origin theory may well have been correct all along (Shriner & Rotimi, 2018). The authors constructed haplotypes from 27 polymorphisms that were in strong linkage disequilibrium with rs334. Through network analysis they then found a common haplotype that correlated collectively with the CAR/Bantu, Cameroon, and Arab/Indian haplotypes and showed that the remaining haplotypes were both derived from this common haplotype. Further, almost all the rs334-carrying samples from the CAR, Kenya, Uganda, and South Africa were of the original rs334 haplotype, suggesting that the mutation pre-dated the Bantu expansions. Based on their analyses, the authors estimated that rs334 first occurred approximately 7,300 years ago and that the survival advantage afforded to heterozygotes during the subsequent years was 15.2%.

Mendelian Selection of rs334

The Shriner study (Shriner & Rotimi, 2018) suggests that from the time that the rs334 c.202A>T mutation first occurred approximately 7,300 years ago, it took approximately 2,400 years before it reached its current equilibrium frequency (12.0%) in malaria-endemic parts of sub-Saharan Africa. It was first suggested that a survival advantage against malaria might be the cause for the selection of rs334 carriers (HbAS; sickle cell trait) more than 70 years ago. During the 1950s and 1960s, a number of investigators including Beet (1946, 1947), Brain (1952), and Allison (1954) noticed a strong correlation within African populations between the prevalence of "sickling" and the endemicity of *P. falciparum* malaria and suggested that this might have been the result of malaria selection. Subsequent studies confirmed that this correlation is seen at a global scale (Livingstone, 1973, 1985) and that, at least in Africa, it is highly statistically significant (Piel et al., 2010). Strong evidence supporting malaria as the agent responsible for this selection comes from numerous epidemiological studies conducted in diverse countries over many years (for example see references Hill et al., 1991; Jallow et al., 2009; Willcox et al., 1983; Williams, Mwangi, Roberts et al., 2005; Williams, Mwangi, Wambua, Alexander et al., 2005). In a recent meta-analysis, Taylor and colleagues showed that HbAS is >30% protective against episodes of uncomplicated clinical malaria and >90% protective against severe and complicated forms of the disease (Taylor, Parobek, & Fairhurst, 2012). More recently, in a very large case-control study that involved more than 28,000 children overall (The Malaria Genomic Epidemiology Network. Reappraisal of known malaria resistance loci in a large multicenter study, 2014), the protective effect of HbAS against all forms of severe malaria was shown to be considerably stronger than that of any other variant in the entire human genome, consistent with overall protection of 86% at a significance level of $P = 1.6 \times 10^{-225}$.

The strong protection afforded by HbAS against malaria means that it also protects against the downstream consequences of malaria, which include other potentially fatal conditions that include invasive bacterial infections (Scott et al., 2011; Uyoga, Macharia, Ndila et al., 2019) and malnutrition (Uyoga, Macharia, Ndila et al., 2019). Consequently, HbAS provides an extraordinary benefit in malaria-endemic environments, where the positive selective survival advantage may well be more than twice as high as that attributable to malaria alone (Scott et al., 2011; Uyoga, Macharia, Ndila et al., 2019). Using a model-based approach based on the current equilibrium frequencies of HbAS, Watson and colleagues recently deduced that in the pre-intervention era, malaria and other conditions that resulted from it were historically responsible for between 15 and 24% of all mortality during childhood in sub-Saharan Africa. It is obvious that any gene reducing that risk would come under substantial positive selective pressure.

Potential Mechanisms for the Malaria Resistance Afforded by HbAS

Despite the overwhelming evidence supporting the strong protective effect of HbAS against all forms of clinical *P. falciparum* malaria, the precise mechanisms for this protection remain unclear (Williams, 2011). Many have been suggested (Table 1.2), some of which are supported by stronger evidence than others. Nevertheless, which of these mechanisms is the most important in nature remains a matter for considerable speculation. Some of the earliest studies in this area showed that erythrocytes from HbAS subjects are vulnerable to sickling when infected by *P. falciparum* parasites *in vitro* and are potentially susceptible, therefore, to an increased rate of removal by the spleen (Luzzatto, Nwachuku-Jarrett, & Reddy, 1970; Roth et al., 1978). In a recent study by Cao and colleagues, this hypothesis was finessed further to invoke a mechanism involving the increased expression of high mannose glycans on the infected red cell surface through a mechanism induced by oxygen stress. Interestingly, the authors also concluded that, unrelated to malaria, the same mechanism is involved in the removal of damaged SCA red blood cells (RBCs) by splenic macrophages, invoking the intriguing possibility that a unifying biological mechanism might be involved in the removal of both parasite-infected HbAS RBCs and effete SCA RBCs that have been damaged by disease-specific mechanisms.

A number of studies have shown that, potentially due to oxidant damage, *P. falciparum* parasites are also less able to grow in HbS-containing erythrocytes *in vitro* (Friedman, 1978, 1979a, 1979b; Friedman, Roth, Nagel, & Trager, 1979a, 1979b; Pasvol, Weatherall, & Wilson, 1978) and are also more vulnerable to removal from circulation by monocytes (Ayi, Turrini, Piga, & Arese, 2004). More recently, it has been suggested that, rather than being entirely innate, the protective effect of HbS might also involve a learned immunological component. For example, in studies conducted in both Kenya (Williams, Mwangi, Roberts et al., 2005) and Uganda (Gong et al., 2012), the degree of protection afforded by HbAS was seen to increase with age. It has been proposed that this might be the result of improved immune responses to proteins expressed on the RBC surface (Cabrera et al., 2005; Marsh, Otoo, Hayes, Carson, & Greenwood, 1989), although the data in support

Table 1.2 Potential mechanisms by which HbAS might protect against *P. falciparum* malaria.

Mechanistic hypotheses	Example observations	References
Reduced growth and multiplication of *P. falciparum* parasites in HbAS RBCs	Malaria infections became established much less frequently in HbAS than in HbAA adult volunteers when inoculated experimentally with *P. falciparum* parasites (two different strains).	Allison (1954)
	P. falciparum growth is reduced in HbAS red cells *in vitro* and is arrested under conditions of low oxygen tension. This probably relates to the polymerization of HbAS haemoglobin when deoxygenated.	Archer et al. (2018); Friedman (1978); Friedman, Roth, Nagel, and Trager (1979b)
Increased clearance of *P. falciparum*-infected RBCs in HbAS individuals	Increased clearance of infected sickled RBCs by the spleen. Early studies suggested this could be mechanical, but a recent study has invoked a mechanism involving high mannose glycan expression on the red cell surface, induced by oxidant stress.	Luzzatto et al. (1970); Mackey and Vivarelli (1954); Miller, Neel and Livingstone (1956)
	More rapidly acquired host immunity and increased phagocytosis of ring-parasitized variant RBCs.	Cao et al. (2021); Cao and Vickers (2021)
Reduced pathophysiological consequences of malaria infections in HbAS individuals	Reduced cytoadherence of infected red cells to endothelial receptors and reduced red cell rosetting.	Carlson, Nash, Gabutti, al-Yaman and Wahlgren (1994); Cholera et al. (2008); Opi et al. (2014); Petersen et al. (2021)
	The above may be explained by impaired trafficking of parasite-specific proteins to the RBC surface.	Chauvet et al., (2021); Cyrklaff et al. (2011); Saelens et al. (2021)
Resistance to all but a few natural *P. falciparum* parasite clones *in vivo*	In a large case-control study, all cases of severe *P. falciparum* malaria in children with either HbAS or HbSS were with parasites carrying one or more of three genetically linked alleles. Such parasites were rare (only ~10%) among individuals without the HbS mutation.	Band et al. (2021)

of this hypothesis are somewhat mixed (Tan et al., 2011). Recent studies have suggested an alternative or additional explanation for the protective advantage of HbS. Expression of the *P. falciparum*-derived molecule PfEMP1 on the surface of HbAS RBCs was reduced in studies conducted *in vitro* (Cholera et al., 2008). PfEMP1 is a key mediator of the cytoadhesion of parasite-infected RBCs to the lining of blood vessels through specific interactions with receptors on the endothelial surface. This process, which is otherwise known as sequestration, is central to the pathophysiology of severe malaria (White, Turner, Day, & Dondorp, 2013). This raises the possibility that protection might relate to the decreased ability of malaria parasite-infected HbAS RBCs to sequester in deep vascular tissues.

This hypothesis is further supported by studies showing that such cells are less able to cytoadhere to a range of endothelial receptors in *in vitro* models (Cholera et al., 2008; Petersen et al., 2021). Subsequent studies have shown that reduced PfEMP1 expression may result from a defect in intracellular transport from the parasite organelle to the red cell surface (Cyrklaff et al., 2011; Saelens et al., 2021). This discovery was echoed in a more recent study by Chauvet and colleagues. On studying the proteome and the phosphoproteome of membrane extracts from both *P. falciparum*-infected and non-infected RBCs, they showed that HbS heterozygous carriage, combined with malaria infection, leads to modulation in the phosphorylation of erythrocyte membrane transporters and skeletal proteins as well as of parasite proteins, concluding that the interactions within membrane protein complexes could be disturbed by altered phosphorylation patterns, disturbing nutrient uptake and cytoadherence to mitigate against severity symptoms.

Finally, in a very recent study it was shown that among children presenting with severe and complicated malaria, the parasites infecting those with the rs334 mutation were genetically quite distinct from the parasites infecting normal children (Band et al., 2021). Virtually all the parasites infecting children with either HbAS or HbSS carried one or more of three linked alleles, which were only seen in a small proportion of the parasites infecting those without the rs334 mutation (Band et al., 2021). Further, parasites carrying these alleles are not found at all in regions where the rs334 mutation is not present (Band et al., 2021). Remarkably, children carrying the rs334 mutation, either as heterozygotes or homozygotes, were almost completely resistant to infections caused by all *P. falciparum* parasites apart from those carrying these specific alleles. This supports the conclusion that rs334 provides total resistance to severe infections caused by the vast majority of other *P. falciparum* strains and that these strains have adapted specifically for their ability to survive in HbS-containing RBCs. This raises the intriguing possibility that Mendelian selection has been at work on multiple levels. Thus, not only has rs334 been selected to its current frequencies because it confers a survival advantage against *P. falciparum* malaria, but, in turn, the same mutation has also resulted in Mendelian selection within *P. falciparum* parasite populations themselves. Further studies investigating the mechanisms that underlie this observation will hopefully provide fresh insights into the evolutionary forces that have led to the selection of these *P. falciparum* alleles in Africa.

Epistasis

Recently, it has been shown that epistasis, or in other words interactions between different genes, has been an important determinant of the geographic distribution of many genetic disorders, including SCA (Miko, 2008). Specifically, the resistance afforded against malaria by HbAS is almost totally lost when it is coinherited with another common haemoglobinopathy, α^+-thalassaemia (Williams, Mwangi, Wambua, Peto et al., 2005). On investigating the potential explanations for this negative epistatic interaction, Opi and colleagues 2014) confirmed the observation from previous reports that *P. falciparum*-infected HbAS RBCs show reduced cytoadhesion, rosetting, and PfEMP1 expression levels compared to normal controls (Cholera et al., 2008). This is thought to relate to the intracellular concentrations of HbS in RBCs from children with these different conditions, which are highest in children with HbAS alone, drop significantly in heterozygotes for α^+-thalassaemia, and drop further still in homozygotes (Opi et al., 2014; Williams, Mwangi, Wambua, Peto et al., 2005). However, they also found that where HbAS was coinherited with α^+-thalassaemia these reductions were reversed, to the degree that malaria-infected RBCs from children carrying both genes showed levels of cytoadhesion, rosetting, and PfEMP1 expression that were indistinguishable from those seen in normal children. Therefore, their study supports the hypothesis that the negative epistasis between HbAS and α^+-thalassaemia observed in epidemiological studies might be explained by host genotype-specific changes in the adhesion properties of malaria-infected RBCs that contribute to parasite sequestration and disease pathogenesis *in vivo*.

Subsequently, through a modelling study based on these and other observations, Penman and colleagues concluded that the complex distribution of various haemoglobinopathies across Africa, the Mediterranean, and South Asia might be explained by interactions that occur between them (Penman, Pybus, Weatherall, & Gupta, 2009). Specifically, they found evidence to support the hypothesis that the patchiness in the population frequencies of rs334 within the Mediterranean might be explained by epistatic interactions between HbAS and the α- and β-thalassaemias. They further hypothesized the converse: that the relatively low prevalence of α-thalassaemia in Africa, in comparison to Southeast Asia, might be explained by the presence of HbS (Penman, Habib, Kanchan, & Gupta, 2011). Taken together, these studies suggest that the evolutionary selection for HbS by malaria is much more complex than previously thought.

Malaria and Sickle Cell Disease

Despite the strong resistance to malaria seen in children with HbAS, it is often said that malaria is a major cause of mortality in African children with SCA (Serjeant, 2005). As already discussed, the protection afforded by HbS against malaria appears to be directly correlated with the concentration of HbS within RBCs – the higher the concentration of intracellular HbS the greater is the degree

of malaria protection (Williams, Mwangi, Wambua, Peto et al., 2005). Consequently, at face value, the increased susceptibility of children with SCA to death
from *P. falciparum* malaria seems counter intuitive. However, in reality, both
facts are probably true: that HbSS is even more strongly protective against the
growth and invasion of *P. falciparum* parasites than HbAS but that this protection
is not complete, and that even light malaria infections can trigger SCA-specific
crises (Uyoga et al., 2022). Anaemic crises are a particular risk in this regard,
whereby malaria infections can precipitate rapid falls in haemoglobin that can
rapidly prove fatal without urgent treatment with blood transfusion and antimalarial drugs. This conclusion is supported by the high mortality that has been observed in children presenting with both SCA and anaemia in a number of settings
(Makani et al., 2011; Uyoga et al., 2022; Williams & Obaro, 2011) and also by
the mortality benefits of prophylaxis with antimalarial drugs (Frimpong, Thiam,
Arko-Boham, Owusu, & Adjei, 2018).

Despite an increased risk of death when children with SCA are infected by
malaria parasites, it appears that they more rarely develop some of the most
common forms of severe malaria that occur in children without the disease,
including cerebral malaria and high-density *P. falciparum* infections (Henrici
et al., 2021; "The World Health Organization. Severe Malaria," 2014). In children without SCA, such infections are classically accompanied by high total
body parasite loads, as indicated by high plasma concentrations of the para-
site-derived protein *P. falciparum* Histidine Rich Protein 2 (PfHRP2) (Dondorp
et al., 2005). In normal children with severe and complicated malaria, plasma
concentrations of PfHRP2 typically exceed 1,000 ng/mL (Hendriksen et al.,
2012). However, values that high were rarely seen among children with SCA and
malaria in two recent studies conducted in Uganda (Henrici et al., 2021; Uyoga
et al., 2022). In a large transfusion trial that included hundreds of children with
SCA and malaria, median levels of PfHRP2 were only 8 ng/mL (Uyoga et al.,
2022), a value similar to those that are typically seen in children without SCA
who have asymptomatic or incidental *P. falciparum* infections (Uyoga et al.,
2021). The most common and important complication of malaria in children
with SCA is severe acute anaemia, most commonly in the presence of only a
relatively low total body parasite load (Uyoga et al., 2022). The fact that malaria
can precipitate such a profound and potentially fatal complication means that in
malaria-endemic regions, it is important that children with SCA are protected
from malaria, preferably by the use of both insecticide-treated bed nets and antimalarial chemoprophylaxis.

The Global Distribution and Current Population Frequencies of the rs334 Mutation

The strong selection for rs334 through the increased malaria survival of heterozygotes means that, historically, SCA was entirely focused on malaria-endemic
regions of the world. The disease occurs most commonly in Africa, the Middle
East, India, and parts of the Mediterranean. Although historically absent from

the Americas, SCA was also introduced to that region during recent centuries as a consequence of the slave trade. As a result, the condition is also now common throughout much of North and South America. The highest population frequencies of rs334 are seen in the band of Africa between the Sahara Desert and the Zambezi River, where malaria transmission has historically been highest. The allele frequency for rs334 typically exceeds 10% throughout most of this region, but balancing selection means that the frequency of 20% is only exceeded in limited areas, which include several parts of Nigeria (Idowu, Mafiana, & Dapo, 2005; Sadek, 1974).

Because the registration of births is incomplete throughout much of Africa, and no countries within the region have yet established comprehensive screening for SCA at birth, it is impossible to know precisely how many children are born with SCA in Africa every year. Similarly, it is also impossible to know the age- and cause-specific mortality rates among this group of children and therefore to estimate the total number of affected people that are currently living on the continent. For these reasons, many such estimates are based on educated guesses, extrapolated from suboptimal data.

Countless population surveys for SCA have been conducted worldwide in the seven decades since the condition was first described. While early studies were largely based on the observation of "sickling" in the presence of reducing agents by use of microscopic methods, more recent studies have employed more accurate phenotypic and molecular approaches that yield information on both heterozygotes and homozygotes. Two scientists, Allison and Livingstone, made particular contributions to the mapping of carrier frequencies from the 1950s onwards, which culminated in the first global database and maps of SCA and other haemoglobinopathies in the mid-1980s (Livingstone, 1985). In 2010, these estimates were significantly refined and updated by Piel and colleagues, who conducted a systematic review of published and unpublished studies that are based on specific criteria and included data from non-biased studies (Piel et al., 2010). From over 40,000 studies reviewed, they identified 278 studies that documented unbiased allele frequencies from 699 specific populations for inclusion in their further analyses. Through a Bayesian geostatistical modelling approach, they were then able to estimate allele frequencies for the entire world at a 10 × 10-km spatial resolution. By overlaying these allele frequency maps onto maps of the historic prevalence of malaria (Lysenko & Semashko, 1968), they were then able to demonstrate a highly significant correlation between the frequency of the two conditions at a global scale (Piel et al., 2010). This study provides some of the strongest evidence to date that the current frequency of rs334 is the result of its Mendelian selection by malaria.

In an extension of this work, the same authors estimated the number of babies born with SCA both globally and nationally. Using their allele frequency maps in concert with United Nations data on national birth rates ("World population prospects: The 2010 revision. http://esa.un.org/ unpp.," 2011), plus data on population densities from the Global Rural Urban Mapping Project (GRUMP) (Guerra et al., 2007), they estimated that a total of 312,302 (IQR 294,307–329,729) babies with

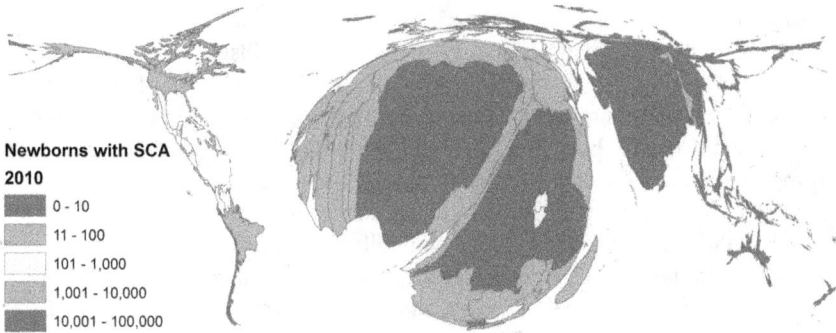

Figure 1.3 The global distribution of SCA in 2010.

SCA were born in 2010 (Piel, Patil et al., 2013). They further estimated that 75.4% of all these births (238,083; IQR 224,003−253,047) occurred in Africa and that the majority of the balance (15.1%; 42,597; IQR 35,022−50,750) were born in India (Piel, Patil et al., 2013). Individually, the top three contributing countries were Nigeria (almost 90,000 births/year), India (>40,000), and the Democratic Republic of Congo (almost 40,000) (Figure 1.3). Extending their estimates into the future, they further predicted that a total of 14,242,000 (95% CI 9,923,600–20,498,500) babies will be born with SCA globally during the 40 years between 2010 and 2050 (Piel, Hay, Gupta, Weatherall, & Williams, 2013).

Mortality among Children Born with SCA in Africa

As stated previously, in the absence of new-born screening programmes and universal vital registration throughout most of Africa, there can be no reliable estimates of mortality among children born with SCA for the whole continent. In the past, it was well recognized that the number of adult patients with SCA in Africa was much lower than that expected based on the assumed numbers that are born with the disease each year. From as early as the 1950s, multiple observers reported an almost complete absence of SCA subjects among surveys of African adults (Edington & Lehmann, 1954; Fleming, Storey, Molineaux, Iroko, & Attai, 1979), while others reported frequencies that were less than 20% of those expected (Akinyanju, 1989; Bernstein, Bowman, & Kaptue Noche, 1980; Jacob, 1957). Such observations suggest that historically, up to 80% or more of all children born with SCA in Africa have been dying, most having never been diagnosed in the first place. Recently, Grosse and colleagues conducted a review of all the published studies conducted in Africa that supported this conclusion. Their study included unselected age-stratified population data for SCA (Grosse et al., 2011) collected through studies conducted throughout Africa since the 1960s. In virtually every report, they found that the population prevalence of SCA declined dramatically with age at a rate that was consistent with an average mortality of 50–90% in children <5 years old.

Such indirect methods for estimating mortality are particularly valuable because they reflect the natural history of SCA in the absence of diagnosis and treatment. Although direct studies observing mortality in cohorts of children with SCA are also important, given that in general they are based on cohorts of children that have already been diagnosed, are attending clinics, and are in receipt of appropriate treatments such as education, vaccination, and infection control, they inevitably yield mortality estimates that are lower. In one such recent study, conducted on the coast of Kenya, Uyoga and colleagues identified 128 children with SCA from among 15,737 infants screened for the condition and followed them until they were five years old (Uyoga, Macharia, Mochamah et al., 2019). Overall, mortality was more than 23 times higher in the children with SCA (58/1,000 person years of observation (PYO); 95% CI 40–86) than in children without the condition (2·4/1,000 PYO; 2·0–2·8). Nevertheless, under-5 mortality among the children with SCA overall (29%) was considerably lower than that based on indirect methods (Grosse et al., 2011), supporting the positive benefits of diagnosis and treatment. Of particular note, for reasons that were not entirely clear, not all of the 128 children diagnosed with SCA through the study agreed to enrol at the clinic for regular treatment (Uyoga, Macharia, Mochamah et al., 2019). The authors noted that the rates of mortality were almost fourfold lower in those who did enrol (29/1,000 PYO) than in those who did not (104/1,000 PYO; Incidence Rate Ratio 0·26, 95% CI 0·11–0·62), such that more than 85% of those attending the clinic survived to the age of five years, a remarkable improvement over historic levels.

Recently, an alternative approach to the estimation of mortality among children with SCA in Africa has been proposed. This approach is based on interviews conducted with the mothers of affected children (Ranque et al., 2022). In a study conducted in SCA clinics in five countries in West Africa, Ranque and colleagues collected mortality data from women with children attending SCA clinics who had also given birth to at least three additional children more than five years previously. Because SCA is an autosomal recessive condition that results from a union between two heterozygous parents, Mendelian principles mean that each child born to such parents has a 25% chance of being affected. The authors applied this logic to inflate the mortality data derived from these mothers to account for the statistical chance that each child, alive or dead, had SCA. Their study suggested that under-5 mortality among children with SCA overall (36.4%; 95% CI 33.4–39.4) was broadly similar to that in the earlier study from Kenya, supporting the conclusion that mortality among affected children across Africa has declined over recent decades.

Causes of Death among Children with SCA in Africa and the Realities of Diagnostics

Given the evidence that child mortality has historically been extremely high in children born with SCA in Africa, it may seem surprising how little is known about the causes. In reality, this is simply a further reflection of the historic neglect that the condition has received until very recently. In the absence of early diagnosis, active follow-up, routine death registration, and routine post-mortems, it is impossible to know the most common causes of death with any certainty. However, it seems likely that historically, invasive bacterial diseases, malaria, and severe anaemia have been among the most important.

Bacterial Diseases in Children with SCA in Africa

Bacterial infections have long been recognized as major causes of morbidity and mortality among children born with SCA worldwide, with the risk rising sharply beyond 3–6 months of age. The causes are numerous, but some of the most important are declining splenic function, defects in complement activation and specific nutrient deficiencies (Booth, Inusa, & Obaro, 2010). It is widely accepted that the first is particularly important, because of the central role of the spleen with regard to protection from capsulated bacteria such as streptococci (Booth et al., 2010). Additionally, the small vessel vaso-occlusion that is a central feature of SCA (Williams & Thein, 2018) leads to areas of ischaemia and microinfarction in organs such as the gut and the bone marrow, which can both breach defences and establish poorly perfused areas of tissue that are conducive to bacterial growth.

A number of organisms, including *Streptococcus pneumoniae, Haemophilus influenzae*, and non-Typhi Salmonella species, were identified as important aetiological agents in seminal studies conducted in the USA (Barrett-Connor, 1971; Diggs, 1967; Powars, Overturf, & Turner, 1983; Robinson & Halpern, 1974) and subsequently mirrored in studies conducted in other parts of the world, including Europe and Jamaica (John et al., 1984). Although the introduction of penicillin prophylaxis and immunization with conjugate vaccines directed against *S. pneumoniae* and *H. influenzae* type b (Hib) has revolutionized the outlook for patients born with SCA in these same regions (Ammann et al., 1977; John et al., 1984), there has long been a paucity of data on the incidence and relative importance of invasive bacterial infections among children with SCA in Africa, where the vast majority of all such children are born (Piel, Patil et al., 2013). Until quite recently, the relative importance of some specific organisms, particularly *S. pneumomiae*, and therefore the need for penicillin prophylaxis and vaccination, was still in question (Kizito, Mworozi, Ndugwa, & Serjeant, 2007; Serjeant, 2005). However, a study from Kenya has since made it very clear that the situation in Africa is no different from that in other regions: that the incidence of invasive bacterial infections among African children with SCA is almost 30 times that in those without the disease, and that the organisms responsible are also the same, the top three culprits being *S. pneumoniae*, non-typhoidal *Salmonella* species, and *H. influenzae* (Williams et al., 2009).

Ramakrishnan and colleagues have since conducted a systematic review and meta-analysis of studies conducted in Africa that indicated a 19-fold risk of invasive bacterial infections in SCA compared to non-SCA children overall, the rates being 36 times higher for *S. pneumoniae* and 13 times higher for *H. influenzae* (Ramakrishnan et al., 2010). In terms of incidence rates, these studies suggest that historically, in the absence of infection prophylaxis, the risk of all cause severe invasive bacterial diseases such as septicaemia and meningitis, among young children with SCA in sub-Saharan Africa, may have been as high as 10% per year (Williams et al., 2009). Given that such infections would have almost certainly have been universally fatal in the pre-antibiotic era, it is obvious that invasive bacterial infections will have played a central role in years gone by.

Notably, highly effective vaccines have been developed in recent years for two of the top three organisms, *S. pneumoniae* and *H. influenzae*, and have now been introduced into extended programmes of immunization throughout the region. Children with SCA will undoubtedly benefit disproportionately from this development, with the result that many more children with SCA will survive to the point at which their diagnosis can be established and result in referral for suitable care. Nevertheless, it remains important that children with SCA are diagnosed as soon as possible, so that they can also be protected from the increased risk of infections through the appropriate use of antibiotic prophylaxis.

Severe Anaemic Episodes

Severe acute anaemia is a second major cause for the high mortality seen historically among children born with SCA in Africa. A common complication of SCA wherever it occurs, there are specific reasons why severe anaemia is more often fatal within the region. First, the absence of new-born screening throughout most of the continent means that it can be very difficult to recognize children with SCA among the many others presenting to health facilities with severe anaemia because of other causes. In many African hospitals, upwards of 10% of all admitted children are severely anaemic and in need of a blood transfusion (Pedro, Akech, Fegan, & Maitland, 2010). Furthermore, the supply of blood for transfusion is often suboptimal within the region, and mortality is particularly high in such circumstances (Maitland et al., 2021).

Finally, as stated above, malaria is a particularly strong precipitating cause of anaemic crises in children with SCA. In a recent multi-centre trial of blood transfusion strategies in Africa, Maitland and colleagues recruited almost three and a half thousand children who had been admitted to hospital in Uganda with haemoglobin levels of <6 g/dL (Uyoga et al., 2022). In the interest of generalizability, they specifically limited recruitment of children with an existing diagnosis of SCA. Nevertheless, when they tested the children recruited at the end of trial, they found that 17% had SCA that had not yet been diagnosed at the point of recruitment. This was despite a background frequency for SCA at birth within the same population of only ~1% (Ndeezi et al., 2016). Similarly, in a surveillance study of almost 19,000 children admitted to hospital in Kenya, Macharia and colleagues found that 31% of the children who had SCA, most diagnosed through the study, were admitted with a haemoglobin level of <5 g/dL (Macharia et al., 2018).

Overall, they found that children with SCA were 58 times more likely to be admitted with anaemia of this severity than were non-SCA children. The incidence of admission to hospital with severe anaemia among children with SCA overall was 17.7/100 PYO and reached 26.1/100 PYO among children 2–13 years old. These rates are significantly higher than those reported from studies conducted in the North. For instance, an incidence of <5/100 PYO was reported in the seminal Cooperative Study of SCA in the USA (Gaston & Rosse, 1982; Gill et al., 1995; Leikin et al., 1989), the difference probably being due to malaria. From such studies, it can be easily appreciated how important severe anaemic episodes will have been historically as a contributing cause of premature death among children with SCA in sub-Saharan Africa.

Further Phenotypes of Specific Relevance to Africa

The clinical complications of SCA have been well described through a number of studies, perhaps most notably the co-operative study in the USA (Gaston & Rosse, 1982; Gill et al., 1995; Leikin et al., 1989) and the long-term cohort study conducted in Jamaica (Serjeant & Serjeant, 2001), and have also been well described in a number of recent reviews (Ware, de Montalembert, Tshilolo, & Abboud, 2017; Williams & Thein, 2018). However, few detailed studies of the clinical epidemiology of SCA have been conducted in Africa that make direct comparisons easy. As a result, it is hard to know whether treatment recommendations developed based on data from these earlier studies are universally relevant to subjects affected by SCA in Africa. There are several theoretical reasons why specific differences in the epidemiology of SCA between Africa and other regions might occur, including environmental factors like malaria, levels of exposure to other infectious diseases (including helminths and other parasites), higher temperatures, and factors related to genetics and under-nutrition. Based on limited data (Macharia et al., 2018; McGann et al., 2018; Olupot-Olupot et al., 2020; Uyoga, Macharia, Mochamah et al., 2019), the incidence rates for many of the most common complications of SCA appear to be broadly similar between the regions; however, significant differences in specific areas, including steady-state haematological and other laboratory values, have been noted in comparative studies conducted in multiple countries (McGann et al., 2018). It has also been suggested that the epidemiology of the condition might differ in a number of important respects. In this regard, two issues of specific interest are the spleen and neurological complications, including strokes and silent cerebral infarcts.

The Spleen

Splenic dysfunction is a central feature of SCA. Children with SCA have morphologically and functionally normal spleens at birth, but through a sequence of vaso-occlusive and ischaemic events, the spleen rapidly becomes fibrotic and atrophic.

It is generally thought that this process of "autosplenectomy" is complete by the age of five years (Pearson, Spencer, & Cornelius, 1969) and is one major reason for the increased risk of invasive bacterial infections in children with SCA. Another life-threatening complication related to the spleen is acute splenic sequestration, a condition that is characterized by the sudden enlargement of the spleen due to pooling of blood, and which is closely associated with rapidly progressive anaemia and hypovolaemia (Brousse et al., 2012). Programmes alerting parents to the signs of splenic sequestration have led to significant declines in mortality from the condition in several regions (Emond et al., 1985).

In high-income countries, splenomegaly in children with SCA is most often transient and is followed by splenic atrophy. In contrast, some authors have observed splenomegaly to be common even past the age of six years among patients with SCA in SSA. For example, in one study conducted in Kenya, palpable splenomegaly was found in 41 of 124 children (33%) with SCA aged 0–14 years (Sadarangani et al., 2009). Although common in all age groups, the peak prevalence was in children aged 6–8 years. Similarly, among more than 600 children in four African countries, McGann and colleagues noted that spleens were palpable in 16%. These observations raise the possibility that the rate at which the spleen involutes in children with SCA might be slower in Africa than in other regions. The determinants of splenomegaly in SCA are not fully understood but probably involve multiple genetic and external factors. Persistently high levels of HbF have been shown to correlate with persistent splenomegaly, and infectious agents may further interfere with spleen size, especially in malaria-endemic countries where hyperreactive malarial splenomegaly is common. In a large Tanzanian cohort with SCA aged 4 months to 47 years (median age 11 years), spleen size was examined in patients with and without malaria parasitaemia (Makani et al., 2010). Palpable splenomegaly was noted in 19.4% of patients with malaria parasitaemia but in only 9.8% of those without, raising the possibility that malaria may be causally related. Despite the potential that important differences may exist between splenic size and function among SCA patients in Africa and other regions, as highlighted in a recent systematic review (Ladu, Aiyenigba, Adekile, & Bates, 2021), there are a paucity of studies describing the contribution of SCD-induced splenic dysfunction to morbidity and infection related mortality in Africa and further studies are therefore required to address this important question.

Strokes and Silent Cerebral Infarcts

Given their huge relevance to quality of life, a final issue of particular importance in the African context is the frequency of strokes and silent cerebral infarcts. Strokes are among the most serious and devastating acute complications of SCA. Based on data from the US Cooperative Study, before the specific interventions were introduced, they occurred at an overall rate of 0.61 episodes/100 PYO (Ohene-Frempong et al., 1998). Strokes can either be infarctive or haemorrhagic, the former being the more common (Ohene-Frempong et al., 1998). The risk of infarctive strokes can be predicted during childhood from velocities in the cerebral blood vessels, measured by Trans-Cranial Doppler (TCD) Ultrasonography (Adams et al., 1992). As a result, TCD is now widely used for screening, and children with high velocities of ≥200 cm/s are considered at high risk of stroke and targeted for preventive treatment using long-term blood transfusion (Adams et al., 1992). In the STOP trial, conducted in the USA, transfusion therapy resulted in a 92% reduction in the risk of overt stroke among children with TCD velocities of ≥200cm/s, and it also reduced the risk of further strokes in children with existing silent infarcts (DeBaun et al., 2014). However, reversion to abnormal TCD velocities and a high risk of further strokes are commonly seen when transfusion therapy is discontinued (Adams, Brambilla, & Optimizing Primary Stroke Prevention in Sickle Cell Anemia Trial, 2005; Lee et al., 2006).

The reliance on TCD monitoring and transfusion therapy for those screening positive as the main stays of stroke prevention present challenges in the African context. First, beyond specific research programmes, few sites have expertise in the use of TCD while, second, long-term transfusion therapy is not realistic for the great majority of affected children within the region. First, the number of blood donations throughout most of the continent falls far short of that recommended by the World Health Organization (WHO, 2016). Second, the risks of transfusion-acquired infections are also substantially higher in Africa than those seen in the North while, third, the unavailability of extended cross-matching presents a substantial risk of alloimmunization (Boateng, Ngoma, Bates, & Schonewille, 2019).

Relatively few studies have been conducted that have assessed the incidence or management of neurological complications among children born with SCA in Africa. Early studies conducted in Nigeria (Izuora, Kaine, & Emodi, 1989) and Kenya (Amayo, Owade, Aluoch, & Njeru, 1992) suggested that the incidence of stroke might be almost twice as high in Africa (1.3/100 PYO) as that reported from studies conducted in the USA (Ohene-Frempong et al., 1998), potentially because of the higher prevalence of key risk factors such as low haemoglobin levels, high white cell counts, and the CAR/Bantu haplotype. However, in the first study of TCD velocities conducted in Africa, Makani and colleagues found that velocities were significantly lower and the number of abnormally high velocities substantially fewer than those reported from other regions (Makani et al., 2009). They hypothesized that this might reflect a survivor bias, that stroke leads to high mortality in the study area, and that at-risk children might therefore have been missing from those sampled. Subsequent studies have found that both stroke and neurological deficits and abnormal TCD velocities are common in children with SCA in multiple settings in Africa. For example, in Nigeria, Lugunju and colleagues found a high prevalence of both stroke (>8%) and conditional (19%) or abnormal (4%) TCD velocities in children attending the SCA clinic at the University College Hospital in Ibadan (Lagunju & Brown, 2012; Lagunju, Sodeinde, & Telfer, 2012), an observation that has since been replicated in other populations (Cox et al., 2014; Galadanci et al., 2017; Soyebi et al., 2014). Similarly, others have found a high prevalence of both silent cerebral infarcts and strokes in imaging studies conducted in multiple populations (Green et al., 2019; Jacob et al., 2020; Kija et al., 2019). Together, such studies underline the importance of the neurological complications of SCA in Africa. Urgent work is needed to identify locally appropriate solutions for both screening and prevention.

Concluding Remarks

While Africa is the global epicentre of SCA, the condition has been widely neglected on the continent for far too long. In recent years, this fact has been recognized both locally and by international organizations such as the World Health Organization ("World Health Organization, Genomics and World Health, Report of the Advisory Committee on Health Research, World Health Organization, Geneva," 2002), the United Nations (United Nations, United Nations Millennium Declaration, resolution 55/2, 2000), the American Society of Hematology (McGann, Hernandez, & Ware, 2017), and the National Institutes of Health in the USA. For the first time, a number of countries within the region have now developed clinical guidelines and are beginning to introduce new-born screening programmes. While major advances have been made in the last 20 years, a great deal remains to be learned about the specifics of SCA in the African context.

References

Adams, R. J., Brambilla, D., & Optimizing Primary Stroke Prevention in Sickle Cell Anemia Trial, I. (2005). Discontinuing prophylactic transfusions used to prevent stroke in sickle cell disease. *N Engl J Med, 353*(26), 2769–2778. https://doi.org/10.1056/NEJMoa050460

Adams, R., McKie, V., Nichols, F., Carl, E., Zhang, D. L., McKie, K., ... Hess, D. (1992). The use of transcranial ultrasonography to predict stroke in sickle cell disease. *N Engl J Med, 326*(9), 605–610.

Akinyanju, O. O. (1989). A profile of sickle cell disease in Nigeria. *Ann N Y Acad Sci, 565*, 126–136. Retrieved from https://pubmed.ncbi.nlm.nih.gov/2672962/

Allison, A. C. (1954). Protection afforded by sickle cell trait against subtertian malarial infection. *British Medical Journal, 1*, 290–295.

Alsultan, A., Alabdulaali, M. K., Griffin, P. J., Alsuliman, A. M., Ghabbour, H. A., Sebastiani, P., ... Steinberg, M. H. (2014). Sickle cell disease in Saudi Arabia: The phenotype in adults with the Arab-Indian haplotype is not benign. *Br J Haematol, 164*(4), 597–604. https://doi.org/10.1111/bjh.12650

Amayo, E. O., Owade, J. N., Aluoch, J. R., & Njeru, E. K. (1992). Neurological complications of sickle cell anaemia at KNH: A five year retrospective study. *East Afr Med J, 69*(12), 660–662.

Ammann, A. J., Addiego, J., Wara, D. W., Lubin, B., Smith, W. B., & Mentzer, W. C. (1977). Polyvalent pneumococcal-polysaccharide immunization of patients with sickle-cell anemia and patients with splenectomy. *N Engl J Med, 297*(17), 897–900.

Archer, N. M., Petersen, N., Clark, M. A., Buckee, C. O., Childs, L. M., & Duraisingh, M. T. (2018). Resistance to Plasmodium falciparum in sickle cell trait erythrocytes is driven by oxygen-dependent growth inhibition. *Proc Natl Acad Sci USA*, *115*(28), 7350–7355. https://doi.org/10.1073/pnas.1804388115

Ayi, K., Turrini, F., Piga, A., & Arese, P. (2004). Enhanced phagocytosis of ring-parasitized mutant erythrocytes. A common mechanism that may explain protection against falciparum-malaria in sickle-trait and beta-thalassemia-trait. *Blood*, *104*, 3364–3371.

Band, G., Leffler, E. M., Jallow, M., Sisay-Joof, F., Ndila, C. M., Macharia, A. W., ... Kwiatkowski, D. P. (2021). Malaria protection due to sickle haemoglobin depends on parasite genotype. *Nature*. https://doi.org/10.1038/s41586-021-04288-3

Barrett-Connor, E. (1971). Bacterial infection and sickle cell anemia. An analysis of 250 infections in 166 patients and a review of the literature. *Medicine*, *50*(2), 97–112.

Beet, E. A. (1946). Sickle cell disease in the Balovale District of Northern Rhodesia. *E African Med J*, *23*, 75–86.

Beet, E. A. (1947). Sickle cell disease in northern Rhodesia. *E African Med J*, *24*, 212–222.

Bernstein, S. C., Bowman, J. E., & Kaptue Noche, L. (1980). Population studies in Cameroon: Hemoglobin S, glucose-6-phosphate dehydrogenase deficiency and falciparum malaria. *Hum Hered*, *30*(4), 251–258.

Boateng, L. A., Ngoma, A. M., Bates, I., & Schonewille, H. (2019). Red blood cell alloimmunization in transfused patients with sickle cell disease in Sub-Saharan Africa: A systematic review and meta-analysis. *Transfus Med Rev*, *33*(3), 162–169. https://doi.org/10.1016/j.tmrv.2019.06.003

Booth, C., Inusa, B., & Obaro, S. K. (2010). Infection in sickle cell disease: A review. *Int J Infect Dis*, *14*(1), e2–e12. https://doi.org/10.1016/j.ijid.2009.03.010

Brain, P. (1952). Sickle-cell anaemia in Africa. *Brit Med J*, *2*, 880.

Brousse, V., Elie, C., Benkerrou, M., Odievre, M. H., Lesprit, E., Bernaudin, F., ... de Montalembert, M. (2012). Acute splenic sequestration crisis in sickle cell disease: Cohort study of 190 paediatric patients. *Br J Haematol*, *156*(5), 643–648. https://doi.org/10.1111/j.1365-2141.2011.08999.x

Cabrera, G., Cot, M., Migot-Nabias, F., Kremsner, P. G., Deloron, P., & Luty, A. J. (2005). The sickle cell trait is associated with enhanced immunoglobulin G antibody responses to *Plasmodium falciparum* variant surface antigens. *J Infect Dis*, *191*(10), 1631–1638.

Cao, H., Antonopoulos, A., Henderson, S., Wassall, H., Brewin, J., Masson, A., ... Vickers, M. A. (2021). Red blood cell mannoses as phagocytic ligands mediating both sickle cell anaemia and malaria resistance. *Nat Commun*, *12*(1), 1792. https://doi.org/10.1038/s41467-021-21814-z

Cao, H., & Vickers, M. A. (2021). Oxidative stress, malaria, sickle cell disease, and innate immunity. *Trends Immunol*, *42*(10), 849–851. https://doi.org/10.1016/j.it.2021.08.008

Carlson, J., Nash, G. B., Gabutti, V., al-Yaman, F., & Wahlgren, M. (1994). Natural protection against severe *Plasmodium falciparum* malaria due to impaired rosette formation. *Blood*, *84*(11), 3909–3914.

Chauvet, M., Chhuon, C., Lipecka, J., Dechavanne, S., Dechavanne, C., Lohezic, M., ... Merckx, A. (2021). Sickle cell trait modulates the proteome and phosphoproteome of Plasmodium falciparum-infected erythrocytes. *Front Cell Infect Microbiol*, *11*, 637604. https://doi.org/10.3389/fcimb.2021.637604

Cholera, R., Brittain, N. J., Gillrie, M. R., Lopera-Mesa, T. M., Diakite, S. A., Arie, T., ... Fairhurst, R. M. (2008). Impaired cytoadherence of *Plasmodium falciparum*-infected erythrocytes containing sickle hemoglobin. *Proc Natl Acad Sci USA*, *105*(3), 991–996.

Cox, S. E., Makani, J., Soka, D., L'Esperence, V. S., Kija, E., Dominguez-Salas, P., ... Kirkham, F. J. (2014). Haptoglobin, alpha-thalassaemia and glucose-6-phosphate dehydrogenase polymorphisms and risk of abnormal transcranial Doppler among patients with sickle cell anaemia in Tanzania. *Br J Haematol, 165*(5), 699–706. https://doi.org/10.1111/bjh.12791

Currat, M., Trabuchet, G., Rees, D., Perrin, P., Harding, R. M., Clegg, J. B., ... Excoffier, L. (2002). Molecular analysis of the beta-globin gene cluster in the Niokholo Mandenka population reveals a recent origin of the beta(S) Senegal mutation. *Am J Hum Genet, 70*(1), 207–223. https://doi.org/10.1086/338304

Cyrklaff, M., Sanchez, C. P., Kilian, N., Bisseye, C., Simpore, J., Frischknecht, F., & Lanzer, M. (2011). Hemoglobins S and C interfere with actin remodeling in *Plasmodium falciparum*-infected erythrocytes. *Science, 334*(6060), 1283–1286. https://doi.org/10.1126/science.1213775

DeBaun, M. R., Gordon, M., McKinstry, R. C., Noetzel, M. J., White, D. A., Sarnaik, S. A., ... Casella, J. F. (2014). Controlled trial of transfusions for silent cerebral infarcts in sickle cell anemia. *N Engl J Med, 371*(8), 699–710. https://doi.org/10.1056/NEJMoa1401731

Diggs, L. W. (1967). Bone and joint lesions in sickle-cell disease. *Clin Orthop, 52*, 119–143.

Dondorp, A. M., Desakorn, V., Pongtavornpinyo, W., Sahassananda, D., Silamut, K., Chotivanich, K., ... Day, N. P. (2005). Estimation of the total parasite biomass in acute falciparum malaria from plasma PfHRP2. *PLoS Med, 2*(8), e204.

Edington, G. M., & Lehmann, H. (1954). A case of sickle cell; Haemoglobin C disease and a survey of haemoglobin C incidence in West Africa. *Trans R Soc Trop Med Hyg, 48*(4), 332–336.

Emond, A. M., Collis, R., Darvill, D., Higgs, D. R., Maude, G. H., & Serjeant, G. R. (1985). Acute splenic sequestration in homozygous sickle cell disease: Natural history and management. *J Pediatr, 107*(2), 201–206.

Fleming, A. F., Storey, J., Molineaux, L., Iroko, E. A., & Attai, E. D. (1979). Abnormal haemoglobins in the Sudan savanna of Nigeria. I. Prevalence of haemoglobins and relationships between sickle cell trait, malaria and survival. *Ann Trop Med Parasitol, 73*(2), 161–172.

Flint, J., Harding, R. M., Clegg, J. B., & Boyce, A. J. (1993). Why are some genetic diseases common? Distinguishing selection from other processes by molecular analysis of globin gene variants. *Hum Genet, 91*(2), 91–117.

Friedman, M. J. (1978). Erythrocytic mechanism of sickle cell resistance to malaria. *Proc Natl Acad Sci USA, 75*(4), 1994–1997.

Friedman, M. J. (1979a). Oxidant damage mediates variant red cell resistance to malaria. *Nature, 280*(5719), 245–247.

Friedman, M. J. (1979b). Ultrastructural damage to the malaria parasite in the sickled cell. *J Protozool, 26*(2), 195–199.

Friedman, M. J., Roth, E. F., Nagel, R. L., & Trager, W. (1979a). *Plasmodium falciparum*: Physiological interactions with the human sickle cell. *Exp Parasitol, 47*(1), 73–80.

Friedman, M. J., Roth, E. F., Nagel, R. L., & Trager, W. (1979b). The role of hemoglobins C, S, and Nbalt in the inhibition of malaria parasite development in vitro. *Am J Trop Med Hyg, 28*(5), 777–780.

Frimpong, A., Thiam, L. G., Arko-Boham, B., Owusu, E. D. A., & Adjei, G. O. (2018). Safety and effectiveness of antimalarial therapy in sickle cell disease: A systematic review and network meta-analysis. *BMC Infect Dis, 18*(1), 650. https://doi.org/10.1186/s12879-018-3556-0

Galadanci, N. A., Umar Abdullahi, S., Vance, L. D., Musa Tabari, A., Ali, S., Belonwu, R., ... DeBaun, M. R. (2017). Feasibility trial for primary stroke prevention in children with sickle cell anemia in Nigeria (SPIN trial). *Am J Hematol*. https://doi.org/10.1002/ajh.24770

Gaston, M., & Rosse, W. F. (1982). The cooperative study of sickle cell disease: Review of study design and objectives. *Am J Pediatr Hematol Oncol*, *4*(2), 197–201.

Gill, F. M., Sleeper, L. A., Weiner, S. J., Brown, A. K., Bellevue, R., Grover, R., ... Vichinsky, E. (1995). Clinical events in the first decade in a cohort of infants with sickle cell disease. Cooperative study of sickle cell disease. *Blood*, *86*(2), 776–783.

Gong, L., Maiteki-Sebuguzi, C., Rosenthal, P. J., Hubbard, A. E., Drakeley, C. J., Dorsey, G., & Greenhouse, B. (2012). Evidence for both innate and acquired mechanisms of protection from Plasmodium falciparum in children with sickle cell trait. *Blood*, *119*(16), 3808–3814. https://doi.org/10.1182/blood-2011-08-371062

Green, N. S., Munube, D., Bangirana, P., Buluma, L. R., Kebirungi, B., Opoka, R., ... Idro, R. (2019). Burden of neurological and neurocognitive impairment in pediatric sickle cell anemia in Uganda (BRAIN SAFE): A cross-sectional study. *BMC Pediatr*, *19*(1), 381. https://doi.org/10.1186/s12887-019-1758-2

Grosse, S. D., Odame, I., Atrash, H. K., Amendah, D. D., Piel, F. B., & Williams, T. N. (2011). Sickle cell disease in Africa: A neglected cause of early childhood mortality. *Am J Prev Med*, *41*(6 Suppl 4), S398–S405. https://doi.org/10.1016/j.amepre.2011.09.013

Guerra, C. A., Hay, S. I., Lucioparedes, L. S., Gikandi, P. W., Tatem, A. J., Noor, A. M., & Snow, R. W. (2007). Assembling a global database of malaria parasite prevalence for the malaria atlas project. *Malar J*, *6*, 17. https://doi.org/10.1186/1475-2875-6-17

Hendriksen, I. C., Mwanga-Amumpaire, J., von Seidlein, L., Mtove, G., White, L. J., Olaosebikan, R., ... Dondorp, A. M. (2012). Diagnosing severe falciparum malaria in parasitaemic African children: A prospective evaluation of plasma PfHRP2 measurement. *PLoS Med*, *9*(8), e1001297. https://doi.org/10.1371/journal.pmed.1001297

Henrici, R. C., Sautter, C. L., Bond, C., Opoka, R. O., Namazzi, R., Datta, D., ... John, C. C. (2021). Decreased parasite burden and altered host response in children with sickle cell anemia and severe anemia with malaria. *Blood Adv*. https://doi.org/10.1182/bloodadvances.2021004704

Henry, E. R., Cellmer, T., Dunkelberger, E. B., ... Eaton, W. A. (2020). Allosteric control of hemoglobin S fiber formation by oxygen and its relation to the pathophysiology of sickle cell disease. *Proc Natl Acad Sci USA*, *117*(26), 15018–15027.

Hill, A. V., Allsopp, C. E., Kwiatkowski, D., Anstey, N. M., Twumasi, P., Rowe, P. A., ... Greenwood, B. M. (1991). Common west African HLA antigens are associated with protection from severe malaria. *Nature*, *352*(6336), 595–600.

Idowu, O. A., Mafiana, C. F., & Dapo, S. (2005). Anaemia in pregnancy: A survey of pregnant women in Abeokuta, Nigeria. *Afr Health Sci*, *5*(4), 295–299. https://doi.org/10.5555/afhs.2005.5.4.295

Ingram, V. M. (1957). Gene mutations in human haemoglobin: The chemical difference between normal and sickle cell haemoglobin. *Nature*, *180*(4581), 326–328.

Italia, K., Kangne, H., Shanmukaiah, C., Nadkarni, A. H., Ghosh, K., & Colah, R. B. (2015). Variable phenotypes of sickle cell disease in India with the Arab-Indian haplotype. *Br J Haematol*, *168*(1), 156–159. https://doi.org/10.1111/bjh.13083

Izuora, G. I., Kaine, W. N., & Emodi, I. (1989). Neurological disorders in Nigerian children with homozygous sickle cell anaemia. *East Afr Med J*, *66*(10), 653–657.

Jacob, G. F. (1957). A study of the survival rate of cases of sickle-cell anaemia. *Br Med J*, *1*(5021), 738–739.

Jacob, M., Stotesbury, H., Kawadler, J. M., Lapadaire, W., Saunders, D. E., Sangeda, R. Z., ... Clark, C. A. (2020). White matter integrity in Tanzanian children with sickle cell anemia: A diffusion tensor imaging study. *Stroke, 51*(4), 1166–1173. https://doi. org/10.1161/STROKEAHA.119.027097

Jallow, M., Teo, Y. Y., Small, K. S., Rockett, K. A., Deloukas, P., Clark, T. G., ... Kwiatkowski, D. P. (2009). Genome-wide and fine-resolution association analysis of malaria in West Africa. *Nat Genet*, 41, 657–665.

John, A. B., Ramlal, A., Jackson, H., Maude, G. H., Sharma, A. W., & Serjeant, G. R. (1984). Prevention of pneumococcal infection in children with homozygous sickle cell disease. *Br Med J (Clin Res Ed)*, *288*(6430), 1567–1570.

Kan, Y. W., & Dozy, A. M. (1978a). Antenatal diagnosis of sickle-cell anaemia by D.N.A. analysis of amniotic-fluid cells. *Lancet, 2*(8096), 910–912.

Kan, Y. W., & Dozy, A. M. (1978b). Polymorphism of DNA sequence adjacent to human beta-globin structural gene: Relationship to sickle mutation. *Proc Natl Acad Sci USA, 75*(11), 5631–5635. https://doi.org/10.1073/pnas.75.11.5631

Kija, E. N., Saunders, D. E., Munubhi, E., Darekar, A., Barker, S., Cox, T. C. S., ... Newton, C. (2019). Transcranial Doppler and magnetic resonance in Tanzanian children with sickle cell disease. *Stroke, 50*(7), 1719–1726. https://doi.org/10.1161/STROKEAHA.118.018920

Kizito, M. E., Mworozi, E., Ndugwa, C., & Serjeant, G. R. (2007). Bacteraemia in homozygous sickle cell disease in Africa: Is pneumococcal prophylaxis justified? *Arch Dis Child, 92*(1), 21–23.

Kulozik, A. E., Wainscoat, J. S., Serjeant, G. R., Kar, B. C., Al-Awamy, B., ... Essan, G. J. (1986). Geographical survey of beta S-globin gene haplotypes: Evidence for an independent Asian origin of the sickle-cell mutation. *Am J Hum Genet, 39*(2), 239–244.

Kurnit, D. M. (1979). Evolution of sickle variant gene. *Lancet, 1*(8107), 104. https://doi. org/10.1016/s0140-6736(79)90093-x

Ladu, A. I., Aiyenigba, A. O., Adekile, A., & Bates, I. (2021). The spectrum of splenic complications in patients with sickle cell disease in Africa: A systematic review. *Br J Haematol, 193*(1), 26–42. https://doi.org/10.1111/bjh.17179

Lagunju, I. A., & Brown, B. J. (2012). Adverse neurological outcomes in Nigerian children with sickle cell disease. *Int J Hematol, 96*(6), 710–718. https://doi.org/10.1007/ s12185-012-1204-9

Lagunju, I., Sodeinde, O., & Telfer, P. (2012). Prevalence of transcranial Doppler abnormalities in Nigerian children with sickle cell disease. *Am J Hematol, 87*(5), 544–547. https:// doi.org/10.1002/ajh.2315210.1002/ajh.23152

Lee, M. T., Piomelli, S., Granger, S., Miller, S. T., Harkness, S., Brambilla, D. J., ... Investigators, S. S. (2006). Stroke prevention trial in sickle cell anemia (STOP): Extended follow-up and final results. *Blood, 108*(3), 847–852. https://doi.org/10.1182/blood-2005-10-009506

Leikin, S. L., Gallagher, D., Kinney, T. R., Sloane, D., Klug, P., & Rida, W. (1989). Mortality in children and adolescents with sickle cell disease. Cooperative study of sickle cell disease. *Pediatrics, 84*(3), 500–508.

Livingstone, F. B. (1973). *Data on the abnormal hemoglobin and glucose-6-phosphate dehydrogenase deficiency in human populations.* Michigan: University of Michigan, Museum of Anthropology.

Livingstone, F. B. (1985). *Frequencies of hemoglobin variants.* New York: Oxford University Press.

Livingstone, F. B. (1989). Who gave whom hemoglobin S: The use of restriction site haplotype variation for the interpretation of the evolution of the beta(S)-globin gene. *Am J Hum Biol,* 1(3), 289–302. https://doi.org/10.1002/ajhb.1310010309

Luzzatto, L., Nwachuku-Jarrett, E. S., & Reddy, S. (1970). Increased sickling of parasitised erythrocytes as mechanism of resistance against malaria in the sickle-cell trait. *Lancet*, *1*(7642), 319–321.

Lysenko, A. J., & Semashko, I. N. (1968). *Itogi Nauki: Medicinskaja Geografija* [in Russian]. (Vol. Geography of malaria. A medico-geographic profile of an ancient disease.) Moscow, Russia: Academy of Science.

Macharia, A. W., Mochamah, G., Uyoga, S., Ndila, C. M., Nyutu, G., Makale, J., ... Williams, T. N. (2018). The clinical epidemiology of sickle cell anemia in Africa. *Am J Hematol*, *93*(3), 363–370. https://doi.org/10.1002/ajh.24986

Mackey, J. P., & Vivarelli, F. (1954). Sickle cell anaemia. *Br Med J*, *1*, 276.

Maitland, K., Kiguli, S., Olupot-Olupot, P., Opoka, R. O., Chimalizeni, Y., Alaroker, F., ... TRACT Stakeholders meeting group. (2021). Transfusion management of severe anaemia in African children: A consensus algorithm. *Br J Haematol*, *193*(6), 1247–1259. https://doi.org/10.1111/bjh.17429

Makani, J., Cox, S. E., Soka, D., Komba, A. N., Oruo, J., Mwamtemi, H., ... Newton, C. R. (2011). Mortality in sickle cell anemia in Africa: A prospective cohort study in Tanzania. *PLoS One*, *6*(2), e14699. https://doi.org 10.1371/journal.pone.0014699

Makani, J., Kirkham, F. J., Komba, A., Ajala-Agbo, T., Otieno, G., Fegan, G., ... Newton, C. R. (2009). Risk factors for high cerebral blood flow velocity and death in Kenyan children with sickle cell anaemia: Role of haemoglobin oxygen saturation and febrile illness. *Br J Haematol*, *145*(4), 529–532.

Makani, J., Komba, A. N., Cox, S. E., Oruo, J., Mwamtemi, K., Kitundu, J., ... Williams, T. N. (2010). Malaria in patients with sickle cell anemia: Burden, risk factors, and outcome at the outpatient clinic and during hospitalization. *Blood*, *115*(2), 215–220. https://doi.org/10.1182/blood-2009-07-233528

Marsh, K., Otoo, L., Hayes, R. J., Carson, D. C., & Greenwood, B. M. (1989). Antibodies to blood stage antigens of *Plasmodium falciparum* in rural Gambians and their relation to protection against infection. *Trans R Soc Trop Med Hyg*, *83*(3), 293–303.

McGann, P. T., Hernandez, A. G., & Ware, R. E. (2017). Sickle cell anemia in sub-Saharan Africa: Advancing the clinical paradigm through partnerships and research. *Blood*, *129*(2), 155–161. https://doi.org/10.1182/blood-2016-09-702324

McGann, P. T., Williams, T. N., Olupot-Olupot, P., Tomlinson, G. A., Lane, A., Luis Reis da Fonseca, J., ... Investigators, R. (2018). Realizing effectiveness across continents with hydroxyurea: Enrollment and baseline characteristics of the multicenter REACH study in Sub-Saharan Africa. *Am J Hematol*, *93*(4), 537–545. https://doi.org/10.1002/ajh.25034

Mears, J. G., Lachman, H. M., Cabannes, R., Amegnizin, K. P., Labie, D., & Nagel, R. L. (1981). Sickle gene. Its origin and diffusion from West Africa. *J Clin Invest*, *68*(3), 606–610. https://doi.org/10.1172/jci110294

Miko, I. (2008). Epistasis: Gene Interaction and phenotype effects. *Nat Educ*, *1*(1), 197.

Miller, M. J., Neel, J. V., & Livingstone, F. B. (1956). Distribution of parasites in the red cells of sickle-cell trait carriers infected with Plasmodium falciparum. *Trans R Soc Trop Med Hyg*, *50*(3), 294–296.

Modiano, D., Bancone, G., Ciminelli, B. M., Pompei, F., Blot, I., Simpore, J., & Modiano, G. (2008). Haemoglobin S and haemoglobin C: 'quick but costly' versus 'slow but gratis' genetic adaptations to Plasmodium falciparum malaria. *Hum Mol Genet*, *17*(6), 789–799. https://doi.org/10.1093/hmg/ddm350

Ndeezi, G., Kiyaga, C., Hernandez, A. G., Munube, D., Howard, T. A., Ssewanyana, I., ... Aceng, J. R. (2016). Burden of sickle cell trait and disease in the Uganda Sickle

Surveillance Study (US3): A cross-sectional study. *Lancet Glob Health, 28*, 1–6. https://doi.org/10.1016/S2214-109X(15)00288-0

Ohene-Frempong, K., Weiner, S. J., Sleeper, L. A., Miller, S. T., Embury, S., Moohr, J. W., … Gill, F. M. (1998). Cerebrovascular accidents in sickle cell disease: Rates and risk factors. *Blood, 91*(1), 288–294.

Olupot-Olupot, P., Wabwire, H., Ndila, C., Adong, R., Ochen, L., Amorut, D., … Williams, T. N. (2020). Characterising demographics, knowledge, practices and clinical care among patients attending sickle cell disease clinics in Eastern Uganda. *Wellcome Open Res, 5*, 87. https://doi.org/10.12688/wellcomeopenres.15847.2

Opi, D. H., Ochola, L. B., Tendwa, M., Siddondo, B. R., Ocholla, H., Fanjo, H., … Williams, T. N. (2014). Mechanistic studies of the negative epistatic malaria-protective interaction between sickle cell trait and alpha-thalassemia. *eBioMedicine, 1*(1), 29–36. https://doi.org/10.1016/j.ebiom.2014.10.006

Pagnier, J., Mears, J. G., Dunda-Belkhodja, O., Schaefer-Rego, K. E., Beldjord, C., Nagel, R. L., & Labie, D. (1984). Evidence for the multicentric origin of the sickle cell hemoglobin gene in Africa. *Proc Natl Acad Sci USA, 81*(6), 1771–1773.

Pasvol, G., Weatherall, D. J., & Wilson, R. J. (1978). Cellular mechanism for the protective effect of haemoglobin S against *P. falciparum* malaria. *Nature, 274*(5672), 701–703.

Pearson, H. A., Spencer, R. P., & Cornelius, E. A. (1969). Functional asplenia in sickle-cell anemia. *N Engl J Med, 281*(17), 923–926. https://doi.org/10.1056/NEJM196910232811703

Pedro, R., Akech, S., Fegan, G., & Maitland, K. (2010). Changing trends in blood transfusion in children and neonates admitted in Kilifi District Hospital, Kenya. *Malar J, 9*, 307. https://doi.org/10.1186/1475-2875-9-307

Penman, B. S., Habib, S., Kanchan, K., & Gupta, S. (2011). Negative epistasis between alpha(+) thalassaemia and sickle cell trait can explain interpopulation variation in South Asia. *Evolution, 65*(12), 3625–3632. https://doi.org/10.1111/j.1558-5646.2011.01408.x

Penman, B. S., Pybus, O. G., Weatherall, D. J., & Gupta, S. (2009). Epistatic interactions between genetic disorders of hemoglobin can explain why the sickle-cell gene is uncommon in the Mediterranean. *Proc Natl Acad Sci USA, 106*(50), 21242–21246. https://doi.org/10.1073/pnas.0910840106

Petersen, J. E. V., Saelens, J. W., Freedman, E., Turner, L., Lavstsen, T., Fairhurst, R. M., … Taylor, S. M. (2021). Sickle-trait hemoglobin reduces adhesion to both CD36 and EPCR by Plasmodium falciparum-infected erythrocytes. *PLoS Pathog, 17*(6), e1009659. https://doi.org/10.1371/journal.ppat.1009659

Piel, F. B., Hay, S. I., Gupta, S., Weatherall, D. J., & Williams, T. N. (2013). Global burden of sickle cell anaemia in children under five, 2010-2050: Modelling based on demographics, excess mortality, and interventions. *PLoS Med, 10*(7), e1001484. https://doi.org/10.1371/journal.pmed.1001484

Piel, F. B., Patil, A. P., Howes, R. E., Nyangiri, O. A., Gething, P. W., Dewi, M., … Hay, S. I. (2013). Global epidemiology of sickle haemoglobin in neonates: A contemporary geostatistical model-based map and population estimates. *Lancet, 381*(9861), 142–151. https://doi.org/10.1016/S0140-6736(12)61229-X

Piel, F. B., Patil, A. P., Howes, R. E., Nyangiri, O. A., Gething, P. W., Williams, T. N., … Hay, S. I. (2010). Global distribution of the sickle cell gene and geographical confirmation of the malaria hypothesis. *Nat Commun, 1*(8), 104. https://doi.org/10.1038/ncomms1104

Powars, D., Overturf, G., & Turner, E. (1983). Is there an increased risk of Haemophilus influenzae septicemia in children with sickle cell anemia? *Pediatrics, 71*(6), 927–931.

Ramakrishnan, M., Moisi, J. C., Klugman, K. P., Iglesias, J. M., Grant, L. R., Mpoudi-Etame, M., & Levine, O. S. (2010). Increased risk of invasive bacterial infections in African people with sickle-cell disease: A systematic review and meta-analysis. *Lancet Infect Dis, 10*(5), 329–337. https://doi.org/10.1016/S1473-3099(10)70055-4

Ranque, B., Kitenge, R., Ndiaye, D. D., Ba, M. D., Adjoumani, L., Traore, H., … Diagne, I. (2022). Estimating the risk of child mortality attributable to sickle cell anaemia in sub-Saharan Africa: A retrospective, multicentre, case-control study. *Lancet Haematol, 9*(3), e208–e216. https://doi.org/10.1016/S2352-3026(22)00004-7

Robinson, M. G., & Halpern, C. (1974). Infections, Escherichia coli, and sickle cell anemia. *JAMA, 230*(8), 1145–1148.

Roth, E. F., Jr., Friedman, M., Ueda, Y., Tellez, I., Trager, W., & Nagel, R. L. (1978). Sickling rates of human AS red cells infected *in vitro* with *Plasmodium falciparum* malaria. *Science, 202*(4368), 650–652.

Sadarangani, M., Makani, J., Komba, A. N., Ajala-Agbo, T., Newton, C. R., Marsh, K., & Williams, T. N. (2009). An observational study of children with sickle cell disease in Kilifi, Kenya. *Br J Haematol, 146*(6), 675–682.

Sadek, S. H. (1974). Sickle cell trait in North Nigeria. *J Trop Med Hyg, 77*(3), 61–64.

Saelens, J. W., Petersen, J. E. V., Freedman, E., Moseley, R. C., Konate, D., Diakite, S. A. S., … Taylor, S. M. (2021). Impact of sickle cell trait hemoglobin on the intraerythrocytic transcriptional program of Plasmodium falciparum. *mSphere, 6*(5), e0075521. https://doi.org/10.1128/mSphere.00755-21

Scott, J. A., Berkley, J. A., Mwangi, I., Ochola, L., Uyoga, S., Macharia, A., … Williams, T. N. (2011). Relation between falciparum malaria and bacteraemia in Kenyan children: A population-based, case-control study and a longitudinal study. *Lancet, 378*(9799), 1316–1323. https://doi.org/10.1016/S0140-6736(11)60888-X

Serjeant, G. R. (2005). Mortality from sickle cell disease in Africa. *BMJ, 330*(7489), 432–433.

Serjeant, G., & Serjeant, B. (2001). *Sickle cell disease* (third ed.). Oxford: Oxford University Press.

Shriner, D., & Rotimi, C. N. (2018). Whole-genome-sequence-based haplotypes reveal single origin of the sickle allele during the holocene wet phase. *Am J Hum Genet, 102*(4), 547–556. https://doi.org/10.1016/j.ajhg.2018.02.003

Soyebi, K., Adeyemo, T., Ojewunmi, O., James, F., Adefalujo, K., & Akinyanju, O. (2014). Capacity building and stroke risk assessment in Nigerian children with sickle cell anaemia. *Pediatr Blood Cancer, 61*(12), 2263–2266. https://doi.org/10.1002/pbc.25216

Steinberg, M. H. (2005). Predicting clinical severity in sickle cell anaemia. *Br J Haematol, 129*(4), 465–481. https://doi.org/10.1111/j.1365-2141.2005.05411.x

Steinberg, M. H., Forget, B. G., Higgs, D. R., & Weatherall, D. J. (2009). *Disorders of hemoglobin: Genetics, pathophysiology, and clinical management* (second ed.). Cambridge: Cambridge University Press.

Tan, X., Traore, B., Kayentao, K., Ongoiba, A., Doumbo, S., Waisberg, M., … Crompton, P. D. (2011). Hemoglobin S and C heterozygosity enhances neither the magnitude nor breadth of antibody responses to a diverse array of Plasmodium falciparum antigens. *J Infect Dis, 204*(11), 1750–1761. https://doi.org/10.1093/infdis/jir638

Taylor, S. M., Parobek, C. M., & Fairhurst, R. M. (2012). Haemoglobinopathies and the clinical epidemiology of malaria: A systematic review and meta-analysis. *Lancet Infect Dis, 12*(6), 457–468. https://doi.org/10.1016/S1473-3099(12)70055-5

The Malaria Genomic Epidemiology Network. (2014). Reappraisal of known malaria resistance loci in a large multicenter study. *Nat Genet, 46*(11), 1197–1204. https://doi.org/10.1038/ng.3107

The World Health Organization. (2014). Severe Malaria. *Trop Med Int Health, 19* (Suppl), 7–131. https://doi.org/10.1111/tmi.12313_2

United Nations, United Nations Millennium Declaration, resolution 55/2. (2000). https://www.preventionweb.net/files/13539_13539ARES552ResolutiononUNMillenniu.pdf.

Uyoga, S., Macharia, A. W., Mochamah, G., Ndila, C. M., Nyutu, G., Makale, J., ... Williams, T. N. (2019). The epidemiology of sickle cell disease in children recruited in infancy in Kilifi, Kenya: A prospective cohort study. *Lancet Glob Health, 7*(10), e1458–e1466. https://doi.org/10.1016/S2214-109X(19)30328-6

Uyoga, S., Macharia, A. W., Ndila, C. M., Nyutu, G., Shebe, M., Awuondo, K. O., ... Williams, T. N. (2019). The indirect health effects of malaria estimated from health advantages of the sickle cell trait. *Nat Commun, 10*(1), 856. https://doi.org/10.1038/s41467-019-08775-0

Uyoga, S., Olupot-Olupot, P., Connon, R., Kiguli, S., Opoka, R. O., Alaroker, F., ... Williams, T. N. (2022). Sickle cell anaemia and severe P. falciparum malaria: A secondary analysis of the transfusion and treatment of African Children Trial (TRACT). *Lancet Child and Adolescent Health, 6*(9), 606–613. https://doi.org/10.1016/S2352-4642(22)00153-5.

Uyoga, S., Wanjiku, P., Rop, J. C., Makale, J., Macharia, A. W., Nyutu, G. M., ... Williams, T. N. (2021). Plasma Plasmodium falciparum histidine-rich protein 2 concentrations in children with malaria infections of differing severity in Kilifi, Kenya. *Clin Infect Dis, 73*(7), e2415–e2423. https://doi.org/10.1093/cid/ciaa1141

Ware, R. E., de Montalembert, M., Tshilolo, L., & Abboud, M. R. (2017). Sickle cell disease. *Lancet, 390*(10091), 311–323. https://doi.org/10.1016/S0140-6736(17)30193-9

White, N. J., Turner, G. D., Day, N. P., & Dondorp, A. M. (2013). Lethal malaria: Marchiafava and Bignami were right. *J Infect Dis, 208*(2), 192–198. https://doi.org/10.1093/infdis/jit116

WHO. (2016). Global status report on blood safety and availability. Retrieved from https://apps.who.int/iris/bitstream/handle/10665/254987/9789241565431-eng.pdf;jsessionid=7648CDE1B0737E3E4FFB55E0CD3CF265?sequence=1

Willcox, M., Bjorkman, A., Brohult, J., Pehrson, P. O., Rombo, L., & Bengtsson, E. (1983). A case-control study in northern Liberia of *Plasmodium falciparum* malaria in haemoglobin S and beta-thalassaemia traits. *Ann Trop Med Parasitol, 77*(3), 239–246.

Williams, T. N. (2011). How do hemoglobins S and C result in malaria protection? *J Infect Dis, 204*(11), 1651–1653. https://doi.org/10.1093/infdis/jir640

Williams, T. N., Mwangi, T. W., Roberts, D. J., Alexander, N. D., Weatherall, D. J., Wambua, S., ... Marsh, K. (2005). An immune basis for malaria protection by the sickle cell trait. *PLoS Med, 2*(5), e128.

Williams, T. N., Mwangi, T. W., Wambua, S., Alexander, N. D., Kortok, M., Snow, R. W., & Marsh, K. (2005). Sickle cell trait and the risk of *Plasmodium falciparum* malaria and other childhood diseases. *J Infect Dis, 192*(1), 178–186.

Williams, T. N., Mwangi, T. W., Wambua, S., Peto, T. E., Weatherall, D. J., Gupta, S., ... Marsh, K. (2005). Negative epistasis between the malaria-protective effects of alpha+-thalassemia and the sickle cell trait. *Nat Genet, 37*(11), 1253–1257. https://doi.org/10.1038/ng1660

Williams, T. N., & Obaro, S. K. (2011). Sickle cell disease and malaria morbidity: A tale with two tails. *Trends Parasitol, 27*(7), 315–320. https://doi.org/10.1016/j.pt.2011.02.004

Williams, T. N., & Thein, S. L. (2018). Sickle cell anemia and its phenotypes. *Annu Rev Genomics Hum Genet, 19*, 113–147. https://doi.org/10.1146/annurev-genom-083117-021320

Williams, T. N., Uyoga, S., Macharia, A., Ndila, C., McAuley, C. F., Opi, D. H., ... Scott, J. A. (2009). Bacteraemia in Kenyan children with sickle-cell anaemia: A retrospective cohort and case-control study. *Lancet, 374*(9698), 1364–1370. https://doi.org/10.1016/S0140-6736(09)61374-X

World Health Organization. (2002). Genomics and world health, report of the Advisory Committee on Health Research, Geneva.

World population prospects: The 2010 revision. (2011). https://population.un.org/wpp/.

2 Laboratory Profile of Sickle Cell Disease

Nwabundo I. Anusim and Ugochi O. Ogu

Introduction

Sickle cell disease (SCD) is an inherited blood disorder caused by a point mutation in the beta-globin gene which results in the expression of an abnormal protein called hemoglobin S. In this point mutation, the normal hydrophilic glutamic acid is substituted with the hydrophobic valine at the sixth residue of the beta-globin gene. In hypoxic situations, hemoglobin (Hb) S polymerizes resulting in an abnormal folding of the red blood cells resulting in a rigid and less soluble sickle red cell. The hallmark of the pathophysiology of SCD is the development of hemolysis via the destruction of the sickle red cells and vaso-occlusion via obstruction of blood flow by the sickle cells (Rees, Williams, & Gladwin, 2010). The degree of hemolytic anemia is determined by the amount and rate of polymerization which in turn depends on the quantity of hemoglobin S, the amount of other hemoglobin variants and the oxygen saturation.

The major variants in SCD are homozygous Hb SS, hemoglobin SC, hemoglobin S/β^0-thalassemia and hemoglobin S/β+-halassemia. However, there are several other rare variants identified in various regions of the world including hemoglobin S/Hereditary Persistence of Fetal Hemoglobin, hemoglobin S/hemoglobin D Punjab or D Los Angeles, hemoglobin S/O-Arab, hemoglobin S/Hemoglobin Lepore, hemoglobin S/hemoglobin E, hemoglobin S/Black($^A\gamma\delta\beta)^0$-thalassemia and the most recently identified hemoglobin S/Haringey (Ogu, Reyes Gil, Tolu, Acharya, & Minniti, 2021).

Considering the significant number of variants with varied presentations and outcomes, it is pertinent to accurately identify these variants as this enables the development of a comprehensive management plan and aids genetic counseling. Here we discuss the diagnostic testing, the rationale behind the diagnostic tests and laboratory profile of the several variants of SCD.

Diagnostic Tests in Sickle Cell Disease

1 Prenatal testing: This is typically performed in pregnant women at risk of having a fetus with hemoglobinopathy. It is a DNA-based testing performed on the specimens obtained from the pre-implanted zygote in first trimester of

DOI: 10.4324/9781003463931-3

pregnancy via chorionic villus sampling, in the second trimester on cells in the amniotic fluid obtained via amniocentesis and after delivery via peripheral blood (Cheung, Goldberg, & Kan, 1996).

2 Complete blood count (CBC) with red blood cell indices: This is a simple inexpensive test with rapid turnaround time. These tests show the degree of anemia, mean corpuscular volume (MCV) and mean corpuscular hemoglobin concentration (MCHC). However, it does not differentiate between the different SCD variants.

3 Blood chemistry: Important values to note that this test may include haptoglobin, lactate dehydrogenase and indirect bilirubin which are indicators of hemolysis. The more significant the numbers, the more polymerization of red blood cells indicating a more severe SCD variant.

4 Peripheral blood smear (PBS): This is an important hematologic test that aids diagnosis. Visualizing the morphology of the red cells can identify the sickle cells and other pathologic cells that aid in differentiating some variants of SCD. It is subject to interobserver variability and interpretation is dependent on the level of skill of the pathologist (de Haan et al., 2020).

5 Sickling prep and turbidity test: These can identify the abnormal hemoglobin S via crystallization and precipitation of the hemoglobin S in sodium metabisulphite or dithionite. The precipitate refracts light and results in a turbid solution. Unfortunately, it is fraught with false negatives especially in newborns with high fetal hemoglobin and individuals with Hb S of <10% and false positives in blood samples with significant erythrocytosis, serum viscosity and leukocytosis. Importantly, it cannot differentiate the SCD variants from sickle cell trait, as the test only indicates sickling due to hemoglobin S but does not quantify the abnormal hemoglobin S (Okwi, Byarugaba, Parkes, & Ocaido, 2010).

6 Hemoglobin electrophoresis: Electrophoresis is a chromatographic technique used to identify hemoglobin variants. This tool entails the use of electrical field in alkaline or acid potential of hydrogen (pH) in cellulose acetate and citrate agar, respectively, to facilitate the migration of electrically charged hemoglobins. It differentiates hemoglobins with different net charges. However, those with the same net charges migrate in the same pattern. For instance, cellulose acetate electrophoresis at an alkaline pH of 8.4 can separate Hb S from other variants except Hb G and Hb D which have the same net charges as hemoglobin S. Similarly, Hb E, Hb O-Arab and Hb C molecules have similar migratory patterns in citrate agar at an alkaline pH. Hence, these variants cannot be differentiated using the cellulose acetate or citrate agar electrophoresis, respectively (Arishi, Alhadrami, & Zourob, 2021).

7 High-performance liquid chromatography (HPLC): This is a highly sensitive and precise test used to identify and quantify the different hemoglobin fractions based on the retention time and peak of the curve. However, it cannot differentiate Hb variants with similar retention pattern. It is the initial testing method of choice, but may be very expensive and not available in most resource-poor centers (Frömmel, 2018).

8 Globin gene analysis: This test provides definitive diagnosis as it detects the exact mutation in the beta-globin gene (Clark & Thein, 2004).

Sickle Cell Disease Variants and Laboratory Profile

Hemoglobin SS Disease (Homozygous Sickle Cell Disease)

Hb SS results from autosomal recessive inheritance of an abnormal hemoglobin S from each parent resulting in a higher degree of hemolysis compared to other variants. Hence the moderate to severe anemia with hemoglobin and hematocrit 8.55 ± 1.33 g/dL and 25.7 ± 4.4%, respectively (Sant'Ana et al., 2017). Due to this chronic ongoing hemolysis, there is polychromasia due to reticulocytosis, but this is not as high as seen in other causes of hemolysis due to the reduced oxygen affinity by the sickle cells thus resulting in normal MCV. In situations where there is macrocytosis, there is relative folate deficiency due to inadequate oral intake or ongoing drug treatment with Hydroxyurea. When the sickle cells undergo oxidative stress, there is an increase in cellular calcium content which activates the calcium potassium transport leading to exit of the potassium which is followed by water resulting in a rigid cell, decreased cell volume and increased hemoglobin concentration which accounts for the increased MCHC (Berda-Haddad et al., 2017). The rigidity of the cells results in endothelial damage and the oxidative stress results in hemolysis and is evident in laboratory results showing anemia, unconjugated hyperbilirubinemia, lactate dehydrogenase and decreased haptoglobin. The peripheral smear is normal in neonatal period but around infancy, the red cells become more sickle cells and Howell jolly bodies are seen in sickle cell patients with functional asplenia. Peripheral blood smear shows anisocytosis and targets cells in addition to the sickle cells (Alvarez, Montague, Marin, O'Brien, & Rodriguez, 2015). In patients on treatment with Hydroxyurea, the hemoglobin F is higher, so the sickling is less apparent. Patients have a higher level Hb S considering they inherit Hb S from each parent, with a small proportion of Hb A2 while Hb A is absent. In the neonatal period, Hb F is high, but it decreases as patients transition from neonatal period to infancy and adolescence. In cellulose acetate electrophoresis at alkaline pH, Hb A and A2 are separated from hemoglobin S while in citrate agar at acid pH, migrating Hb D is separated form Hb S.

Hemoglobin SC Disease

Hb SC disease results from inheritance of Hb C and Hb S from each parent. Hb C occurs due to substitution of lysine for glutamic acid at the sixth amino acid position of the beta-globin gene. The hemoglobin concentration is higher, 10.12–11.82 g/dL, than those of patients with Hb SS (Aleluia et al., 2017).

Like Hb S, the Hb C activates the potassium chloride pathway resulting in the exit of potassium from the cells followed by water and this leads to intracellular dehydration, increased red cell rigidity, formation of Hb C crystals and subsequent destruction in the spleen and this may contribute to sickling noted in these patients (Fabry, Kaul, Raventos-Suarez, Chang, & Nagel, 1982). The intracellular dehydration results in an elevated MCHC in the range of 24.60–28.67 fL while the red cell destruction leads to a mild anemia with elevated hemolytic parameters but are less pronounced compared to Hb SS due to longer survival of Hb SC red cells (Aleluia et al., 2017). The peripheral smear shows less of sickle cells than seen in homozygous SCD, target cells, microcytosis and straight edged six-sided Hb C crystals. Hb S and Hb C are inherited in equal proportions in hemoglobin SC disease with an absence of Hb A on iso-electric focusing (Moll & Orringer, 1997) In cellulose acetate electrophoresis on alkaline pH, Hb C will migrate with Hb A_2, Hb E and Hb O-Arab. While in citrate agar on acid pH, Hb C can be separated from Hb A_2 (Rodak, Fritsma, & Doig, 2011). High-performance liquid chromatography can distinguish other co-migratory variants.

Hemoglobin S/ß⁰-Thalassemia

In this SCD variant, in addition to the Hb S mutation, there are mutations in the beta-globin gene that cause complete loss (β^0) of the beta-globin chain. The peripheral smear shows microcytosis, hypochromia and sickled cells. On hemoglobin electrophoresis almost all the hemoglobin is Hb S with Hb A_2 of about 4–6% present and Hb A is absent. The complete blood count may show hemoglobin ranges between 8 and 10 g/dL with anMCV of 60–75 fL but the hemoglobin has also been observed to fall into lower ranges, similar to Hb SS disease (Figueiredo, 2015).

Hemoglobin S/ß⁺-Thalassemia

In this SCD variant, there is partial beta-globin ($\beta+$) synthesis resulting in vari-able amount of Hb A. This Hb A dilutes the amount of Hb S leading to a decrease in the amount of Hb S polymerization, sickling of the red cells, hemolysis and vaso-occlusive crisis. The peripheral blood smear shows microcytosis, targets cells and rarely, sickle cells. Hemoglobin electrophoresis has both Hb A and Hb S present with majority of it being Hb S. The Hb A may range from <5% to45%, with higher levels of Hb A usually associated with a milder phenotype (Figue-iredo, 2015).

Hemoglobin S/Hereditary Persistence of Fetal Hemoglobin

Hereditary persistence of fetal hemoglobin (HPFH) results from failure of the physiologic switch from fetal hemoglobin Hb F to adult hemoglobin Hb A. El-evated Hb F in combination with Hb S ameliorates the laboratory and clinical find-ing in patients with this variant of SCD. However, this protection wanes with aging (Tolu et al., 2020). The CBC shows a higher hemoglobin concentration and a lower MCV, an average of 12.6 g/dL and 74.9fL, respectively, while chemistry shows a lower total bilirubin compared to sickle cell anemia (Steinberg, 2020). Electropho-resis shows an average Hb F level of 32.9%. In infancy, it is difficult to differentiate Hb S/HPFH from sickle cell anemia due to the high Hb F. Gene globin analysis would be ideal in situations that Hb F persists after two years of age, for definitive diagnosis (Ngo et al., 2012).

Hemoglobin S/Hemoglobin D Punjab (Hemoglobin S/Hemoglobin D Los Angeles

Hemoglobin D Punjab occurs due to a mutation in the beta-globin gene that results from substitution of glutamine for glutamic acid at the 121st amino acid position of the beta-globin gene. The complete blood count shows a hemoglobin concentration is between 7 and 9.2 g/dL, an MCV 99.6–99.9 fL, MCH 35.1 and 37.1 g/dL. Peripheral smear shows sickle cells, some macrocytes, Howell jolly bodies, pappenheimer bodies and large platelets. On cellulose acetate electrophoresis at alkaline ph, hemoglobin S and D-Punjab show same mobility while on citrate agar in acid ph, these two hemoglobins are separated (Ali, Jain, Agarwal, & Kumar, 2020; Lund, Chakravorty, Toma, & Bain, 2015).

Hemoglobin S/O-Arab

Hemoglobin O-Arab occurs as due to a mutation in the beta-globin gene in which there is a substitution of glutamic acid for lysine at position 121. Hb S/O-Arab form of SCD is severe with hemoglobin concentration varying between 6.1 and 9.9 g/dL, MCV between 64 and 91 fL and reticulocyte count is 1.2–10.3%. The peripheral smear is similar to sickle cell anemia with sickled cells, polychromasia, Howell jolly body, target cells and nucleated red cells. In cellulose acetate electrophoresis at alkaline ph, Hb O-Arab comigrates with Hb C while in citrate agar at acid ph Hb O-Arab migrates close to Hb S (Milner et al., 1970).

Hemoglobin S/Hemoglobin E

Hemoglobin E results from the replacement of Glutamic acid by Lysine in codon 26th codon of the beta-globin gene. The complete blood count in Hb S/E disease shows a hemoglobin range of 7.8–8 g/dL and MCV 66.9–114 fL. On the cellulose acetate electrophoresis on agar gel at alkaline pH (8.6), Hb E comigrates with Hb A2, Hb C and Hb O-Arab. Hemoglobin electrophoresis shows Hb S in the 50% range, and Hb E percentage in the 20–30s range (Basumatary, Baruah, Sarma, & Sarmah, 2021; Dani & Shrikhande, 2007; Masiello et al., 2007).

Hemoglobin S/Black($^{A}\gamma\delta\beta)^{0}$-Thalassemia

This is a rare form of SCD which results from large deletions in the gamma, delta (HBD) and beta-globin gene (HBB) and known as HbS-Sicilian $(\delta\beta)^{0}$-Thalassemia. The heterozygous combination with hemoglobin S is known to run a varied course with some patients having benign course and others having a complicated course. The hemoglobin range is 8.3–14.7 g/dL, with reticuolcytosis, MCV 65–84.3 fL and total bilirubin 0.2–1.6. The peripheral smear shows anisocytosis, poikilocytosis, microcytosis, targets cells and rare sickled forms (Cancio et al., 2017; Onimoe & Smarzo, 2017).

Table 2.1 Hemoglobin patterns in major types of sickle cell disease.

	Genotype	Newborn screen	Hb A (%)	Hb A2 (%)	Hb F (%)	Hb S (%)	Hb C (%)
Normal	AA	FA	95–98%	<3.5	<2	0	0
Sickle cell trait	AS	FAS	~60	<3.5	<2	~40	0
Homozygous sickle cell disease	SS	FS	0	<3.5	<5	>90	0
Sickle-beta zero thalassemia	$S\beta^0$	FS	0	3.5–7	2–15	85–95	0
Sickle-beta plus thalassemia	$S\beta+$	FSA	10-30	3.5–7	2–10	65–90	0
Hb SC disease	SC	FSC	0	<3.5	1–5	~45	~45

Hemoglobin S/Haringey

Hb Haringey results from replacement of glutamic acid by glycine on codon 43 of the beta-globin gene. Hb S/Haringey variant of SCD has only been reported once in the literature, an incidental finding in a patient during an admission for acute pancreatitis (Ogu et al., 2021). Based on current knowledge, it usually runs a benign course. Asymptomatic avascular necrosis of the bilateral hips was the only sickle-related complication observed incidentally during abdominal imaging for pancreatitis. The hemoglobin range was between 11 and 13 g/dL, with reticulocytosis of 40,000–130,000 while LDH and total bilirubin were within normal limits. Peripheral blood smear revealed no sickle cells but numerous targets cell and inclusion bodies as seen in hemoglobin C. High-performance liquid chromatography and hemoglobin electrophoresis revealed Hb S of 39.7%, Hb F of 0.5% and Hb Haringey of 49.2% that migrated in the Hb A2 window (Ogu et al., 2021).

Table 2.1 describes the hemoglobin patterns in the major variants of SCD. Hemoglobin A2 is an important parameter used to differentiate Hb SS from the sickle beta thalassemias. The upper limit of normal value for Hb A2 is 3.5, and an elevated A2 favors sickle/beta-zero thalassemia or sickle/beta-plus thalassemia. However, caution must be exercised with interpretation, as while significantly elevated A2 levels of 6–7 range are most likely due to the sickle beta thalassemias, lower levels of >3.5 to 4–5 ranges could occur in both homozygous SS and the sickle beta thalassemias (personal observation of patients with genetically confirmed SCD genotypes and their corresponding laboratory Hb A2 values, unpublished data). In difficult cases when not accompanied by microcytosis and there is a diagnostic dilemma between Hb SS and sickle beta zero thalassemia, beta-globin sequencing is useful, especially for genetic counseling.

References

Aleluia, M. M., Fonseca, T. C. C., Souza, R. Q., Neves, F. I., da Guarda, C. C., Santiago, R. P., ... Gonçalves, M. S. (2017). Comparative study of sickle cell anemia and hemoglobin SC disease: Clinical characterization, laboratory biomarkers and genetic profiles. *BMC Hematol, 17*, 15. https://doi.org/10.1186/s12878-017-0087-7

Ali, W., Jain, M., Agarwal, S., & Kumar, A. (2020). A case of hemoglobin sickle-D Punjab. *Indian J Hematol Blood Transfus*, *36*(1), 205–207. https://doi.org/10.1007/s12288-019-01179-6

Alvarez, O., Montague, N. S., Marin, M., O'Brien, R., & Rodriguez, M. M. (2015). Quantification of sickle cells in the peripheral smear as a marker of disease severity. *Fetal Pediatr Pathol*, *34*(3), 149–154. https://doi.org/10.3109/15513815.2014.987937

Arishi, W. A., Alhadrami, H. A., & Zourob, M. (2021). Techniques for the detection of sickle cell disease: A review. *Micromachines (Basel)*, *12*(5). https://doi.org/10.3390/mi12050519

Basumatary, N., Baruah, D., Sarma, P. K., & Sarmah, J. (2021). Compound heterozygosity for hemoglobin S and hemoglobin E in a family of proto-Australoid origin: A case report. *J Med Case Rep*, *15*(1), 386. https://doi.org/10.1186/s13256-021-02974-4

Berda-Haddad, Y., Faure, C., Boubaya, M., Arpin, M., Cointe, S., Frankel, D., … Dignat-George, F. (2017). Increased mean corpuscular haemoglobin concentration: Artefact or pathological condition? *Int J Lab Hematol*, *39*(1), 32–41. https://doi.org/10.1111/ijlh.12565

Cancio, M. I., Aygun, B., Chui, D. H. K., Rothman, J. A., Scott, J. P., Estepp, J. H., & Hankins, J. S. (2017). The clinical severity of hemoglobin S/Black ((A) γδβ)(0)-thalassemia. *Pediatr Blood Cancer*, *64*(11). https://doi.org/10.1002/pbc.26596

Cheung, M. C., Goldberg, J. D., & Kan, Y. W. (1996). Prenatal diagnosis of sickle cell anaemia and thalassaemia by analysis of fetal cells in maternal blood. *Nat Genet*, *14*(3), 264–268. https://doi.org/10.1038/ng1196-264

Clark, B. E., & Thein, S. L. (2004). Molecular diagnosis of haemoglobin disorders. *Clin Lab Haematol*, *26*(3), 159–176. https://doi.org/10.1111/j.1365-2257.2004.00607.x

Dani, A. A., & Shrikhande, A. V. (2007). Double heterozygous for hemoglobin S and hemoglobin E – a case report from central India. *Indian J Hematol Blood Transfus*, *23*(3–4), 119–121. https://doi.org/10.1007/s12288-008-0012-0

de Haan, K., Ceylan Koydemir, H., Rivenson, Y., Tseng, D., Van Dyne, E., Bakic, L., … Ozcan, A. (2020). Automated screening of sickle cells using a smartphone-based microscope and deep learning. *NPJ Digit Med*, *3*, 76. https://doi.org/10.1038/s41746-020-0282-y

Fabry, M. E., Kaul, D. K., Raventos-Suarez, C., Chang, H., & Nagel, R. L. (1982). SC erythrocytes have an abnormally high intracellular hemoglobin concentration. Pathophysiological consequences. *J Clin Invest*, *70*(6), 1315–1319. https://doi.org/10.1172/jci110732

Figueiredo, M. S. (2015). The compound state: Hb S/beta-thalassemia. *Rev Bras Hematol Hemoter*, *37*(3), 150–152. https://doi.org/10.1016/j.bjhh.2015.02.008

Frömmel, C. (2018). Newborn screening for sickle cell disease and other hemoglobinopathies: A short review on classical laboratory methods-isoelectric focusing, HPLC, and capillary electrophoresis. *Int J Neonatal Screen*, *4*(4), 39. https://doi.org/10.3390/ijns4040039

Lund, K., Chakravorty, S., Toma, S., & Bain, B. J. (2015). Compound heterozygosity for hemoglobins S and D. *Am J Hematol*, *90*(9), 842. https://doi.org/10.1002/ajh.24095

Masiello, D., Heeney, M. M., Adewoye, A. H., Eung, S. H., Luo, H. Y., Steinberg, M. H., & Chui, D. H. (2007). Hemoglobin SE disease: A concise review. *Am J Hematol*, *82*(7), 643–649. https://doi.org/10.1002/ajh.20847

Milner, P. F., Miller, C., Grey, R., Seakins, M., DeJong, W. W., & Went, L. N. (1970). Hemoglobin O arab in four negro families and its interaction with hemoglobin S and hemoglobin C. *N Engl J Med*, *283*(26), 1417–1425. https://doi.org/10.1056/nejm197012242832601

Moll, S., & Orringer, E. P. (1997). Hemoglobin SC disease. *Am J Hematol*, *54*(4), 313. https://doi.org/10.1002/(SICI)1096-8652(199704)54:4%3C313::AID-AJH9%3E3.0.CO;2-Y

Ngo, D. A., Aygun, B., Akinsheye, I., Hankins, J. S., Bhan, I., Luo, H. Y., ... Chui, D. H. (2012). Fetal haemoglobin levels and haematological characteristics of compound heterozygotes for haemoglobin S and deletional hereditary persistence of fetal haemoglobin. *Br J Haematol*, *156*(2), 259–264. https://doi.org/10.1111/j.1365-2141.2011.08916.x

Ogu, U. O., Reyes Gil, M., Tolu, S. S., Acharya, S. A., & Minniti, C. P. (2021). First report of compound heterozygosity for Hb S (HBB: c.20A>T) and Hb Haringey (HBB: c.131A>G). *Hemoglobin*, *45*(2), 136–139. https://doi.org/10.1080/03630269.2021.1926276

Okwi, A. L., Byarugaba, W., Parkes, A., & Ocaido, M. (2010). The reliability of sickling and solubility tests and peripheral blood film method for sickle cell disease screening at district health centers in Uganda. *Clin Mother Child Health*, *7*. https://doi.org/10.4303/cmch/C101947

Onimoe, G., & Smarzo, G. (2017). HbS-Sicilian (δβ)(0)-thalassemia: A rare variant of sickle cell. *Case Rep Hematol*, *2017*, 9265396. https://doi.org/10.1155/2017/9265396

Rees, D. C., Williams, T. N., & Gladwin, M. T. (2010). Sickle-cell disease. *Lancet*, *376*(9757), 2018–2031. https://doi.org/10.1016/s0140-6736(10)61029-x

Rodak, B. F., Fritsma, G. A., & Doig, K. (2011). *Hematology: Clinical principles and applications*. Saunders.

Sant'Ana, P. G., Araujo, A. M., Pimenta, C. T., Bezerra, M. L., Junior, S. P., Neto, V. M., ... Pinheiro, M. B. (2017). Clinical and laboratory profile of patients with sickle cell anemia. *Rev Bras Hematol Hemoter*, *39*(1), 40–45. https://doi.org/10.1016/j.bjhh.2016.09.007

Steinberg, M. H. (2020). Fetal hemoglobin in sickle hemoglobinopathies: High HbF genotypes and phenotypes. *J Clin Med*, *9*(11). https://doi.org/10.3390/jcm9113782

Tolu, S. S., Reyes-Gil, M., Ogu, U. O., Thomas, M., Bouhassira, E. E., & Minniti, C. P. (2020). Hemoglobin F mitigation of sickle cell complications decreases with aging. *Am J Hematol*, *95*(5), E122–E125. https://doi.org/10.1002/ajh.25759

3 Pre-implantation Genetic Diagnosis for Prevention of Sickle Cell Disorder

Current Trends and Barriers

Annette Akinsete

Introduction

"An ounce of PREVENTION is worth a ton of CURE".
"Prevention is BETTER than CURE".
"Prevention is CHEAPER and BETTER than CURE".

Above are popular maxims that underscore the importance of PREVENTION. In the field of medicine, much of ill health can be prevented and prevention is indeed vital to improving individual as well as population health. This is particularly true for chronic conditions such as sickle cell disease (SCD) – long and drawn out as they are, placing tremendous pressure on individual, family and state finances and inimical to quality of life and longevity.

SCD is the most common form of inherited blood disorders. It is a condition associated with shortage of blood and severe pain, as well as complications such as stroke in children, chronic leg ulcers and hip joint degeneration. There are also psycho-social challenges for both the patients and their families, quality of life is poor and life expectancy less than the general population. In a 2014 study of autopsy findings and pattern of mortality in Nigerian SCD patients, the mean age at death was found to be 21 years (Ogun et al., 2014).

In addition, depression and anxiety are common in SCD and, as can be imagined, these impact the patients' lives negatively. In a 2008 study titled "Depression and Anxiety in Adults with Sickle Cell Disease: The PiSCES Project (Pain in Sickle Cell Epidemiology Study)", 27.6% of the 232 subjects surveyed were depressed and 6.5% had anxiety disorder. Depressed subjects had pain on significantly more days than non-depressed subjects and on non-crisis days, depressed subjects had higher mean pain, distress from pain and interference from pain. Both depressed and anxious subjects had poorer functioning. The anxious patients had more pain, distress from pain and interference from pain on non-crisis days and used opioids more often (Smith et al., 2015). If there is any one disease therefore, requiring prevention intervention, it is SCD. Fortunately, with advancement in technology and medicine, SCD can now be prevented through a number of interventions, including Pre-implantation Genetic Diagnosis (PGD).

DOI: 10.4324/9781003463931-4

Definitions

It is important to differentiate between PGD and PGT-A (Pre-implantation Genetic Testing – Aneuploidy) – also known as PGS (Pre-implantation Genetic Screening). PGD refers specifically to when one or both genetic parents have a known genetic abnormality and testing is performed on an embryo to determine if it also carries a genetic abnormality. In contrast, PGS refers to the technique whereby embryos from presumed chromosomally normal genetic parents are screened for aneuploidy (Nordica Fertility Centre, 2015). Also, while PGD detects specific disorders with a high probability of being passed down to offspring – such as SCD – PGT-A/PGS does not. PGT-A/PGS is used for the determination of the chromosomal status of In Vitro Fertilization (IVF) embryos by screening all 23 pairs of human chromosomes (Dayal et al., 2022).

PGD is the testing of embryos produced through IVF for genetic defects, in which testing is carried out prior to the implantation of the fertilized egg within the uterus. PGD may also be performed on eggs prior to fertilization. Examples of post-conception diagnostic procedures are amniocentesis and Chorionic Villus Sampling (CVS). PGD provides an alternative to these diagnostic procedures which are often followed by the difficult decision of pregnancy termination, in the event that the outcomes are unfavourable.

PGD is currently the only option available for eliminating the high risk of having a child with a genetic disease prior to implantation.

Aneuploidy: Aneuploidy refers to the presence of an extra chromosome or a missing chromosome and is the most common form of chromosomal abnormality (Mandal, 2019).

Pre-implantation Genetic Testing (PGT): Some authors have described PGT as an early form of PGD, where abnormal embryos are identified, thereby allowing transfer of genetically normal embryos. The technology has become an integral part of Assisted Reproductive Technology (ART) procedures (Parikh et al., 2018).

Assisted Reproductive Technology (ART): The International Committee for Monitoring Assisted Reproductive Technology (ICMART) and the World Health Organization (WHO)-revised glossary of ART terminology (2009) have defined ART as all treatments or procedures that include the in vitro handling of both human oocytes and sperm or of embryos for the purpose of establishing a pregnancy. This includes, but is not limited to, IVF and embryo transfer, gamete intrafallopian transfer, zygote intrafallopian transfer, tubal embryo transfer, gamete and embryo cryopreservation, oocyte and embryo donation, and gestational surrogacy. ART does not include assisted insemination (artificial insemination) using sperm from either a woman's partner or a sperm donor (Zegers-Hochschild et al., 2009).

In Vitro Fertilization (IVF)

According to the American Society for Reproductive Medicine (ASRM), IVF is a method of assisted reproduction involving a complex series of procedures, in which a man's sperm and a woman's eggs are combined outside of the body in a laboratory dish. One or more fertilized eggs (embryos) may be transferred into the woman's uterus, where they may implant in the uterine lining and develop. IVF is the most effective form of ART (Mayo Clinic, 2021).

One of Nigeria's foremost practitioners in this field, Professor Oladapo Ashiru OFR, described IVF as fertilization achieved outside of the body, involving ovulation induction, oocyte retrieval, sperm preparation, oocyte stripping, insemination and fertilization in a culture dish and, finally, embryo transfer. Oocyte retrieval and embryo transfer processes are carried out under ultrasound guidance. Without the development of IVF, PGD would not be possible (Ashiru & Akinyanju, 2018).

Evolution/History of PGD

Historically, the development of PGT technology dates back to 1890 with Walter Heape's experiments of successfully transferring embryos in the Belgian Hare doe rabbits (Davidson, 2023).

Indeed, in a 1937 manuscript, in the *New England Journal of Medicine*, Dr. John Rock predicted that human IVF, gender selection and gestational carriers would be utilized in reproductive science. He stated that one day, science will allow for parents to obtain sons or daughters "according to specification", foreshadowing the ability to screen out detrimental disease states with PGD (Franasiak et al., 2008).

Work in animal models as well as implementation of a number of techniques in human embryology in the 1960s and the 1980s paved the way for the application of PGD in human reproduction, so that a pioneer in the person of the American embryologist and geneticist, Alan Handyside, came along and was the first to use the approach in 1989 to test for the presence of the gene defects responsible for cystic fibrosis, an X-linked disease. Handyside, later in 1990, carried out biopsies on IVF embryos, removing one or two cells from each embryo. The biopsy procedure was performed three days after fertilization. Of three couples who volunteered for the procedure, one woman had two embryos that were fertilized normally and were negative for the cystic fibrosis gene. The woman underwent an embryo transfer with the normal embryo and gave birth to a healthy female who was free of cystic fibrosis and was not a carrier of the gene defects. The results of the trial proved that single-gene diseases could be identified prior to implantation, marking an important development for families who are affected by inherited genetic mutations (Davidson, 2023).

PGD for Sickle Cell Disease

PGD for SCD is simply the process of choosing one's child's Haemoglobin Genotype before pregnancy, employing the process of IVF. The father's sperm is collected and injected into the mother's previously retrieved eggs within a sterile container. The haemoglobin genotypes of the resultant embryos undergo DNA analysis, after amplification by Polymerase Chain Reaction (PCR). The couple can then have unaffected embryos (i.e. with Hb AA, AS, AC) implanted into the mother's womb. PGD is particularly desired by couples at risk (i.e. Hb AS married to Hb SS) – who have a 50% chance of having an Hb SS-affected child with each pregnancy (Ashiru & Akinyanju, 2018).

Preliminary Work before PGD for Sickle Cell Disease

To go through PGD for sickle cell anaemia (SCA), DNA samples from family members must be obtained to build a probe. This probe which contains specific genetic information received from the collected DNA will be used to test the cells biopsied from the embryos. DNA samples are required only from the direct family members (siblings or parents of the two partners). The PGD probe preparation takes 8–10 weeks. Professor Ashiru's Medical Art Centre in Lagos, Nigeria, collaborates with the world-renowned Genetics institute – Genesis Genetics – pioneers of PGD for inherited, genetic abnormalities. With the Collaborating Centre, results of the PGD are usually received within ten days – indicating which embryos are Hb SS, Hb AS or Hb AA. So today in Nigeria, sickle cell carrier couples (Hb AS and Hb AS) can now screen their embryos before conception to avoid or prevent getting a sickle cell baby (Hb SS). Although the process is quite expensive, it is hoped that various groups – including the government – can come to the financial aid of couples in need of PGD (Ashiru & Akinyanju, 2018).

Barriers to PGD

The reliability of PGD is well established. With the extremely low error rate, it can generally be considered safe. The principal drawbacks to PGD include the relatively high cost, access, availability, knowledge or awareness about the procedure and legal controls.

Cost of PGD

PGD is a complex procedure that requires considerable laboratory and clinical work, including Pre-IVF screening, ovarian stimulation monitoring, anaesthesia for egg retrieval, egg retrieval procedure, fertilization by ICSI and culture of the embryos, trophectoderm biopsy of blastocysts, vitrification (freezing) of the embryos, DNA testing, frozen embryo transfer and medications.

The cost therefore can be significant anywhere in the world and constitutes equally significant barrier to access.

The average cost of PGD in the US is $20,000–$25,000 (Advanced Fertility Center of Chicago, 2022), while in the United Kingdom, it ranges between $15,000 and $25,000 (Centre for Reproductive and Genetic Health, 2022) and in India, it is, on average, $10,000 (Iswarya Fertility Centre, 2022). In Nigeria, the cost ranges from $10,000 to $15,000 (Fertility Hub Nigeria, 2022), while in South Africa, it is on average $10,000 (Carzis et al, 2019).

In a review of data from the Genetic Counselling Department Register at the National Sickle Cell Centre/Sickle Cell Foundation Nigeria, out of the 256 couples-at-risk counselled between January and December 2019, 216 said they would NOT like to have PGD to prevent sickle cell in their offspring because "it was too expensive". But all 216 of them responded in the affirmative when asked if they would go for the procedure, were they to be sponsored (Sickle Cell Foundation Nigeria, 2019). This is understandable in a country where most treatment is paid for out-of-pocket and health insurance remains rudimentary.

Knowledge/Awareness and Attitude

A survey conducted by the Genetics and Public Policy Center, Washington, DC, USA, about two decades ago, found that only 24% of the general public in the United States had heard of PGD (Winkelman et al., 2015).

Similarly, the review of the Genetic Counselling data at the National Sickle Cell Centre (Sickle Cell Foundation Nigeria) revealed poor knowledge of PGD among the couples counselled. Out of the 256 couples counselled between January and December 2019, only three had heard about PGD (1.2%); 253 (98.8%) had never heard about PGD (Sickle Cell Foundation Nigeria, 2019).

A 2013 study of the perspectives of the US population towards the use of PGD in various clinical scenarios suggested that knowledge of PGD did not appear to have changed appreciably over the previous decade despite the increased utilization of PGD within IVF and advancements within the field. While awareness of PGD within the United States was comparable to that in other developed countries, individuals familiar with PGD (knowledge/awareness of PGD) were more supportive of the use of PGD to screen for genetic diseases, suggesting that further education and outreach may help inform the public and provide the knowledge upon which opinion can be formed more accurately (Winkelman et al., 2015).

In the same 2013 study, majority of the US population supported PGD to identify genetic diseases. Similar levels of support for PGD have been seen in populations outside the United States including Europe and Asia. Although the majority of respondents supported PGD for genetic diseases, most did not support PGD for diseases that manifest late in life (Winkelman et al., 2015).

Not unexpectedly, the data from Sickle Cell Foundation Nigeria showed that after the 253 couples who had never heard about PGD were provided information about PGD, 247 (96.5%) of them indicated they would like to go for the procedure.

Availability of PGD

Despite the growing popularity of PGD, it remains a relatively scarce or rare procedure in many parts of the world – to some extent, due to restrictions, laws, ethical, moral and religious considerations. In some countries, PGD is permitted and regulated by law, in some others, it is permissible under professional guidelines, but in some countries, PGD is completely prohibited by law.

Countries where PGD is permitted and regulated by law: Belgium, Denmark, Estonia, France, Greece, Iceland, India, Netherlands, New Zealand, Norway, Spain, South Australia (State) Victoria Australia (State) and South Africa.

Countries in which PGD is permissible under professional guidelines: Canada, Israel, Japan, Singapore, South Africa and the United Kingdom.

Some countries in which PGD is prohibited by law: Austria, Germany, Italy, Switzerland and Western Australia (Knoppers et al, 2006).

The United States: Unlike in many European countries, PGD is not regulated in the United States. As a result, PGD may be used for any condition for which genetic testing is available – at the discretion of fertility specialists and their patients.

Over 75% of fertility clinics in the United States offer PGD, and approximately 4–6% of IVF procedures utilize PGD annually (Winkman et al., 2015).

Africa: The expertise and capacity for PGD exist only in a few countries in Africa, including Nigeria, Ghana and South Africa. PGD is offered by only three known entities in Nigeria. These are The Bridge Clinic (with centres in Lagos, Abuja and Port Harcourt), Nordica Clinics (with centres in Lagos and Asaba) and The Medical Art Centre in Lagos.

In South Africa, fertility clinics provide PGD for prevention of genetic disorders, such as SCD, but gender selection is not allowed – it is illegal according to the National Health Act.

Ghana has a few fertility centres currently offering PGD for prevention of SCD, including RUMA Fertility and Specialist Hospital Ltd, Ebony IVF and Holy Trinity Medical Centre – all in Accra (RUMA Fertility & Specialist Hospital Ghana, 2022).

There is no evidence of policies or guidelines or laws regulating PGD in Nigeria and Ghana; officials of the Federal Ministry of Health, Abuja, Nigeria were interviewed as part of preparation for this project. Nevertheless, at Sickle Cell Foundation Nigeria, Genetic Counsellors list PGD as one of the options available to couples at risk of having children with SCD. It is also taught as part of the Foundation's bi-annual, Genetic Counselling Training Course that is attended by participants from all over Africa.

Ethical Considerations

While the application of PGD to help prevent SCD and other genetic disorders might seem clearly beneficial, the technique has also been used for more controversial purposes. In the United States, PGD is also widely offered for sex selection; a 2017 study showed that 72.7% of US fertility clinics offer sex selection, and 83.5% of those clinics offer sex selection for couples without infertility. Furthermore, there are concerns that PGD could be used to select for traits such as hair colour, height and athletic ability. The reason PGD can be employed for "nonmedical" purposes in the United States is because there are no legal limitations on the use of the technique. It can be used for any condition for which genetic testing is available at the discretion of fertility treatment clinicians and their patients. By contrast, many European countries have rigid legal structures that determine for what indications PGD is permissible (Bayefsky, 2018).

In a number of other countries, such as the United Kingdom and Canada, PGD is specifically prohibited for non-medical purposes by statute (Jones & Cohen, 2007).

Therefore, although it raises new possibilities, PGD has also become associated with considerable controversy due to ethical, legal and socio-cultural issues around it. Other scholars have also lent their voices to these ethical considerations, noting that they include the status of the embryo (the moral and legal status of early human life) and the interests and duties of the parents, considerations of equitable access, as well as the impact of the technology on families, women and physicians' duties.

In some countries, cases for PGD are first reviewed by experts, who take into consideration the specific genetic disease and the seriousness of the condition and then make recommendations as to whether the procedure should be approved. The Pre-implantation Genetic Diagnosis International Society was formed in 2002 to provide multidisciplinary research and education in the PGD arena and to advance the science of PGD (Davidson, 2023).

Religion and PGD

In a 2016 survey in Malaysia, in-depth interviews were conducted on religious scholars from three different religious organizations in the Klang Valley, Malaysia. Findings showed that Christian scholars were very skeptical of the long-term use of PGD because of its possible effect on the value of humanity and the parent-children relationship. This differed from Islamic scholars, who viewed PGD as God-given knowledge in medical science to further help humans understand medical genetics. For Buddhist scholars, PGD was considered to be new medical technology that could be used to save lives, avoid suffering and bring happiness to those who need it (Olesen et al., 2016).

On its part, the Roman Catholic Church has explicitly placed limitations on the use of PGD, as the technology results in the destruction of several embryos. PDG is manifestly contrary to the respect of every human life from the very moment of conception that is defended by the Catholic Magisterium and, thus, morally unacceptable (Institute of Clinical Bioethics. Editorial, 2014).

Recommendations

Over the years, the utilization of PGD worldwide has increased. Paradoxically though, despite sub-Saharan Africa (SSA) having the highest burden of SCD in the world, this region has the least access to PGD for prevention of the condition in the world. It is imperative that countries in SSA come on board the PGD wagon for improved individual and population health, as SCD presents low hanging fruits for success of healthcare interventions in the region. This will take strong political will and intentionally prioritizing SCD as a public health problem. Already, WHO (AFRO) recognizes the severity of the prevalence of SCD and has produced a Framework Strategy for SCD in the region. This framework is being adopted by member states accordingly. But to what extent are member states implementing the Strategy? This is where Advocacy Groups, including Non-Governmental Organisations (NGOs) such as Sickle Cell Foundation Nigeria and Sickle Cell Foundation Ghana, have a role to play. These NGOs need to hold governments accountable by ensuring that governments fund and implement Sickle Cell Prevention and Control programmes in the various countries.

Regulation of the practice of PGD is vital. Governments and other stakeholders need to come up with the necessary protocols, policies and guidelines, and legal frameworks that will guide the practice of PGD. Religious institutions and human rights groups must also sit at the table. This is particularly important in SSA where religion and religious organizations constitute powerful social forces of influence in the lives of everyday people.

Still on the subject of access, there is a need to educate the public about PGD and its availability. This will improve access, although there are still considerations of cost. Further research is required in order to improve the speed of diagnosis and make the PGD process less expensive.

Technology continues to advance in all areas and the future does appear to be bright. There are now discussions and research around Non-invasive Pre-implantation Testing techniques – although they are currently in experimental stages.

References

Advanced Fertility Center of Chicago (2022). PGD and IVF costs – What is the cost for preimplantation genetic diagnosis? https://advancedfertility.com/fertility-treatment/affording-care/pgd-cost/ (accessed February 2, 2022).

Ashiru O., Akinyanju O. (2018). Prenatal diagnosis and preimplantation diagnosis of sickle cell disorder: *Sickle Cell Bullet.* 10(2).

Bayefsky M. (2018). Who should regulate preimplantation genetic diagnosis in the United States? *AMA J Ethics.* https://journalofethics.ama-assn.org/article (accessed February 2, 2022).

Carzis B., Wainstein T., Gobetz L., Krause A. (2019). Review of 10 years of preimplantation genetic diagnosis in South Africa: Implications for a low-to-middle-income country. *J Assist Reprod Genet.* https://doi.org/10.1007/s10815-019-01537-3

Centre for Reproductive and Genetic Health (CRGH). https://crgh.co.uk/ (accessed February 2, 2022).

Davidson M. R. (2023, March 20). *Preimplantation genetic diagnosis. Encyclopedia Britannica.* https://www.britannica.com/science/preimplantation-genetic-diagnosis

Dayal M. B., Taylor L., Miller M. E. (Updated December 7, 2022). Pre-implantation Genetic Diagnosis: *Medscape.* https://emedicine.medscape.com/article/273415-overview?form=fpf (accessed January 31, 2024).

Fertility Hub Nigeria. https://www.fertilityhubnigeria.com/ (accessed February 2, 2022).

Franasiak J., Richard T., Scott R. T. (2008). A Briefbrief history of preimplantation genetic diagnosis and preimplantation genetic screening. *Virtual Acad Genet.* https://ivf-worldwide.com/cogen/oep/pgd-pgs/history-of-pgd-and-pgs.html (accessed February 2, 2022).

Institute of Clinical Bioethics. Editorial (January 6, 2014). Is pre-implantation genetic diagnosis (PGD) acceptable for Catholics? https://sites.sju.edu/icb/is-pre-implantation-genetic-diagnosis-pgd-acceptable-for-catholics/(accessed February 2, 2022).

Iswarya Fertility Centre. https://www.iswaryafertility.com/ (accessed February 2, 2022).

Jones H. W., Cohen J. (2007). Preimplantation genetic diagnosis. *Letter.* https://doi.org/10.1016/j.fertnstert.2007.01.080

Knoppers B. M., Bordet S., Isasi R. M. (2006). Preimplantation genetic diagnosis: An overview of socio-ethical and legal considerations. *Annu Rev Genom Human Genet.* 7: 201–221. https://doi.org/10.1146/annurev.genom.7.080505.115753 (accessed February 1, 2022).

Mandal A. (2019). Chromosomal abnormalities. *News Medical Life Sciences.* https://www.news-medical.net/health/Chromosomal-Abnormalities.aspx (accessed January 21, 2024).

Mayo Clinic (September 10, 2021). In Vitro Fertilisation (IVF). https://www.mayoclinic.org/tests-procedures/in-vitro-fertilization/about/pac-20384716

Ogun G. O., Ebili H., Kotila T. R. (2014). Autopsy findings and pattern of mortality in Nigerian sickle cell disease patients. *Pan Afr Med J.* https://doi.org/10.11604/pamj.2014.18.30.4043

Olesen A., Nor S. N., Amin L. (2016). Religious scholars' attitudes and views on ethical issues pertaining to pre-implantation genetic diagnosis (PGD) in Malaysia. *J Bioethical Inquiry.* 13: 419–429. https://doi.org/10.1007/s11673-016-9724-2

Parikh F. R., Athalye A. S., Naik N. J., Naik D. J., Sanap R. R., Madon P. F. (2018). Preimplantation genetic testing: Its evolution, where are we today? *J Hum Reprod Sci.* 11(4): 306–314. https://doi.org/10.4103/jhrs.JHRS_132_18

Preimplantation Genetic Diagnosis (PGD) or Screening(PGS) (April 22, 2015). https://nordicalagos.org/preimplantation-genetic-diagnosis-pgd-or-screeningpgs/

RUMA Fertility & Specialist Hospital, Ghana. https://thewvg.com/vendor/ruma-fertility-and-specialist-hospital-ltd/ (accessed January 29, 2022).

Sickle Cell Foundation Nigeria (2019). Information Brochure. https://www.sicklecellfoundation.com/wp-content/uploads/2019/02/Information-Brochure_Sept-2017_Edited.pdf (accessed January 31, 2024)

Smith W. R., McClish D. K., Dahman B. A., Levenson J. L., Aisiku I. P., Citero V., Victor E., Bovberg V. E., Roberts J. D., Penberthy L. T., Roseff S. D. (2015). Daily home opioid use in adults with sickle cell disease: The PiSCES project. *J Opioid Manag.* https://doi.org/10.5055/jom.2015.0273

Winkelman W. D., William D., Missmer S. A., Myers D., Ginsburg E. S. (2015). Public perspectives on the use of preimplantation genetic diagnosis. *J Assist Reprod Genet.* 32(5): 665–675. https://doi.org/10.1007/s10815-015-0456-8

Zegers-Hochschild F., Adamson G. D., de Mouzon J., Ishihara O., Mansour R., Nygren K., Sullivan E., Vanderpoel S. (2009). International Committee for Monitoring Assisted Reproductive Technology (ICMART) and the World Health Organization (WHO) revised glossary of ART terminology, 2009. *Special Contribution.* 92(5): 1520–1524. https://doi.org/10.1016/j.fertnstert.2009.09.009

4 The State of Newborn Screening for Sickle Cell Disease in Low- and Middle-income Countries

Baba Inusa, Juliana Olufunke Lawson,
Livingstone Dogara and Lewis Hsu

Chapter on Newborn Screening – Why?

Sub-Saharan Africa (SSA) and India are the cradle of sickle cell disease (SCD) accounting for over 85% of the world's 300–400,000 annual live births with the disorder (Ghafuri et al., 2020; Weatherall, 2010). Six of the seven countries with the largest of burden of disease are from SSA which include Nigeria, Democratic Republic of Congo, Tanzania, Uganda, Angola, and Cameroon and Nigeria leading with about 150,000 births per year (Piel et al., 2013, 2014). India is the world's third highest with incidence of over 40,000 SCD live births annually (Piel et al., 2013). The increasing burden of SCD in high-income countries is due to several factors including migration and the incidence of SCD is increasing in the US, over 1,000, France over 400, and the UK between 250 and 300 affected live births per year (Inusa & Colombatti, 2017; Streetly et al., 2009, 2018).

Definition of NBS

Newborn screening (NBS) may be defined as the process by which infants and newborn babies are tested for congenital or inherited disorders that result in serious lifelong disability, death, or chronic complications if not treated shortly after birth (El-Hattab, Almannai, & Sutton, 2018; Kayton, 2007; Wilcken, 2011). The treatment may not necessarily prevent disability but ameliorate the full-blown features or prevent death and the conditions may include genetic, metabolic, physical, or functional affecting the lives of infants (Therrell et al., 2015; Zimmer, 2020). The overall goal is to identify those affected early, with the purpose of instituting therapy prior to the onset of clinical features and thereby improve their quality of life and improve survival (Hinton et al., 2017; Wilcken, 2011). To achieve this, a set of approaches are required to identify asymptomatic individuals in a defined population followed by confirmatory test followed by the institution of appropriate therapeutic strategies (Berry, 2015). When all infants are tested for disorder irrespective of individual characteristics such as race but based entirely on the age of the infant irrespective of gestation this is referred to as Universal NBS (Kayton, 2007; Remec et al.,

DOI: 10.4324/9781003463931-5

2021). Universal NBS is the recommended method in majority of European countries (Frömmel, Brose, Klein, Blankenstein, & Lobitz, 2014; Lobitz et al., 2018; Runkel et al., 2020; Streetly, Maxwell, & Campbell, 1998). With Selective NBS programme, the method used by France, Scotland, and Wales, infants are identified as high risk as determined by parental characteristics or based on screening blood tests (Brousse, Allaf, & Benkerrou, 2021; Diallo et al. 2018). The policy choice between Universal NBS and Selective NBS is not a straight-forward economic justification but also includes equity and logistics (Grosse, 2005; McGann et al. 2015). Screening of infants may take place from birth up to but not including one year (Modell et al., 1999; Streetly, Latinovic, Hall, & Henthorn, 2009).

NBS for Sickle Cell Disease and Survival Outcomes

There is growing evidence to support the fact that implementation of NBS for SCD followed by comprehensive care reduces the occurrence of life-threatening complications (e.g., sepsis, splenic sequestration crisis) as well as under-five mortalities (Frempong & Pearson, 2007; Melorose, Perroy, & Careas, 2015). Effective follow-up treatment including Penicillin V and vaccination (pneumococcal and *Haemophilus influenzae*) contributes to the reduction in morbidity and mortality (Nottage et al., 2013; Vichinsky, 1991). Therefore, the implementation of NBS for SCD followed by the early institution of compre-hensive care is recognized as the most effective tool in improving the survival of SCD) (Frempong & Pearson, 2007; L.G.C., S., C.A., & M.E.G., 2015). NBS is reported to reduce mortality of infants born of SCD by a factor of ten in in a ten-year period (de Montalembert, 2002; El-haj & Hoppe, 2018; Watson, Lloyd-Puryear, & Howell, 2022). The disparity in the survival of infants born with SCD between high income countries and low- and middle-income coun-tries remains very wide; while the US and the UK reported that over 94% sur-vive into adulthood (Gardner et al., 2016; Quinn, Rogers, & Buchanan, 2004; Telfer et al., 2007), a recent report based on DHIS data in Nigeria reported that less than 50% of babies would survive beyond five years. Nigeria (Berger et al., 2022) and our group also reported a 50% increased mortality (Inusa, Popoola, & Wonkam, 2017). The establishment of infrastructure and appropriate paren-tal education for NBS for low- and middle-income countries is of paramount importance in efforts to reduce excess SCD-related deaths from 90% to 5% (Archer et al., 2022; Grosse et al., 2011; Obaro et al., 2016; Tubman et al., 2022) (Table 4.1).

In this chapter, we will explore some of the characteristics of success and limita-tions and the need for national policy and leveraging foreign funding support for NBS for SCD. We will explore the role of the primary and community healthcare structures in Africa. We will propose the adaptation/modification of implementa-tion and monitoring tools from high-income settings for current and future pro-grammes for NBS for SCD in the Africa and India.

Table 4.1 Summary of the level of public health infrastructure and excess mortality considered per income class and for each of the four scenarios tested.

Scenario	Low-/middle-income countries (GNI$_{pc}$≤US$12,275)		High-income countries (GNI$_{pc}$>US$12,275)	
	General level of public health infrastructures for under-five children with SCA	Excess mortality in under-five children with SCA	General level of public health infrastructures for under-five children with SCA	Excess mortality in under-five children with SCA
Scenario 1	Poor access to public health infrastructures	90%	Good access to public health infrastructures	10%
Scenario 2	Good access to public health infrastructures	50%	Specific interventions for children with SCA (e.g., diagnosis, treatment)	5%
Scenario 3	Specific interventions for children with SCA (e.g., diagnosis, treatment)	10%	Universal screening programme (optimum)	0%
Scenario 4	Universal screening programme	5%	Universal screening programme (optimum)	0%

Source: Peil F.B., Hay S.I., Weatherall D.J., and Williams T.N. (2013). Global Burden of Sickle Cell Anaemia in Children under Five, 2010–2050: Modelling Based on Demographics, Excess Mortality, and Interventions (Plos Medicine) https://doi.org/10.1371/journal.pmed.1001484.t002.

Historical Perspectives

Historical of Newborn Screening and Sickle Cell Disease

Global Perspectives

NBS was first introduced in the 1960s with phenylketonuria (PKU) when Robert was able to identify asymptomatic babies using bacterial inhibition test. This was later refined as an inexpensive and reliable simple test for mass screening. The first NBS was reported by *Metters* in London (Metters & Yawson, 1970); then it was introduced in *Jamaica* in 1973 and New York in 1975 (El-Hattab et al., 2018; Therrell et al., 2015). Universal NBS was implemented in the US in 2006 (Daniel et al., 2019; Frömmel et al., 2014; Therrell et al., 2015). In the UK while NBS was implemented for SCD as early as 1984 in parts of London, universal NBS in the England was implemented between 2002 and 2006 following the establishment of a national screening programme (Daniel et al., 2019; Streetly et al., 2018; Zeuner et al., 1999). The introduction of NBS for SCD in 50 states of the US in 2006 is the result of different factors including the 1972 sickle cell act by President Richard Nixon in 1972, the work of pioneers like Charles Whitten and the National Sickle Cell Association (now Sickle Cell Disease Association of America) community-based organizations (Hinton et al., 2017; Minkovitz et al. 2016). In the UK, while different boroughs such as Lambeth, South and Lewisham in South London introduced universal screening for SCD from 1984, it was not until 2002–2005 when national sickle cell screening committee was set up under leadership of Allison Streetly that the programme was rolled across England. Scotland and Wales currently offer targeted screening based on the family origin antenatal questionnaire and at-risk babies are identified for screening at birth (Almeida, Henthorn, & Davies, 2001). Other European countries with national NBS programmes are France, Netherlands, and Germany while Cuba and Brazil also offer national NBS for SCD. The feasibility of implementing newborn SCD screening has been tested in India, Malta, Italy, and Canada. Italia et al. tested over 5,000 babies in Gujarat region screened using high-performance liquid chromatography with 0.67% HbSS, 0.23% sickle cell beta thalassaemia and emphasizing the presence of severe SCD phenotypes in India (Italia et al., 2011). Even though Jamaica was a global pioneer of NBS for SCD but now is reportedly testing less than 40% of babies for SCD compared to England and the US where universal screening occurs (Almeida et al., 2001; King, Reid, King, & Reid, 2014; Runkel et al., 2020).

Africa Perspectives

The situation is more precarious in Africa where not one country has yet adopted a national policy for NBS for SCD. This is despite that fact that NBS for other genetic disorders is not new in Africa, the first NBS for PKU in Egypt occurred in 1991, hypothyroidism and other metabolic disorders in 1996. The first national policy for NBS programme was introduced for hypothyroidism in 2003 and PKU added in 2015 (El-attar et al., 2022; Temtamy, 2017). On the other hand, there is yet to be a national policy for NBS for SCD in Africa even though the incidence is high in some regions (Moez & Younan, 2016). The implementation of NBS for SCD has been limited to institutional or regional community-based programmes, even though successful leading hundreds of thousand babies screened, none has been rolled out nationally yet. Ghana and Benin Republic were the leading countries to introduce NBS as well as DRC Congo but none has resulted in national rollout yet (Archer et al., 2022; Therrell et al., 2020; Tshilolo et al., 2008). The programme in Ghana was instituted in 1991 with over 25-year history screening involving about 40 birth centres and by 2020 had screened over 500,000 babies for SCD (Ohene-frempong & Oduro, 1993). Rahimy et al. in Benin republic implemented screening in two major cities and enrolled 85% in comprehensive care and over 80% still being followed up after five years (Rahimy, 2009). Therrell et al. (2020) reported from the First Pan African Workshop on Newborn Screening that was convened in June 2019 in Rabat, Morocco that NBS for SCD in Angola tested over 300,000 babies for SCD and enrolled over 1,000 SCD babies with 96% enrolment in treatment centres (Therrell et al. 2020). However, the Angolan programme funded through Chevron-Baylor College of Medicine partnership has not been sustained. Other NBS pilots were also reported in DRC (2006), Mali (2013) Nigeria (2009–2011), Tanzania (2009), and Uganda (2019) (Archer et al., 2022; Kuznik, Habib, Munube, & Lamorde, 2016).

Examples of Foreign Funding Support for NBS for SCD in Africa

There have been increasing efforts to implement NBS and comprehensive care in partnerships with a foreign technical and infrastructure funding support (CONSA, SPARCO, ARISE), Consortium On Newborn Screening (CONSA) was instituted by the American Society of Hematology in 7-African countries to implement a standardized screening and offer early intervention for children with SCD (Green et al., 2016, 2022). The programme aims to evaluate the effectiveness of the intervention, cultural adaptation with the goal of achieving a sustainable initiative for the continent. SPARCO (Sickle cell Pan-African Consortium) aims to involve 20 sites in 15 countries in Africa with the main objective of developing a sickle cell database and implement standard of care for sickle cell management. African Research and Innovative initiative for Sickle cell Education (ARISE), funded by European Union Horizon (2020), supports training of research and technical staff in SCD, including laboratory capacity, clinical and community management, using staff exchange between Africa and Europe (Strunk et al., 2020). ARISE, while not funded to undertake NBS, supports the development of human capacity through skills acquisition, institutional partnerships aimed to improving the environment such as laboratory Quality Assurance, standard operating procedures, and the application of appropriate management protocols for paediatrics, Transition from *paediatric to adult and the management of adults with SCD* (see ARISE work packages, Figure 4.1). ARISE has embarked on conducting "train the trainer" workshops for diagnosis, blood transfusion, clinician care and community health workers' role in NBS for SCD and investigated the role of implementation science approaches (Inusa et al., 2018) (Figure 4.2).

Pitfalls in NBS for SCD in Sub-Saharan Africa

A recent qualitative assessment of some of the pilot programmes in six countries, namely, Angola, Ghana, DRC Congo, Nigeria, Liberia, and Tanzania (Archer et al., 2022) identified some of the challenges limiting success in Africa. This paper *identified four themes – governance and structure, funding, technical and cultural barriers, and enhancers for achieving* sustainable NBS programmes in Africa.

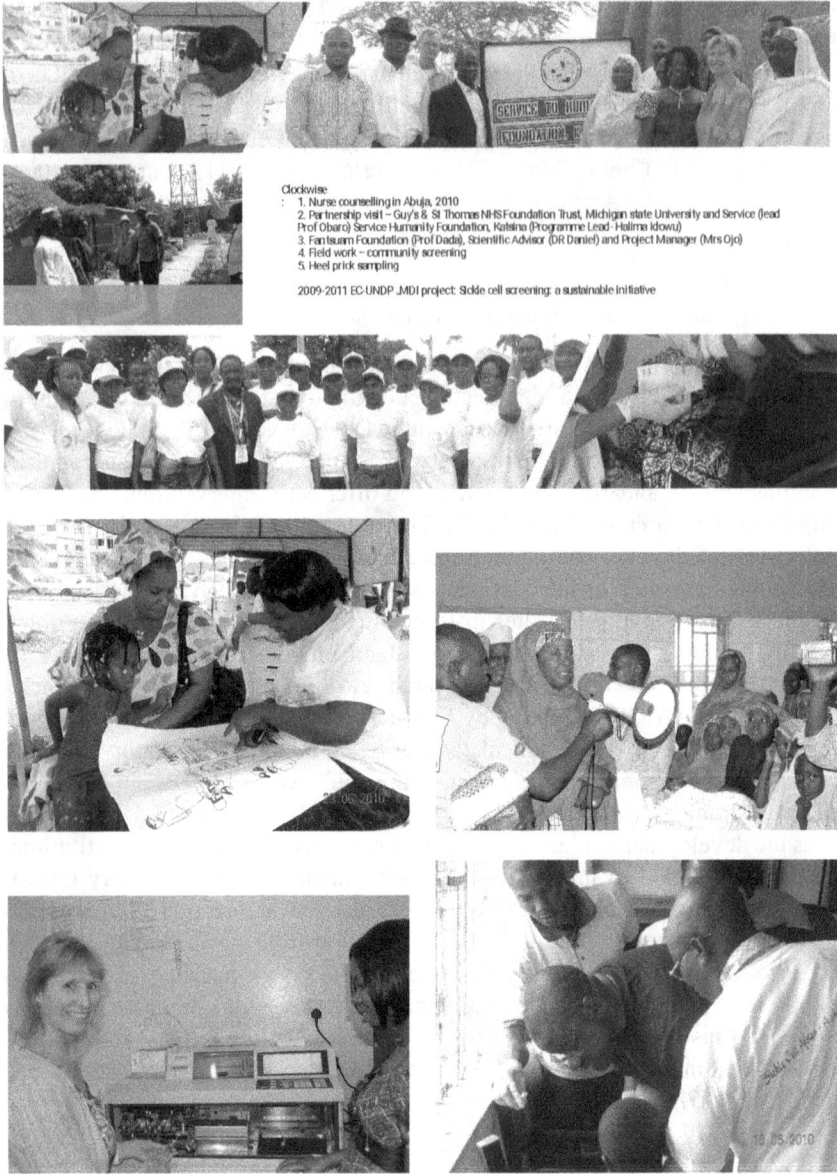

Clockwise
: 1. Nurse counselling in Abuja, 2010
  2. Partnership visit – Guy's & St Thomas NHS Foundation Trust, Michigan state University and Service (lead Prof Obaro) Service Humanity Foundation, Katsina (Programme Lead - Halima Idowu)
  3. Fantsuam Foundation (Prof Dada), Scientific Advisor (DR Daniel) and Project Manager (Mrs Ojo)
  4. Field work – community screening
  5. Heel prick sampling

2009-2011 EC-UNDP JMDI project: Sickle cell screening: a sustainable initiative

Figure 4.1 Sensitization visits to traditional leaders in 2020 prior to pilot screening project.

Primary Theme I: Structural and Governance Aspects

The survey reported that the programmes that engaged the 'state or national governments' early in the planning stage were likely to become sustainable beyond the funding cycle. The absence of late government input was identified as major setback and resulted in the termination of the pilot. The nature of government

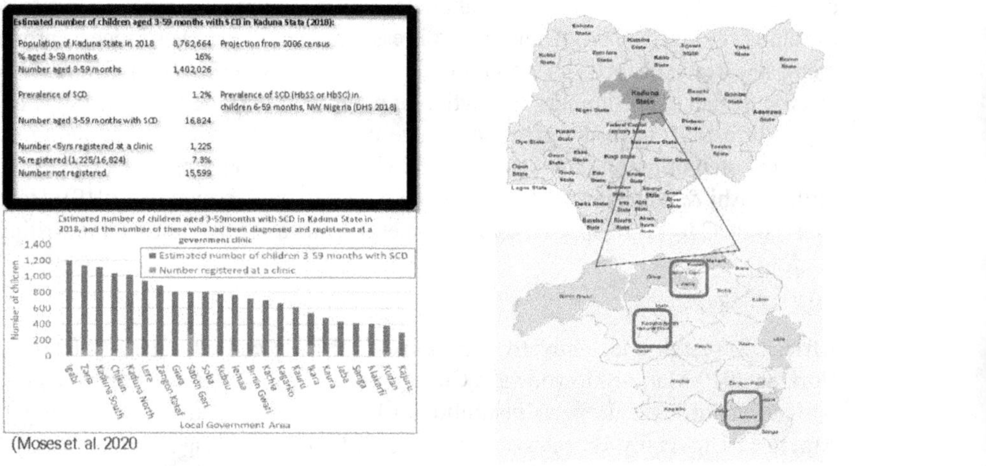

(Moses et. al. 2020)

Figure 4.2 Preliminary survey data of newly registered patients in public health institutions in Kaduna state showing a gap between the projected numbers and actual patients attending treatment centres. ARISE project (Mamman et al., 2020; Strunk et al., 2020).

involvement was also important, and all programmes were based at public health institutions and minimal partnership with private health services.

CASE SCENARIO 1

EC-UNDP joint migration initiative project 2009–2011 (Nations, 2010) – "Sickle cell cohort study: a sustainable pilot scheme" (Daniel, Obaro, Dada, Lawson, & Inusa, 2011; Obaro et al., 2016). These activities required the mobilization and consent of parents and caregivers for participation in the project. Leveraging their proximity to target communities, and relying on an awareness raising campaign, Nigerian partners succeeded in (a) obtaining authorizations (i.e., from village chiefs, State government to conduct the study; (b) obtaining parents' consent to enrol infants in the screening programme; and (c) engaging community health workers (doctors, nurses and midwifes) to empower beneficiaries to manage the disease – showing community sensitization and result of annual registration of new patients in Kaduna.

Primary Theme II: Technical Aspects

The study observed that successful workflow required for sample collection, storage, transportation, and reporting of the results essential to provide the desired confidentiality is complex. This involves multiple staff to be trained and retained within the services. A few challenges were observed, and, in some cases, the diagnostic laboratories were in different countries or different states and over 7-hour car drive. In some situations, in the region, access to some communities is seasonal, making it difficult to transfer samples to remote laboratories. The capabilities for data collection were variable where majority were paper based, Ghana had developed a digital App (A mobile application) for use during sample collection in the clinic setting. The provision of data is essential for advocacy, service improvement, and research. All the programmes except the Nigerian (HPLC) used isoelectric focusing. Preliminary evaluation of point-of-care (POC) tests [lateral-flow, paper diffusion], have the great advantage of immediate results, eliminating the laborious step of finding the family 1–2 weeks after they have returned home after birth (Arishi & Alhadrami, 2021; Therrell et al. 2020; Nnodu et al., 2019). However, no POC tests are approved for commercial sale as of the time of this writing.

CASE SCENARIO 2

African Research and Innovative Initiative for Sickle cell education (ARISE) is Horizon 2020 Marie-Sklowdowska Curie staff exchange programme between four African countries, European institutions (the UK, Italy, France, and Portugal), American University Beirut, and University Illinois at Chicago for the development of human capacity in various skills including implementation science, research, community training, counselling and clinical care as well as strengthening haematological laboratories in Africa (see Figure 4.3).

Primary Theme III: Cultural Aspects

The programmes that were surveyed undertook community engagement activities at different stages of implementation such as meeting with community leaders, focus group events, and membership of steering committees to ensure acceptability of the programmes. Some of the concerns were anxiety about receiving results and issues around stigma or poor knowledge about SCD. Both communities and

ARISE project

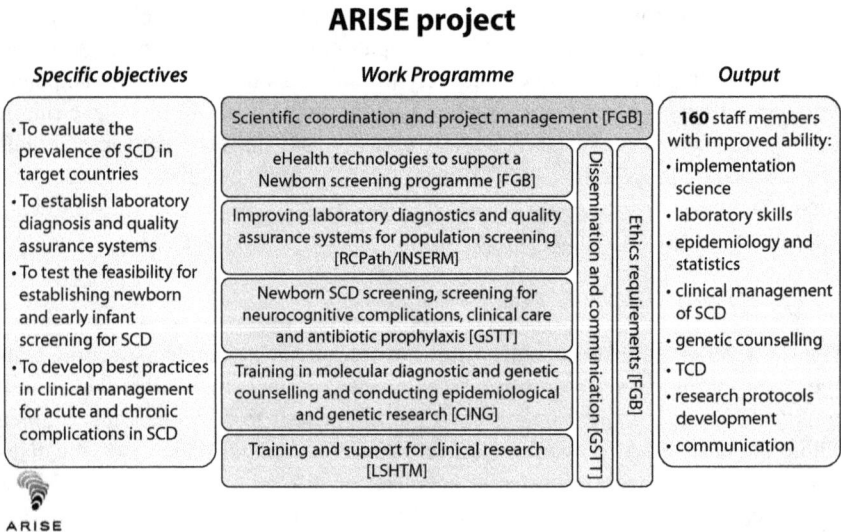

Figure 4.3 Arise project.

medical systems recognize that some of these issues in SCD have already been addressed in the screening and care of perinatal HIV/AIDS and other maternal-child health issues. Community awareness can be raised by volunteer community mobilizers, who are familiar with traditional rulers, elders, and other key opinion leaders. Health educational materials can be largely pictorial, transcending languages and reaching populations with low literacy. Training the primary health centre personnel can involve the primary health centres and midwives, conserving the resources of hospitals and tertiary care centres. Role-playing skits and specific protocols are developed for train-the trainer programmes, which also allow these key stakeholders to highlight barriers and facilitators for NBS. Informal transportation networks can be used for patients or for blood samples.

Primary Theme IV: Financial Aspects

All six programmes relied on external funding from forewing partners. The professional interviewed were concerned that the fact that there is little local, state, and national partner funding meant that the chance of achieving a sustainable and expanded programme was very minimal. While external funding was seen as a stimulus for success, the lack of local financial support was a major setback for success.

Two key implementation strategies are: (1) aligning SCD NBS and care with existing healthcare systems, (2) stakeholder engagement to adapt SCD to local needs. Improved SCD care should improve national mortality statistics for children and mother, which has indirect economic implications. Recent analyses of the health economics of SCD suggest that the costs of NBS and follow-up care have a "return on investment" of greater economic productivity for the patients and families (Hernandez & Howard, 2021; Kuznik et al., 2016).

CASE SCENARIO 2 – CONSA

- American Society of Hematology–funded 7-country in sub-Saharan consortium (CONSA) for implementation research on newborn SCD screening and early clinical intervention.
- The primary objectives are to determine SCD birth incidence and effectiveness of early standardized care for preventing under five mortality (Tubman et al., 2022).

Blood Sample Management

In low-resource setting *blood sample collection* from infants and subsequent *blood sample management* leading up to disclosure of result to the family can be challenging. It is important to constantly review the staff undertaking sample collection to ensure quality blood spots for laboratory testing. This needs to be the role of dedicated staff, commonly nurses of midwives or in some cases laboratory technicians. Because majority of the testing laboratories may be located far from the blood collection sites, a system to ensure safe and *secure transportation system* is needed and the medium for sample storage, e.g., twinning the process with HIV blood screening "Riders for Health" as used in Zambia and Kaduna state, Nigeria. The pathway of sample management in the laboratory, analysis, result verification, and reporting need to be consistent to ensure that the result is given to the correct family in a timely manner, and they are supported with counselling and can afford treatment and care.

Characteristics of Successful Programmes

Ten Principles of WHO Public Health Screening

The WHO recommendation in Wilson and Jungner 1968 is still relevant and applies based on the central idea for early disease detection as the path to successful treatment and prevention of complications and premature death (Ding & Han, 2022; Dobrow, Hagens, Chafe, Sullivan, & Rabeneck, 2018; Hsu, Green, Ivy et al., 2016; Mighton et al., 2022). They referred to the ten recommendations as collective principles and recommend for public health programmes:

- *The condition sought should be an important health problem.* The fact that SCD is a public health programme for many countries in SSA has been made by the WHO over 20 years ago, yet it remains an aspiration rather than a reality.
- *There should be an accepted treatment for patients with recognized disease.* Effectiveness of SCD treatment including *Prophylactic treatments* (Penicillin, Vaccination, antimalaria therapy), disease *modifying therapies* (hydroxyurea treatment has been used for over 30 years and recently new therapies such as L-Glutamine (2017), Crizanlizumab (2019), Voxelotor (2019)) and curative therapies such *as* bone marrow transplantation and gene therapy (Kanter & Falcon, 2021; Migotsky, Beestrum, & Badawy, 2022; Nottage et al., 2013).
- *Facilities for diagnosis and treatment should be available.* It is necessary to ensure functioning of treatment clinic facility before embarking on NBS for SCD (Ohene-Frempong, personal communication). Otherwise, laboratory diagnosis is only a step-in pathway of care. This must be accompanied by a tight process from sample collection, sample transportation to testing centres, and rapid turnover of result and patient referral to treatment centres.
- *There should be a recognizable latent or early symptomatic stage.* Due to the high foetal haemoglobin (HbF), babies are asymptomatic in the first 5–6 months and programmes recommended that those identified are referred to treatment by 3 months.
- *There should be a suitable test or examination.* The dried blood spot was first used in the early 1970s and there are different methods available to analyse samples.
- *The test should be acceptable to the population.* Most of the programmes in Africa are welcomed by the community raising unfulfilled expectations (Hinton et al., 2017).
- *The natural history of the condition*, including development from latent to declared disease, should be adequately understood.
- *There should be an agreed policy on whom to treat as patients.* All sickle cell syndromes from homozygous disease (HbSS) to double heterozygous states (HbSC, HbSbeta thalassaemia +/o and HbSE) are amenable to prophylactic treatment even though the role of hydroxyurea may be limited in double heterozygous states (Nottage et al., 2013).

- *The cost of case-finding* (including diagnosis and treatment of patients diagnosed) should be economically balanced in relation to possible expenditure on medical care.
- *Case-finding should be a continuing process* and not a "once and for all" project. This emphasizes the role of national and state policies to ensure that programmes are sustainable. This can only be achieved when NBS implementation funding is not entirely dependent on foreign institutions, and it is driven together with indigenous service providers in equitable manner.

Criteria for Programme Monitoring and Evaluation

The system for NBS requires multidisciplinary and multi-sectorial input to succeed. The essence of screening is to provide treatment, and this may be at primary, secondary, and tertiary as well as community based. The care pathway therefore includes primary/community health workers, public and private hospitals all must be engaged in a meaningful manner to close the loop for patient care. Therefore, the framework proposed by Hinton et al. of primary drivers for outcomes, outcome measures, and the proportion achieved as shown in Table 4.2 (Hinton et al., 2017; Meyers, Durlak, & Wandersman, 2012).

Table 4.2 Primary drivers, outcome measures, and percentages – related to SCD framework (Hinton et al., 2017).

Primary outcome drivers	Rapid and reliable detection and diagnosis	Provision of evidence-based care	Coordination and integration of services	Improvement, discovery, and innovation
Outcome measures	Detection by NBS Confirmation of SCD using secondary and molecular tests	Prevention of major disease-related mortality and morbidities Growth and development	Patient-centred engagement and satisfaction Primary care, secondary and community providers	Patients enrolled in registries, clinical trials, improvements in outcomes
Measures concept percentages	#/of HbSS, HbSC, HbS-beta thalassemia detected at birth Prompt confirmation with definitive diagnosis	Penicillin V, malaria, follow-up care – stroke, renal, pulmonary function testing Clinical database Public health/ Education databases	Counselling and SC gene assessment for hemoglobinopathies provided by genetic counsellors	Proportion enrolled in SCD registries, databases, and critical care processes with statistically meaningful, educational, and public health records

Primary Drivers and Outcome Measures

Primary Outcomes of Care of SCD

The goals of comprehensive care are both the prevention of complications and re-duction of mortality in SCD, to provide optimal health outcome. These include the number of children developing infections, malaria, stroke, acute chest syndrome or other lung disease, or iron overload from transfusion therapy.

The potential data sources include birth registries, immunization clinics and maternity services which many be incorporated into short-term and medium- to long-term databases. Other data sources include education records, primary and clinic registers.

a   Morbidity and mortality data may be assessed using proxies such as attendance at the primary care, accident and emergencies hospital admissions and community-based data.
b   There is a need to review data and assess disparities.

Rapid and Reliable Detection and Diagnosis (Detection and Diagnosis)

There is a growing array of diagnostic methodology to be adopted for newborn infants with different degrees of precision – specificity and sensitivity, costs, and ease of application. (Knapkova, Hall, & Loeber, 2018).

- ISOELECTRIC FOCUSING: This is based on the principle that Hb molecules travel across a pH gradient until they reach their isoelectric points where the net charge is zero. In addition to its ability to identify the different variants of HB, it also has the following advantages. Detect HbS and HbA easily in a high concentration of HbF, requires only small volume of the sample, able to use dried blood spot (DBS). *Disadvantages:* expensive, requires highly trained staff to interpret the results.
- HIGH-PERFORMANCE LIQUID CHROMATOGRAPHY: Migration of the different variant in this technique is based on their retention time as they interact with the stationary medium. In addition to its ability to identify the different variant of Hb, it is a more reliable technique when monitoring patients under Blood Transfusion and HU treatment; it has better sensitiv-ity than electrophoresis and fully automated. *Disadvantages:* high cost and not sustainable in many low- and middle-income countries. Inability to dif-ferentiate variants with same retention time and too expensive for most low resource setting.
- LATERAL FLOW IMMUNOASSAY. This technique uses several portable platforms in biomedical detection of SCD such as: Sickle Cell SCAN: uses polyclonal antibodies on lateral flow chromatographic immunoassay against HbS, HbC, HbA to detect different variants of SCD qualitatively. It is fast and affordable.

Validity of this assay has been confirmed in a study that showed a sensitivity and specificity of 98.4% and 98.6%, respectively. It also demonstrated that the detection of HbC and HbC is not affected by HbF.

Disadvantages: misinterpretation of results due to visual reading. Cross reactivity of the polyclonal antibody. Another assay using this technique includes **Hemo-TypeSC assay** (Arishi & Alhadrami, 2021)

Provision of Evidence-Based Care for SCD (Inati, 2009)

Prophylaxis – Penicillin V
Immunization
Malaria prevention
Stroke screening
Hydroxyurea
Specialist joint clinics – Pulmonary, Nephrology, and Neurology
Growth and development monitoring

Coordination and Integration

Linkage to Services and Care: The immediate benefit of NBS is the timely initiation of evidence-based interventions. In our framework example, one such intervention would include the provision of prophylactic penicillin for infants with SCD. Linkages to services and care extend beyond a single intervention to include access to primary and subspecialty services and other resources to achieve primary outcomes of care (Hsu, Green, Ivy et al., 2016). Family-centred engagement and satisfaction with the experience of care are other important measures of whether a patient and family relate to an integrated and inclusive healthcare system providing patient-centred engagement and satisfaction that incorporates primary and community health workers clinics, secondary hospital care supported by linked specialist provision and guidelines (Green et al., 2016).

Continuous Improvement of Care, Discovery, and Innovation

MECHANISM FOR CONTINUOUS IMPROVEMENT OF CARE,
DISCOVERY, AND INNOVATION

Monitoring is a key public health function; measurement is also an essential element of high-performing healthcare systems. Measures related to this driver could include whether a registry or other surveillance system is in place, the proportion of children with a condition in that registry, the timeliness and accuracy of that information, and the extent to which the data are used for quality improvement and discovery (McCormick, Osei-Anto, & Martinez, 2021).

Registry and Database: The number of patients entering clinical trials and whether clinical outcomes are improvement in care. Therefore, the programme requires continuous audit and re-audit and adjust implementation based on local or national need in response to data.

Monitoring and Evaluation

Monitoring and Evaluating the Outcomes of NBS for SCD as Proposed by Hinton et al. (2017)

They presented a framework defining specific health comes using the concept of Drivers and outcome measures: it is a useful tool that facilitates programme evaluation to determine what data is existing and whether there are gaps. This provides the motivation for getting additional data collection and it is built on a driver diagram with a vision to support the delivery of a comprehensive programme. It is useful for monitoring and evaluation and hence improvement of services and drives research. Key additions from the field of implementation science are stakeholder empowerment and assessments of readiness.

This framework, built on a driver diagram, also provides a vision for a comprehensive approach to monitor and continuously improve the NBS system as opportunities arise for better outcomes through new measures and improved treatments in the US and could be used by other nation's NBS programmes.

Outcome Measures

Outcome measures, which in this case ought to:

a   assess the traditional metrics of *mortality* and *morbidity, proxy measures* such as preventable healthcare utilization (hospitalizations, emergency department visits), measures of harm associated with treatment, developmental and social-emotional outcomes, and family experience of care; and
b   *identify potential disparities in* these outcomes among individuals or groups.

Summary and Recommendations

NBS programmes for screening congenital and inherited disorders at birth were first introduced in the early 1960s firstly the antibacterial testing for PKU. NBS for SCD was first implemented in Jamaica in 1973 followed by the US.

The key to success for programme has been the establishment of national policy in advance of the introduction of NBS for SCD. This is the pattern of the most successful national programmes in the US, the UK, Brazil, and a growing number of European countries.

The programmes that are driven through research or foreign funders have limited reach and none has resulted in nationally rollout implementation.

The challenge facing such initiatives is well described in the qualitative study by Archer by *identifying four themes – governance and structure, funding, technical and cultural barriers, and enhancers for achieving* sustainable NBS programmes in Africa. The lesson from these earlier initiatives is useful for the ongoing programmes including the US- and EU-funded projects. The importance for national programmes to comply with the *WHO recommendation Wilson and Jungner 10 steps of a screening programme and ensure that there is an agreed policy on whom to treat as patients* and the *cost of case-finding* (including diagnosis and treatment of patients diagnosed) should be economically balanced in relation to possible expenditure on medical care. The practical aspects of providing adequate diagnostic platform with sufficient technical support is emphasised. The authors have proposed better alignment of donor programmes within countries to ensure better coordination to avoid the tendency for researchers working in silos. It is necessary that SCD programmes in Sub-Saharan Africa and other LMICs countries implement sustainable national screening programmes that are embedded in the public health systems, affordable and accessible to the majority.

Effective programme monitoring and evaluation is possible by adapting a framework of Primary Drivers for outcome and outcome measures percentages to assess the proportion of infants being referred to treatment centres and are being maintained over specified period, e.g., two years, five years, or ten years and long-term outcomes

Acknowledgement

1 Mrs Bola Ojo, N253 Programme manager and co-founder Sickle cell cohort research foundation (www.scorecharity.com)
2 Dr Yvonne Daniel, Scientific Adviser, N253 Scientific adviser and chief scientist
3 Professor John Dada and Professor Stephen Obaro for their expert advise

References

Almeida, A. M., Henthorn, J. S., & Davies, S. C. (2001). Neonatal screening for haemoglobinopathies: The results of a 10-year programme in an English health region. *British Journal of Haematology*, *112*(1), 32–35. https://doi.org/10.1046/j.1365-2141. 2001.02512.x

Archer, N. M., Inusa, B., Makani, J., Nkya, S., Tshilolo, L., Tubman, V. N., ... Ohene-Frempong, K. (2022). Enablers and barriers to newborn screening for sickle cell disease in Africa: Results from a qualitative study involving programmes in six countries. *BMJ Open*, *12*(3). https://doi.org/10.1136/bmjopen-2021-057623

Berger, G., Louis, S., Dioulde Ba, S. M., Diagne, I., de Yopougon, C., Adjoumani, I. L., ... Tshilolo, L. (2022). Estimating the risk of child mortality attributable to sickle cell anaemia in sub-Saharan Africa: A retrospective, multicentre, case-control study. *Articles Lancet Haematol*, *9*(3), e208–e216. https://doi.org/10.1016/S2352-3026(22)00004-7

Berry, S. A. (2015). Newborn screening. *Clinics in Perinatology*, *42*(2), 441–453. https://doi.org/10.1016/j.clp.2015.03.002

Brousse, V., Allaf, B., & Benkerrou, M. (2021). Newborn screening for sickle cell disease in France. *Medecine/Sciences*, *37*(5), 482–490. https://doi.org/10.1051/medsci/2021056

Daniel, Y., Elion, J., Allaf, B., Badens, C., Bouva, M. J., Brincat, I., ... Gulbis, B. (2019). Newborn screening for sickle cell disease in Europe. *International Journal of Neonatal Screening*, 1–12. https://doi.org/10.3390/ijns5010015

Daniel, Y., Obaro, S., Dada, J., Lawson, J. O., & Inusa, B. P. D. (2011). Use of HbA2 as a discriminator for S/Beta thalassaemia in a Nigerian setting. *Blood*, *118*(21), 4206.

de Montalembert, M. (2002). Management of children with sickle cell anemia: A collaborative work. *Archives of Pediatrics, 9*(11), 1195–1201.

Diallo, D. A., Guindo, A., Touré, B. A., Sarro, Y. S., Sima, M., Tessougué, O., ... Dorie, A. (2018). [Targeted newborn screening for sickle-cell anemia: Sickling test (Emmel test) boundaries in the prenatal assessment in West African area]. *Revue d'Épidémiologie et de Santé Publique, 66*(3), 1–2. https://doi.org/10.1016/j.respe.2018.02.007

Ding, S., & Han, L. (2022). Newborn screening for genetic disorders: Current status and prospects for the future. *Pediatric Investigation, 6*(4), 291–298. https://doi.org/10.1002/ped4.12343

Dobrow, M. J., Hagens, V., Chafe, R., Sullivan, T., & Rabeneck, L. (2018). Consolidated principles for screening based on a systematic review and consensus process. *CMAJ, 190*(14), E422–E429. https://doi.org/10.1503/cmaj.171154

Ducrocq, R., Pascaud, O., Bévier, A., Finet, C., Benkerrou, M., & Elion, J. (2001). Strategy linking several analytical methods of neonatal screening for sickle cell disease. *Journal of Medical Screening, 8*(1), 8–14. https://doi.org/10.1136/jms.8.1.8

EC-UN Joint Migration and Development Initiative. (2010). https://www.local2030.org/library/192/The-JMDI-Handbook.pdf (accessed 31 January 2024).

El-attar, E. A., Mohamed, R., Elkaffas, H., Aglan, S. A., Naga, I. S., Nabil, A., & Abdallah, H. Y. (2022). Genomics in Egypt. *Current Status and Future Aspects, 13*(May), 1–22. https://doi.org/10.3389/fgene.2022.797465

El-haj, N., & Hoppe, C. C. (2018). Newborn Screening for SCD in the USA and Canada throughout. *International Journal of Neonatal Screening.* https://doi.org/10.3390/ijns4040036

El-Hattab, A. W., Almannai, M., & Sutton, V. R. (2018). Newborn screening: History, current status, and future directions. *Pediatric Clinics of North America, 65*(2), 389–405. https://doi.org pcl.2017.11.013

European Union Horizon. (2020). ARISE, An interagency and multidisciplinary staff exchange programme. https://www.ariseinitiative.org/arise-project/project-description/ (accessed 31 January 2024).

Frempong, T., & Pearson, H. A. (2007). Newborn screening coupled with comprehensive follow-up reduced early mortality of sickle cell disease in Connecticut. *Connecticut Medicine, 71*(1), 9–12.

Frömmel, C., Brose, A., Klein, J., Blankenstein, O., & Lobitz, S. (2014). Newborn Screening for Sickle Cell Disease: Technical and Legal Aspects of a German Pilot Study with 38, 220 Participants. *BioMed Research International.* https://doi.org/10.1155/2014/695828

Gardner, K., Douiri, A., Drasar, E., Allman, M., Mwirigi, A., Awogbade, M., & Thein, S. L. (2016). Survival in adults with sickle cell disease in a high-income setting. *Blood.* https://doi.org/10.1182/blood-2016-05-716910

Ghafuri, D. L., Abdullahi, S. U., Jibir, B. W., Gambo, S., Bello-Manga, H., Haliru, L., ... Debaun, M. R. (2020). World health organization's growth reference overestimates the prevalence of severe malnutrition in children with sickle cell anemia in Africa. *Journal of Clinical Medicine, 9*(1). https://doi.org/10.3390/jcm9010119

Green, N. S., Mathur, S., Kiguli, S., Makani, J., Fashakin, V., LaRussa, P., ... Mupere, E. (2016). Family, community, and health system considerations for reducing the burden of pediatric sickle cell disease in Uganda through newborn screening. *Global Pediatric Health, 3.* https://doi.org/10.1177/2333794x16637767

Green, N. S., Zapfel, A., Nnodu, O. E., Franklin, P., Tubman, V. N., Chirande, L., ... Novelli, E. M. (2022). The consortium on newborn screening in Africa for sickle cell disease: Study rationale and methodology. *Blood Advances, 6*(24), 6187–6197. https://doi.org/10.1182/bloodadvances.2022007698

Grosse, S. D. (2005). Does newborn screening save money? The difference between cost-effective and cost-saving interventions. *Journal of Pediatrics, 146*(2), 168–170. https://doi.org/10.1016/j.jpeds.2004.10.015

Grosse, S. D., Odame, I., Atrash, H. K., Amendah, D. D., Piel, F. B., & Williams, T. N. (2011). Sickle cell disease in Africa: A neglected cause of early childhood mortality. *American Journal of Preventive Medicine, 41*(6 Suppl.4), S398–S405. https://doi.org/10.1016/j.amepre.2011.09.013

Hernandez, A., Kiyaga, C., Howard, T., Ssewanyana, I., Ndeezi, G., Aceng, J., Ware, R. (2021). Operational analysis of the national sickle cell screening progreamme in the Republic of Uganda. *African Journal of Laboratory Medicine, 10*(1), 1–8. https://doi.org/10.4102/ajlm.v10i1.1303

Hernandez A. G., Kiyaga C., Howard T. A., Ssewanyana I., Ndeezi G., Aceng J. R., & Ware R. E. (2020). Trends in sickle cell trait and disease screening in the Republic of Uganda, 2014–2019. *Tropical Medicine & International Health, 26*(1), 23–32. https://doi.org/10.1111/tmi.13506

Hinton, C. F., Homer, C. J., Thompson, A. A., Williams, A., Hassell, L., Feuchtbaum, L., ... Brown, C. (2017). On the road to measuring its promise A framework for assessing outcomes from newborn screening: on the road to measuring its promise. *Molecular Genetics and Metabolism, 118*(4), 221–229. https://doi.org/10.1016/j.ymgme.2016.05.017

Hsu, L. L., Green, N. S., Ivy, E. D., Neunert, C., Smaldone, A., Johnson, S., ... Martin, M. (2016). Community health workers as support for sickle cell care: A white paper. *American Journal of Preventive Medicine, 51*(1 Suppl 1), S87–S98. doi:10.1016/j.amepre.2016.01.016

Inati, A. (2009). Recent advances in improving the management of sickle cell disease. *Blood Reviews, 23*(Suppl 1), S9–S13. https://doi.org/10.1016/S0268-960X(09)70004-9

Inusa B., Daniel Y., Lawson J., Dada J., Matthews C., Momi S. S., Obaro K. (2015). Sickle Cell Disease Screening in Northern Nigeria: The Co-Existence of B-Thalassemia Inheritance. *Pediatrics & Therapeutics, 5*:3 DOI: 10.4172/2161-0665.1000262

Inusa B. P. D., & Colombatti R. (2017). European migration crises: The role of national hemoglobinopathy registries in improving patient access to care. *Pediatric Blood & Cancer, 64*(7). https://doi.org/ 10.1002/pbc.26515. doi:10.1002/pbc.26515

Inusa, B. P. D., Anie, K. A., Lamont, A., Dogara, L. G., Ojo, B., Ijei, I., ... Hsu, L. (2018). Utilising the 'Getting to Outcomes®' Framework in community engagement for development and implementation of sickle cell disease newborn screening in Kaduna state, Nigeria. *International Journal of Neonatal Screening, 4*(4), 33.

Inusa, B., Popoola, J., & Wonkam, A. (2017). Sickle cell disease. *New England Journal of Medicine, 377*(3). https://doi.org/10.1056/NEJMc1706325

Italia, Y. M., Colah, R. B., Ghosh, K. K., Rajwadi, H. P., Mehta, V. I., Raicha, B. K., ... Krishnamurti, L. (2011). Newborn screening for sickle cell disease in a tribal area of south Gujarat, India. *American Journal of Hematology, 86*(10).

Therrell, B. L., Jr., Lloyd-Puryear, M. A., Ohene-Frempong, K., Ware, R. E., Padilla, C. D., Ambrose, E. E., ... faculty and speakers at the First Pan African Workshop on Newborn Screening, Rabat, Morocco, June 12–14, 2019. (2020). Empowering newborn screening programs in African countries through establishment of an international collaborative effort. *Journal of Community Genetics, 11*(3), 253–268. https://doi.org/10.1007/s12687-020-00463-7

Kanter, J., & Falcon, C. (2021). Gene therapy for sickle cell disease: Where we are now? *Hematology (United States), 2021*(1). https://doi.org/10.1182/hematology.2021000250

Kayton, A. (2007). Newborn screening: A literature review. *Neonatal Network: NN, 26*(2), 85–95. https://doi.org/10.1891/0730-0832.26.2.85

King, L., Reid, M., King, L., & Reid, M. (2014). Newborn screening for sickle cell disease in Jamaica: A review – Past, Present and Future Tamizaje Neonatal para la Enfermedad de Células Falciformes en Jamaica: Una Revisión – Pasado, Presente y Futuro. *West Indian Medical Journal*, *63*(2). https://doi.org/10.7727/wimj.2013.107

King, L. G., Bortolusso-Ali, S., Cunningham-Myrie, C. A., Reid, M. E. (2015). Impact of a Comprehensive Sickle Cell Center on Early Childhood Mortality in a Developing Country: The Jamaican Experience. *Journal of Pediatrics*, *167*(3), 702–5.e1. doi:10.1016/j.jpeds.2015.06.028

Knapkova, M., Hall, K., & Loeber, G. (2018). Reliability of neonatal screening results. *International Journal of Neonatal Screening*, *4*(3), 28. https://doi.org/10.3390/ijns4030028

Kuznik, A., Habib, A. G., Munube, D., & Lamorde, M. (2016). Newborn screening and prophylactic interventions for sickle cell disease in 47 countries in sub-Saharan Africa : A cost- effectiveness analysis. *BMC Health Services Research*. https://doi.org/10.1186/s12913-016-1572-6

Lobitz, S., Telfer, P., Cela, E., Allaf, B., Angastiniotis, M., Backman Johansson, C., … Colombatti, R. (2018). Newborn screening for sickle cell disease in Europe: Recommendations from a Pan-European consensus conference. *British Journal of Haematology*, *183*(4), 648–660. https://doi.org/10.1111/bjh.15600

Mamman, M., Scott, S., Milligan, P., Inusa, B., Dabo, Y., Yusuf, R., Bako, A., Ahmad, H., Shariason, A. & Igbah, F. (2020). HemaSphere Abstract Book for the 15th Annual Sickle Cell & Thalassaemia & 1st EHA European Sickle Cell Conference, 32–33.

McCormick, M., Osei-Anto, H. A., & Martinez, R. M. (2021). *Addressing sickle cell disease. Addressing Sickle Cell Disease*. https://doi.org/10.17226/25632

Melorose, J., Perroy, R., & Careas, S. (2015). Evidence-based management of sickle cell disease. Expert panel report, 2014. *U.S. Department of Health and Humand Services. NIH*, *1*. https://doi.org/10.1017/CBO9781107415324.004

McGann, P. T., Grosse, S. D., Santos, B., de Oliveira, V., Bernardino, L., Kassebaum, N. J., … Airewele, G. E. (2015). A Cost-Effectiveness analysis of a pilot neonatal screening program for sickle cell anemia in the Republic of Angola. *The Journal of Pediatrics*, *167*(6), 1314–1319. https://doi.org/10.1016/j.jpeds.2015.08.068

Metters, J. S., Huntsman, R., Yawson, G. (1970). The use of the cord blood sample for the detection of sickle cell anaemia in the newborn. *The Journal of Obstetrics and Gynaecology of the British Commonwealth*, *77*(10), 935–938. https://doi.org/10.1111/j.1471-0528.1970.tb03430.x

Meyers, D. C., Durlak, J. A., & Wandersman, A. (2012). The quality implementation framework: A synthesis of critical steps in the implementation process. *American Journal of Community Psychology*, *50*(3–4), 462–480. https://doi.org/10.1007/s10464-012-9522-x

Minkovitz, C. S., Grason, H., Ruderman, M, Casella, J. F. (2016). Newborn screening programs and sickle cell disease: A public health services and systems approach. *American Journal of Preventive Medicine*, *51*(1 Suppl 1), S39–S47. https://doi.org/10.1016/j.amepre.2016.02.019

Mighton, C., Shickh, S., Aguda, V., Krishnapillai, S., Adi-Wauran, E., & Bombard, Y. (2022). From the patient to the population: Use of genomics for population screening. *Frontiers in Genetics*, *13*(October), 1–21. https://doi.org/10.3389/fgene.2022.893832

Migotsky, M., Beestrum, M., & Badawy, S. M. (2022). Recent advances in sickle-cell disease therapies: A review of Voxelotor, Crizanlizumab, and L-glutamine. *Pharmacy*, *10*(5), 123. https://doi.org/10.3390/pharmacy10050123

Modell, B., Petrou, M., Layton, M., Varnavides, L., Slater, C., Ward, R. H., … Davies, S. C. (1999). Haemoglobinopathies in Europe: Health & migration policy perspectives. *Health Technology Assessment*, *55*(3), F161–F167. https://doi.org/10.1136/fn.79.3.F161

Moez, P., & Younan, D. N. A. (2016). High prevalence of haemoglobin S in the closed Egyptian community of Siwa Oasis. *Journal of Clinical Pathology*, *69*(7), 632–636. https://doi.org/10.1136/jclinpath-2015-203199

Nnodu, O., Isa, H., Nwegbu, M., Ohiaeri, C., Adegoke, S., Chianumba, R., ... Adekile, A. (2019). HemoTypeSC, a low-cost point-of-care testing device for sickle cell disease: Promises and challenges. *Blood Cells, Molecules, and Diseases*. https://doi.org/10.1016/J.BCMD.2019.01.007

Nottage, K. A., Hankins, J. S., Smeltzer, M., Mzayek, F., Wang, W. C., Aygun, B., & Gurney, J. G. (2013). Hydroxyurea use and hospitalization trends in a comprehensive pediatric sickle cell program. *PLoS ONE*, *8*(8), 1–5. https://doi.org/10.1371/journal.pone.0072077

Obaro, S. K., Daniel, Y., Lawson, J. O., Hsu, W.-W., Dada, J., Essen, U., ... Inusa, B. P. D. (2016). Sickle-cell disease in Nigerian children: Parental Knowledge and Laboratory Results. *Public Health Genomics*, *19*(2). https://doi.org/10.1159/000444475

Ohene-frempong, K., & Oduro, J. (1993). Screening newborns for sickle cell disease in Ghana. Submitted by Kwaku Ohene-Frempong. Suppression of the olivocochlear reflex: A Neurotoxic adverse effect of vincristine. Submitted by Helen Kosmidis. Transplantation for the treatment of thalassemia : The G.

Piel, F. B., Patil, A. P., Howes, R. E., Nyangiri, O. A., Gething, P. W., Dewi, M., ... Hay, S. I. (2013). Global epidemiology of sickle haemoglobin in neonates: A contemporary geo-statistical model-based map and population estimates. *The Lancet*, *381*(9861), 142–151. https://doi.org/10.1016/S0140-6736(12)61229-X

Piel, F. B., Tatem, A. J., Huang, Z., Gupta, S., Williams, T. N., & Weatherall, D. J. (2014). Global migration and the changing distribution of sickle haemoglobin: A quantitative study of temporal trends between 1960 and 2000. *The Lancet Global Health*. https://doi.org/10.1016/S2214-109X(13)70150-5

Quinn, C. T., Rogers, Z. R., & Buchanan, G. R. (2004). Survival of children with sickle cell disease. *Blood*, *103*(11), 4023–4027. https://doi.org/10.1182/blood-2003-11-3758

Rahimy, M. C., Gangbo, A., Ahouignan, G., Alihonou, E. (2009). Newborn screening for sickle cell disease in the Republic of Benin. *Journal of Clinical Pathology*, *62*(1), 46–48. doi:10.1136/jcp.2008.059113

Remec, Z. I., Trebusak Podkrajsek, K., Repic Lampret, B., Kovac, J., Groselj, U., Tesovnik, T., ... Debeljak, M. (2021). Next-generation sequencing in newborn screening: A review of current state. *Frontiers in Genetics*. https://doi.org/10.3389/fgene.2021.662254

Runkel, B., Klüppelholz, B., Rummer, A., Sieben, W., Lampert, U., Bollig, C., Markes, M., Paschen, U., & Angelescu, K. (2020). Screening for sickle cell disease in newborns: A systematic review. *Systematic Reviews*, *9*(1):250. https://doi.org/10.1186/s13643-020-01504-5

Streetly, A., Maxwell, K., & Campbell, B. (1998). Coordinated neonatal screening pro-gramme for haemoglobin disorders is needed. *BMJ*, *316*(7135), 937–937. https://doi.org/10.1136/bmj.316.7135.937

Streetly, A., Latinovic, R., Hall, K., & Henthorn, J. (2009). Implementation of universal newborn bloodspot screening for sickle cell disease and other clinically significant haemo-globinopathies in England: Screening results for 2005-7. *Journal of Clinical Pathology*, *62*(1), 26–30. https://doi.org/10.1136/jcp.2008.058859

Streetly, A., Sisodia, R., Dick, M., Latinovic, R., Hounsell, K., & Dormandy, E. (2018). Evaluation of newborn sickle cell screening programme in England: 2010–2016. *Arch Dis Child*, *103*(7), 648–653. https://doi.org/10.1136/archdischild-2017-313213

Strunk, C., Campbell, A., Colombatti, R., Andemariam, B., Kesse-Adu, R., Treadwell, M., & Inusa, B. P. D. (2020). Annual academy of sickle cell and thalassaemia (ASCAT)

conference: A summary of the proceedings. *BMC Proceedings, 14*(Suppl 20), 1–27. https://doi.org/10.1186/s12919-020-00204-1

Telfer, P., Coen, P., Chakravorty, S., Wilkey, O., Evans, J., Newell, H., ... Kirkham, F. (2007). Clinical outcomes in children with sickle cell disease living in England: A neonatal cohort in East London. *Haematologica, 92*(7), 905–912.

Temtamy, S. (2019). The development of human genetics at the national research centre, Cairo, Egypt: A story of 50 year. *Annual Review of Genomics and Human Genetics, 20,* 1–19. https://doi.org/10.1146/annurev-genom-083118-01520

Therrell, B. L., Lloyd-Puryear, M. A., Ohene-Frempong, K., Ware, R. E., Padilla, C. D., Ambrose, E. E., ... Watson, M. S. (2020). Empowering newborn screening programs in African countries through establishment of an international collaborative effort. *Journal of Community Genetics, 11*(3). https://doi.org/10.1007/s12687-020-00463-7

Therrell, B. L., Padilla, C. D., Loeber, J. G., Kneisser, I., Saadallah, A., Borrajo, G. J. C., & Adams, J. (2015). Current status of newborn screening worldwide: 2015. *Seminars in Perinatology, 39*(3), 171–187. https://doi.org/10.1053/j.semperi.2015.03.002

Tshilolo, L., Kafando, E., Sawadogo, M., Cotton, F., Vertongen, F., Ferster, & Gulbis, B. (2008). Neonatal screening and clinical care programmes for sickle cell disorders in sub-Saharan Africa: Lessons from pilot studies. *Public Health, 122*(9), 933–941. https://doi.org/10.1016/j.puhe.2007.12.005

Tubman, N., Chirande, L., Kiyaga, C., Green, N. S., Zapfel, A., Nnodu, O. E., ... Berliner, N. (2022). The consortium on newborn screening in Africa for sickle cell disease : Study rationale and methodology. *Blood Advances, 6*(24), 6187–6197. https://doi.org/10.1182/bloodadvances.2022007698

Vichinsky, E. P. (1991). Comprehensive care in sickle cell disease: Its impact on morbidity and mortality. *Seminars in Hematology, 28*(3), 220–226.

Watson, M. S., Lloyd-Puryear, M. A., & Howell, R. R. (2022). The progress and future of US newborn screening. *International Journal of Neonatal Screening, 8*(3), 1–25. https://doi.org/10.3390/ijns8030041

Weatherall, D. J. (2010, June). The inherited diseases of hemoglobin are an emerging global health burden. *Blood.* https://doi.org/10.1182/blood-2010-01-251348

Wilcken, B. (2011). Newborn screening: How are we travelling, and where should we be going? *Journal of Inherited Metabolic Disease, 34*(3), 569–574. https://doi.org/10.1007/s10545-011-9326-4

Wjdan, A., Hani, A., Mohammed, Z. (2021). Techniques for the detection of sickle cell disease: A review. *Micromachines (Basel), 12*(5), 519. https://doi.org/10.3390/mi12050519

Zeuner, D., Ades, A. E., Karnon, J., , Brown J., Dezateux, C., & Anionwu, E. (1999). Antenatal and neonatal haemoglobinopathy screening in the UK: Review and economic analysis. *Health Technology Assessment, 3*(11), i–v, 1–186.

Zimmer, K. P. (2020). Newborn screening: Still room for improvement. *Deutsches Arzteblatt International, 118*(7), 99–100. https://doi.org/10.3238/arztebl.m2021.0008

5 Routine Comprehensive Care for Children with SCD

Nnenna Ukachi Badamosi

Introduction

Sickle cell disease is a group of inherited autosomal recessive disorders of hemoglobin, characterized by the presence of hemoglobin S, leading to impaired oxygenation and sickling of red blood cells under a variety of stressful conditions. Homozygous hemoglobin S disease results in sickle cell anemia, whereas other forms of sickle cell disease occur when hemoglobin S is co-inherited with another mutated hemoglobin such as hemoglobin C or hemoglobin D (Sundd et al., 2019). The sickle hemoglobin mutation results in the substitution of glutamic acid with valine in the sixth position of the beta globin chain, leading to formation of rigid hemoglobin polymers within the red cells under de-oxygenated conditions, forming a sickle shape. These sickle red cells lead to microvascular occlusion, hemolysis and shortened red cell life spans. Sickle cell disease is characterized by repeated cycles of red cell sickling, vaso-occlusion, hemolytic anemia and oxidative stress leading to vasculopathy, endothelial damage and multi-systemic inflammatory complications over time (*Eurorad.Org*, 2019). Landmark studies over the past several decades have led to increased life expectancy in patients, where sickle cell disease is no longer a debilitating disease of childhood. As a result, advancements in routine preventative care have continued to improve quality of life in children and young adults, where potentially life-threatening complications can be identified and successfully mitigated.

This chapter provides healthcare personnel with an overview of routine care provided by a comprehensive sickle cell team from the newborn period through late adolescence, prior to adult care transition.

Routine Care in Early Childhood (0–5 Years of Age)

Newborn Screening and Establishing Care

A newborn screening program is integral to successful preventative care of infants and children with sickle cell disease. Infants with sickle cell disease can be identified and referred as soon as possible to a hematologist or a comprehensive sickle cell center for management.

DOI: 10.4324/9781003463931-6

The comprehensive care team should include a pediatric hematologist, an advanced practice provider (nurse practitioner or physician assistant), a nurse clinician, a social worker, a psychologist and a genetic counselor, when available.

An initial visit with the hematologist involves establishing a rapport between provider and family and introduction to the comprehensive care team, confirming the diagnosis on newborn screening with additional testing if needed, and providing a baseline understanding of the sickle cell disease diagnosis, complications and prognosis. Subsequent follow-up visits may be scheduled every 2–4 months depending on the genotypic diagnosis and level of parental comfort.

The education of the parent(s) of a newborn with sickle cell disease is often multi-layered and involves empathy, social support, genetic counseling and deconstruction of any pre-existing myths or beliefs that may have been held about sickle cell disease. The families are educated about the initial complications and how they may present, such as dactylitis, fever, splenic sequestration and anemia. They are counseled on the onset of vaso-occlusive symptoms, typically after the first six months of life and provided with return precautions for urgent complications such as fever, sequestration or symptomatic anemia. Families are also educated about available treatment options and when they can be initiated, such as hydroxyurea therapy in infancy. Finally, patients are initiated on antibiotic prophylaxis to prevent pneumococcal infections.

Antibiotic Prophylaxis

The use of antibiotic prophylaxis has been pivotal in changing life expectancy and clinical course of sickle cell disease and is now accepted as standard of care (Falletta et al., 1995; Gaston et al., 1986). Septicemia and pneumonia from pneumococcal disease used to be a leading cause of mortality in children with sickle cell disease resulting in an average life expectancy of 14 years prior to the penicillin prophylaxis studies and the routine use of antibiotics (Chaturvedi & DeBaun, 2016). Children with sickle cell disease remain at high risk for invasive bacteremia due to functional asplenia. Therefore, one of the goals of a successful newborn screening program is for early identification and initiation of penicillin or one of its alternatives (amoxicillin, erythromycin) as soon as a sickle cell diagnosis is established (Cober & Phelps, 2010).

Initial recommendations for prophylaxis were initially limited to children with more severe sickle cell anemia (homozygous hemoglobin S and compound heterozygous hemoglobin S-beta zero genotypes); however clinical practice now routinely includes children with all sickle cell genotypes. Recommended dosing is typically 125 mg twice daily in children under three years and 250 mg in children older than 3. Most common adverse effects include diarrhea and transient maculopapular rash. True allergic reaction to penicillin is uncommon, in which case erythromycin may be used. Discontinuation of antibiotic prophylaxis is recommended around age 5, after completion of routine childhood pneumococcal vaccine series and two doses of the pneumococcal polysaccharide vaccine, as described below (Falletta et al., 1995).

Vaccines

Routine childhood vaccines vary by region and are recommended to cover the prevailing vaccine-preventable infectious diseases. In the United States, the Centers for Disease Control and Prevention (CDC) outline vaccine recommendations for children to include a series of pneumococcal conjugate vaccines before age 5 (CDC, 2022). In Sub-Saharan Africa, pneumococcal vaccine recommendations may be based on availability, infection prevalence, or guided by the World Health Organization (WHO). The latest pneumococcal conjugate vaccine is a four-dose series that covers 13 common serotypes of *Streptococcus pneumoniae* (PCV-13). The CDC guidelines also offer recommendations for extended pneumococcal vaccine coverage in patients with functional asplenia or impaired immunity. This pneumococcal polysaccharide vaccine which covers 23 serotypes (PPSV-23) should therefore administered at age 2 and age 5 in children with sickle cell disease. The use of routine pneumococcal vaccines has further helped reduce the incidence of invasive pneumococcal infections in children under five with sickle cell disease.

In the United States, meningococcal conjugate vaccines are typically administered in later childhood and adolescence. However, in children in sickle cell disease, as well as in many Sub-Saharan countries, the meningococcal vaccines may be administered as early as nine months of age (CDC, 2022).

Regional bacteremic infections in African children with sickle cell disease are often attributed to streptococcal, hemophilus and salmonella infections (Williams et al., 2009). The vaccine schedule in Nigeria recommends the completion of PCV-10 and Hib vaccine series and by 14 weeks of life, to cover infections by *Streptococcus pneumoniae* and *Haemophilus influenzae* type b, respectively. Salmonella prevention efforts should include discussions on safe food hygiene, oral-fecal contamination and consumption of raw foods.

Initiation of Disease-Modifying Therapy

Hydroxyurea, or hydroxycarbamide, is a ribonucleotide reductase inhibitor and potent inducer of fetal hemoglobin that is approved for the management of sickle cell disease (Agrawal et al., 2014; McGann & Ware, 2015; Tshilolo et al., 2019; Ware, 2013). The increased production of fetal hemoglobin within red cells helps inhibit sickle hemoglobin polymerization and increase their resilience against sickling and hemolysis. The precise mechanism of action of hydroxyurea is unknown, but it has been demonstrated to have several beneficial effects in sickle cell in addition to fetal hemoglobin induction, such as decreasing neutrophil count and pro-inflammatory milieu, decreasing red cell adhesion and improving red cell deformability (Verma et al., 2018). Hydroxyurea is also used in a wide range of diseases including neoplasms. In sickle cell disease, it has been shown to decrease frequency of vaso-occlusive episodes including acute chest syndrome, improve anemia and decrease need for transfusions and decrease the risk of stroke in children with abnormal transcranial Doppler (TCD) ultrasounds (Charache et al., 1995; Hasson et al., 2019; Lagunju et al., 2015; Lefèvre et al., 2008).

Hydroxyurea initiation is recommended around nine months of age, at which time natural production of gamma globin ramps down and fetal hemoglobin levels progressively decrease. Recommended dosing starts at 20 mg/kg and may be increased as tolerated up to 35 mg/kg. Most common adverse effects include dose-dependent neutropenia and thrombocytopenia, risk of infection or bleeding, hair loss and macrocytosis. Neutropenia is reversible with dose adjustment or temporary cessation of hydroxyurea. Additional manufacturer warnings with long-term use of hydroxyurea include myelosuppression, embryo-fetal toxicity in both males and females, vasculitic toxicity and pulmonary toxicity.

Management of Acute Complications

The complications of sickle cell disease evolve with age and tend to begin after natural fetal hemoglobin production decreases. In young children, clinically concerning complications include dactylitis, fever and infection, and symptomatic anemia from splenic sequestration, aplastic crisis or hemolytic crisis. As children get older, other complications such as priapism and acute chest syndrome may occur. Dactylitis is usually the first symptom of vaso-occlusion and may present after 6–12 months of age. In these children, symptoms include swelling of hands or feet, mild fever, irritability and unwillingness to crawl, walk or be carried. Mild cases of dactylitis may be managed at home with over-the-counter analgesics and anti-inflammatory drugs as long as no clinically significant fever is recorded (101°F or 38.4°C).

Young infants and children can also present with fever at any age, along with other symptoms such as upper respiratory infection, poor feeding or dactylitis. Although a low-grade fever commonly accompanies vaso-occlusive events, a clinically concerning fever (101°F or 38.4°C) warrants emergent evaluation at a healthcare facility as it may be one of the earliest signs of bacteremia or septicemia. A thorough workup for the fever should include a blood culture, hemoglobin and reticulocyte count. In the United States, standard of care also involves initiation of intravenous or intramuscular broad-spectrum antibiotics (e.g. third-generation cephalosporin) within hours of emergency room presentation and after blood culture is obtained to provide empiric coverage for pneumococcal infection. Patients of all ages are also particularly susceptible to infections with *Salmonella* spp. that may lead to acute gastroenteritis and osteomyelitis. Depending on the infant's clinical status, inpatient observation vs. close outpatient follow-up may be required to ensure negative blood cultures and clinical improvement. Empiric antibiotic coverage may be discontinued after 48 hours if no bacteremia is identified, and infant is clinically well.

The duration of fever precautions depends on parental comfort and reliability for close follow-up, frequency of febrile infections, and compliance with recommended vaccines and scheduled appointments. In fully vaccinated children with reliable families and access to close follow-up, fever precautions may be discontinued after 12–24 months of age.

Symptomatic anemia from splenic sequestration is a common complication in infants and young children. Splenic enlargement occurs frequently in setting of infections such as viral upper respiratory or gastrointestinal infections. In addition, early hydroxyurea use has been associated with preservation of splenic function and reversal of auto-infarction in sickle cell disease (Hankins et al., 2008; Huang et al., 2003; Nottage et al., 2014). Parents should be taught how to feel for splenic enlargement and to present to emergency if symptoms of sequestration are present such as tenderness to palpation, pallor, fatigue, tachycardia or poor feeding. Mild jaundice due to hemolysis is also a common feature in children as they get older. Clinically significant jaundice should include acute deepening of scleral ictera associated with pallor, fatigue and poor breathing. Symptomatic anemia may also be seen in an aplastic crisis, most commonly due to parvovirus-B19 infection. Regardless of cause, symptomatic anemia requires emergent evaluation for blood counts and red cell transfusion to prevent hypovolemic shock and eventual mortality. Parents are also educated on baseline hemoglobin or hematocrit levels so they can help identify acute anemia by significant drops in hemoglobin (2g/dL or more) or hematocrit (6% or more), respectively (*Evidence-Based Management of Sickle Cell Disease: Expert Panel, 2014*).

Priapism is an unwanted and painful erection affecting boys and men with sickle cell disease. It may present at any age, as a stuttering event or as a sustained painful event lasting several hours. Prompt recognition and management of painful episodes can help provide symptomatic relief and prevent long-term vascular damage to the penis (Olujohungbe & Burnett, 2013). Conservative management may be initiated at home with warm sitz baths, frequent urination and anti-inflammatory drugs. Use of alpha-adrenergic agents like pseudo-ephedrine (over-the-counter vs. prescription) or beta-agonists like terbutaline may also provide relief for recurrent episodes. Episodes lasting more than four hours require emergent evaluation and possible urologic intervention to preserve long-term fertility.

Acute Chest Syndrome

Acute chest syndrome (ACS) is a life-threatening complication and one of the leading causes of mortality in early childhood. It results from vaso-occlusion and intravascular sickling within pulmonary vessels due to underlying hypoxia, acidosis or infection, leading to a vicious cycle of endothelial injury, ischemia and impaired oxygen exchange (Friend & Girzadas, 2022). It is diagnosed radiographically as a new onset lobar infiltrate with fever and respiratory symptoms in a child with sickle cell disease. In children, it typically arises in the setting of underlying respiratory infection or pneumonia, and children with underlying asthma or reactive airway disease are at higher risk. It is also commonly seen in the first 48–72 hours after onset of a severe vaso-occlusive pain crisis in an inpatient setting. The concomitant use of intravenous fluids and narcotics may lead to transient pulmonary edema and decreased respiratory drive, respectively, which may contribute to the pathophysiology of ACS. Management involves preventative measures such as the use of incentive spirometry in hospitalized patients or patients with asthma, judicious use of intravenous fluids and narcotics, and empiric management of fever and pneumonia to cover pneumococcal and atypical bacteria (e.g., *Mycoplasma pneumoniae* and *Chlamydophila pneumoniae*). In addition, the early use of red cell transfusion (simple vs. exchange) quickly improves oxygen-carrying capacity within the lungs and can halt the cycle of intra-pulmonary sickling leading to clinical improvement.

Initiation of Stroke Screening

Stroke is a potentially disabling complication in sickle cell disease, with high risk of recurrence and mortality. The pathophysiology of stroke in children with sickle cell disease is multifactorial and includes anemia, hypoxic-ischemic injury and progressive endothelial damage within the internal carotid arteries and the circle of Willis from chronic intravascular hemolysis of sickling red cells (Fasano et al., 2015; Switzer et al., 2006). In adults, a higher frequency of hemorrhagic strokes may be seen with peak incidence of hemorrhagic strokes occurring in the third decade (Ohene-Frempong et al., 1998). Around 10% of children and young adults under 20 with sickle cell disease will develop a stroke without intervention (Verduzco & Nathan, 2009). Stroke risk is highest in children with sickle cell anemia (hemoglobin SS) and occurs most frequently in the first ten years of life, with a peak incidence of first stroke between ages 2 and 5 (Ohene-Frempong et al., 1998). Silent strokes are more common and can occur in 20–40% of patients with sickle cell anemia, and recurrent strokes are likely to occur in the first two years in up to 25% of patients.

The TCD ultrasound emerged from the Stroke Prevention Trial in Sickle Cell Anemia (STOP) as a valid screening tool to identify patients at high risk for ischemic strokes (Naffaa et al., 2015). The TCD measures timed average maximum velocity (TAMV) of blood flow in the internal carotid and middle cerebral arteries. TAMV measurements of 200 centimeters per second (cm/s) or higher are considered abnormal and associated with a high stroke risk. The TCD screening is initiated in children starting at two years of age and repeated annually if normal. Abnormal TCDs are watched more closely with initiation of hydroxyurea in untreated patients, and initiation of chronic transfusions in patients already on hydroxyurea (Chou et al., 2020; *Evidence-Based Management of Sickle Cell Disease: Expert Panel*, 2014)

Routine Care in Mid–Late Childhood (6–12 Years)

Health Maintenance and School Precautions

By age 6, most children in the United States have completed their routine and extended vaccine series and have discontinued antibiotic prophylaxis. Fever and infection remain a clinical concern but require less emergent evaluation in older children who are fully vaccinated and able to communicate their symptoms, or in whom a clear source of infection is identified. Health maintenance in this age group involves catching up on any missing vaccines including the five-yearly pneumococcal conjugate booster and the meningococcal series, when applicable, ensuring hydroxyurea compliance as children get older, and offering therapy to those who have not yet started treatment. In addition, voxelotor, a newly approved polymerization inhibitor, may be offered to children five years and older for significant anemia. In addition, parents continue to be educated about the evolving complications of sickle cell disease as children get older.

The comprehensive team and social worker provide psychosocial support for families and children in school by providing educational letters to teachers and coaches on school and sports participation. In the United States, additional accommodations may be made at school including frequent breaks at school and extended time for testing. School age children with sickle cell disease may be at higher risk for developmental disorders and require regular screening through their pediatrician and/or sickle cell center (Gyamfi et al., 2021). The social worker may liaise with pediatrician and school to communicate results of developmental screening tests and appropriate resources to support students. Participation in sports and physical activities is strongly encouraged for overall health, with precautions against contact sports like boxing, wrestling or American football due to risk for splenic injury.

Management of Vaso-Occlusive Episodes

As episodes of dactylitis become less frequent, overt episodes of vaso-occlusive crises, or VOCs, may begin to occur in this age group. Parents and children are taught to recognize signs of vaso-occlusion such as severe pain, especially in extremities, that may be associated with a low-grade fever. They are also taught to identify and avoid triggers which may lead to more frequent episodes such as dehydration, stress, fever or infection and temperature extremes. Parents are given instructions on home management to include hydration and rest, anti-inflammatory drugs and occasional use of oral narcotics. Frequent vaso-occlusive episodes warrant a review of treatment options including initiation of hydroxyurea or escalation of dose for improved VOC management. In addition, newer therapies may be offered that are indicated for frequent VOCs such as oral L-glutamine therapy.

Prevention of Acute Complications

In addition to the complications discussed above, hepatobiliary complications may become more common at this age. Asymptomatic gall stones are frequently found in sickle cell disease with increasing frequency due to age (Sarnaik et al., 1980). In about 10% of patients, these stones may become symptomatic and present with right upper quadrant pain and hyperbilirubinemia exacerbated by dehydration or greasy foods. Acute cholecystitis may result from obstructed stones and presents with fever, worsening jaundice and right upper quadrant pain. While occasional gallstones may be managed conservatively, acute cholecystitis requires emergent evaluation and intervention. Intrahepatic stones are a less common complication and may occur with or without co-existing gall stones. Patients are counseled on triggers that may exacerbate gall stone symptoms and may be started on ursodiol (ursodeoxycholic acid) for decreased biliary secretion and improved biliary drainage.

Intrahepatic sequestration is a rare form of red cell sequestration that presents with acute right upper quadrant pain in addition to elevated bilirubin and liver transaminases, anemia and thrombocytopenia (Ogu et al., 2021). It may occur in the setting of splenic sequestration or intrahepatic stones in an acutely ill patient. Management includes transfusion, ursodiol and supportive care.

Although renal complications also increase in frequency with age, acute renal failure is uncommon in childhood. One of the first manifestations of renal sickle cell disease is isosthenuria and inability to concentrate urine. Many young patients therefore present with enuresis and bedwetting symptoms. This is complicated by the need for proper hydration to decrease VOCs. As many as 70% of children with sickle cell disease between ages 6 and 8 may present with nocturia, when compared to 40% of the general population (Field et al., 2008). Renal function tests and urine analysis may be normal in these patients, and renal ultrasound will likely reveal no gross abnormalities. Conservative measures may be used in management such as alarms and nightly water restriction. Desmopressin is a selective vasopressin receptor agonist that has been used for enuresis when conservative management fails.

Stroke Screening and Management

Chronic transfusions have been extensively demonstrated to prevent recurrent strokes in sickle cell disease, as well as primary strokes in children with two or more abnormal TCD screens (Adams et al., 1998; DeBaun, 2011). In children who have no imaging-identified neuropathy and normalized TCDs after years of transfusion, hydroxyurea may be offered as a non-inferior alternative for stroke prevention (Lefèvre et al., 2008). Annual stroke screenings are continued annually until around age 16, when the cranial acoustic windows for Doppler measurement slowly close. In patients who are started or who remain on chronic transfusions, it is important to screen for and prevent secondary complications such as alloimmunization and iron overload.

Transfusional iron overload occurs more quickly in patients who receive simple transfusions or when exchange blood transfusions are unavailable. Such patients require frequent assessment of iron stores (ferritin) as well as magnetic resonance-based (MR) quantification of hepatic iron levels when feasible. In the absence of MR, a ferritin level >500 micrograms/liter is an indication to start iron chelation therapy. Iron chelation therapy may be oral (deferasirox, deferiprone) or parenteral (deferoxamine).

Alloimmunization is a potentially serious complication of transfusion therapy and should be avoided as much as possible. In addition to safe transfusion practices, extended phenotypic typing and matching of blood units against major and minor antigens is recommended to decrease likelihood of alloantibody formation and delayed hemolytic transfusion reactions (Chou et al., 2020; *Evidence-Based Management of Sickle Cell Disease: Expert Panel*, 2014).

Screening for End-Organ Damage

Screening for early signs of end-organ damage is also recommended in this age group in addition to routine health maintenance and screening for iron overload in transfused patients.

Sickle retinopathy is an uncommon complication that occurs in higher frequency in patients with hemoglobin SC disease. Universal ophthalmology screening and dilated eye exams are recommended annually in children aged 10 and older.

Pulmonary complications: Asthma is a common comorbidity in children with sickle cell disease and often increases frequency of acute chest syndrome. In addition, some children may present with persistently low oxygen saturations (<92% while awake) or reported sleep apnea. Pulmonology follow-up is recommended for patients with recurrent ACS, comorbid asthma or persistently low saturations. Pulmonary hypertension (PH) is a potential cause of morbidity in older teenagers and adults. Associations include recurrent ACS episodes, left ventricular diastolic dysfunction and chronic hemolytic anemia. Tricuspid regurgitant jet velocities (TRVs) on echocardiogram that are above 2.5 cm/s may suggest PH but definite diagnosis is made by cardiac catheterization. Screening is not routinely recommended unless patients are symptomatic.

Cardiovascular complications are common in sickle cell disease and may be detected on routine physical examination. Many patients with sickle cell anemia (hemoglobin SS) have compensatory cardiomegaly and left ventricular hypertrophy. As such, a systolic murmur is detectable in many patients. A change in the quality of the murmur, arrhythmia or exercise intolerance may warrant cardiology referral and evaluation.

Gastrointestinal complaints are common in the sickle cell patient population. Constipation may be encountered frequently in children who require frequent use of narcotics. Diarrhea may be seen in relation to use of oral antibiotics in younger children or intravenous antibiotics in older children. Vaso-occlusive crises may present with abdominal pain, as constipation often serves as a trigger for VOC. In addition, patients may present with epigastric pain and discomfort from frequent use of non-steroidal anti-inflammatory drugs. Hepatobiliary complications such as gall stones and intrahepatic sequestration have already been discussed. Routine screening for gastrointestinal and hepatic complications is not recommended.

Renal complications apart from isosthenuria that are routinely screened for include proteinuria and/or microscopic hematuria starting at age 10. Proteinuria or microalbuminuria is common and may represent early renal ischemic disease resulting in tubular and medullary dysfunction (Ogu et al., 2021). Management of proteinuria involves early initiation of angiotensin-converting enzyme (ACE) inhibitors and similar agents that offer renal protection and prevent progression of renal disease. Hematuria occurs less often and may be seen in setting of acute ischemia and renal papillary necrosis. In addition, iron chelation therapy may lead to tubular necrosis and hematuria. Occasionally, kidney stones may cause hematuria. Hematuria is usually transient and improves with increased hydration. Hypertension is a common comorbidity in sickle cell disease and may exacerbate underlying renal complications. Aggressive management of hypertension is recommended to include use of nephro-protective anti-hypertensives. End-stage renal disease requiring renal replacement therapy and/or renal transplant may occur in older adults with sickle cell disease if not properly managed.

Musculoskeletal complications like avascular necrosis (AVN) and osteonecrosis become more frequent in older children and young adults. Screening is symptomatic, with imaging and referral to orthopedics for persistent hip or joint pain or decreased range of motion. Early AVN may be treated conservatively, whereas progressive AVN may require joint replacement therapy.

Reproductive health in children and young adults with sickle cell disease is important as they head into puberty. Puberty may be delayed by 1–2 years in adolescents with sickle cell disease. In girls, menstrual cycles may be irregular and/or heavy and may potentiate iron deficiency anemia or trigger vaso-occlusive episodes. In boys, priapism may become more frequent or painful. Parental and child education important to manage these complications as they arise.

Routine Care in Adolescence (13–18 Years)

Health Education

The adolescent age group of patients present with unique challenges that may increase morbidity from sickle cell disease. In addition to social and societal challenges such as peer pressure, feeling of invincibility, and other psychosocial challenges, these patients become more aware of their chronic illnesses and the challenges associated with it. In this group of patients, daily medication adherence becomes challenging as parents slowly transfer responsibility for medications to their children. Compliance with routine clinic visits may also decrease as their schedules get busier, in addition to increased utilization of emergency room and acute care facilities. Anxiety and depression may be seen more frequently in adolescent patients and use of rescue opioid therapy for acute pain episodes may increase with concomitant decrease in hydroxyurea use.

In adolescents, health education priorities must shift from parent to patient in order to improve self-awareness and self-efficacy in dealing with a lifelong illness. Many sickle cell centers create dedicated transition programs to address some of the challenges in this population.

Medication Management and Compliance

Adolescents are educated on techniques to stay compliant with their daily medications such as hydroxyurea or chelation therapy in transfused patients, to avoid long-term effects. Peer mentoring and support groups are helpful in improving compliance and support. In addition, compliance with routine appointments and preventative screenings is encouraged to minimize emergency department and acute care visits.

Management of Chronic Pain

Adolescent patients with sickle cell disease frequently present with chronic pain that is distinctly different from acute painful vaso-occlusive episodes. Chronic pain may be defined as ongoing near-daily pain lasting six months or more (Osunkwo et al., 2020). The underlying pathophysiology of chronic pain is complex and may result from progressive bone and joint ischemia and infarctive damage, chronic inflammation and nerve damage, as well as opioid-induced central sensitization over time. The resulting pain complex can result in a vicious cycle of hyperalgesia, opioid tolerance and increased opioid-induced side effects, leading to more acute care utilization, hospitalization and increased frustration for both patients and providers. Many young patients with sickle cell disease are labeled as drug-seeking due to frequent acute care visits, and unfortunately, current therapies do not sufficiently address this challenging complication.

One of the strategies to address chronic pain in a routine care visit is by creating a comprehensive pain plan. A multidisciplinary team consisting of a hematologist, psychologist, anesthesiologist/pain physician and social worker should work collaboratively with patient to create their individualized pain plan. This pain plan should be a portable document that is presented at every acute care visit and addresses patient-specific pain control and opioid needs as well as other comorbidities that may be contributing to pain. For example, in patients with progressive or underlying renal disease, a pain plan must specifically exclude non-steroidal anti-inflammatory drugs, and in patients with hepatic complications, acetaminophen should be excluded. Adjunct therapies like gabapentin, anxiolytics and serotonin-reuptake inhibitors should be included in plan based on patient-specific symptoms. A potential barrier to comprehensive pain plans is that in the setting of the opioid epidemic and its abuse potential, providers may be uncomfortable with giving high doses of opioids despite patient's pain tolerance level. As a result, pain episodes are inadequately controlled and may lead to recurrent visits or prolonged hospitalizations. Ongoing patient and provider education is needed to better manage acute presentations of pain, while researchers continue to explore safer alternatives to opioid therapy.

A newly approved p-selectin inhibitor, crizanlizumab, may also be helpful in managing frequent pain episodes in adolescents and young adults aged 16 or older. It is administered intravenously once a month and may be used in addition to hydroxyurea therapy.

Preparation for Adult Transition

The transition period in adolescents and young adults (aged 19–25) is high-risk for loss to follow up and increased mortality (Aduloju et al., 2008). Therefore, the transition to adult care should be an organized patient-centered process that involves education, monitoring and close follow-up. Helping the patient identify an adult hematologist that specializes in sickle cell care and equipping them with knowledge about their individual medical histories is crucial to successful outcomes. It is also important to follow patients closely to ensure appointments are made and kept and a proper handoff to receiving adult hematologist until their care is established.

References

Adams, R. J., McKie, V. C., Hsu, L., Files, B., Vichinsky, E., Pegelow, C., Abboud, M., Gallagher, D., Kutlar, A., Nichols, F. T., Bonds, D. R., Brambilla, D., Woods, G., Olivieri, N., Driscoll, C., Miller, S., Wang, W., Hurlett, A., Scher, C., … Waclawiw, M. (1998). Prevention of a first stroke by transfusions in children with sickle cell anemia and abnormal results on transcranial Doppler ultrasonography. New England Journal of Medicine, 339(1), 5–11. https://doi.org/10.1056/NEJM199807023390102

Aduloju, S. O., Palmer, S., & Eckman, J. R. (2008). Mortality in sickle cell patient transitioning from pediatric to adult program: 10 years grady comprehensive sickle cell center experience. Blood, 112(11), 1426. https://doi.org/10.1182/blood.V112.11.1426.1426

Agrawal, R. K., Patel, R. K., shah, V., Nainiwal, L., & Trivedi, B. (2014). Hydroxyurea in sickle cell disease: Drug review. Indian Journal of Hematology & Blood Transfusion, 30(2), 91–96. https://doi.org/10.1007/s12288-013-0261-4

American Society of Hematology 2020 guidelines for sickle cell disease: Transfusion support | Blood Advances | American Society of Hematology. (2020). Retrieved May 30, 2022, from https://ashpublications.org/bloodadvances/article/4/2/327/440607/American-Society-of-Hematology-2020-guidelines-for

CDC. (2022, February 17). Immunization Schedules for 18 & Younger. Centers for Disease Control and Prevention. https://www.cdc.gov/vaccines/schedules/hcp/imz/child-adolescent.html

Charache, S., Terrin, M. L., Moore, R. D., Dover, G. J., Barton, F. B., Eckert, S. V., McMahon, R. P., & Bonds, D. R. (1995). Effect of hydroxyurea on the frequency of painful crises in sickle cell anemia. Investigators of the multicenter study of hydroxyurea in sickle cell anemia. The New England Journal of Medicine, 332(20), 1317–1322. https://doi.org/10.1056/NEJM199505183322001

Chaturvedi, S., & DeBaun, M. R. (2016). Evolution of sickle cell disease from a life-threatening disease of children to a chronic disease of adults: The last 40 years. American Journal of Hematology, 91(1), 5–14. https://doi.org/10.1002/ajh.24235

Chou, S. T., Alsawas, M., Fasano, R. M., Field, J. J., Hendrickson, J. E., Howard, J., Kameka, M., Kwiatkowski, J. L., Pirenne, F., Shi, P. A., Stowell, S. R., Thein, S. L., Westhoff, C. M., Wong, T. E., & Akl, E. A. (2020). American Society of hematology 2020 guidelines for sickle cell disease: Transfusion support. Blood Advances, 4(2), 327–355. https://doi.org/10.1182/bloodadvances.2019001143

Cober, M. P., & Phelps, S. J. (2010). Penicillin prophylaxis in children with sickle cell disease. The Journal of Pediatric Pharmacology and Therapeutics, 15(3), 152–159.

DeBaun, M. R. (2011). Secondary prevention of overt strokes in sickle cell disease: Therapeutic strategies and efficacy. Hematology. American Society of Hematology. Education Program, 427–433. https://doi.org/10.1182/asheducation-2011.1.427

Eurorad.org. (2019). Eurorad – Brought to You by the ESR. Retrieved May 30, 2022, from https://www.eurorad.org/case/16842

Falletta, J. M., Woods, G. M., Verter, J. I., Buchanan, G. R., Pegelow, C. H., Iyer, R. V., Miller, S. T., Holbrook, C. T., Kinney, T. R., & Vichinsky, E. (1995). Discontinuing penicillin prophylaxis in children with sickle cell anemia. Prophylactic penicillin study II. The Journal of Pediatrics, 127(5), 685–690. https://doi.org/10.1016/s0022-3476(95)70154-0

Fasano, R. M., Meier, E. R., & Hulbert, M. L. (2015). Cerebral vasculopathy in children with sickle cell anemia. Blood Cells, Molecules & Diseases, 54(1), 17–25. https://doi.org/10.1016/j.bcmd.2014.08.007

Field, J. J., Austin, P. F., An, P., Yan, Y., & DeBaun, M. R. (2008). Enuresis is a common and persistent problem among children and young adults with sickle cell anemia. Urology, 72(1), 81–84. https://doi.org/10.1016/j.urology.2008.02.006

Friend, A., & Girzadas, D. (2022). Acute Chest Syndrome. In StatPearls. StatPearls Publishing. http://www.ncbi.nlm.nih.gov/books/NBK441872/

Gaston, M. H., Verter, J. I., Woods, G., Pegelow, C., Kelleher, J., Presbury, G., Zarkowsky, H., Vichinsky, E., Iyer, R., & Lobel, J. S. (1986). Prophylaxis with oral penicillin in children with sickle cell anemia. A randomized trial. The New England Journal of Medicine, 314(25), 1593–1599. https://doi.org/10.1056/NEJM198606193142501

Gyamfi, J., Lee, J. T., Islam, F., Opeyemi, J., Tampubolon, S., Ojo, T., Qiao, Y., Mai, A., Vieira, D., & Peprah, E. (2021). Characterization of neurological complications among children with sickle cell disease in the United States: Findings from the 2007–2018 National Health Interview Survey (NHIS). Blood, 138, 1909. https://doi.org/10.1182/blood-2021-148849

Hankins, J. S., Helton, K. J., McCarville, M. B., Li, C.-S., Wang, W. C., & Ware, R. E. (2008). Preservation of spleen and brain function in children with sickle cell anemia treated with hydroxyurea. Pediatric Blood & Cancer, 50(2), 293–297. https://doi.org/10.1002/pbc.21271

Hasson, C., Veling, L., Rico, J., & Mhaskar, R. (2019). The role of hydroxyurea to prevent silent stroke in sickle cell disease: Systematic review and meta-analysis. Medicine, 98(51), e18225. https://doi.org/10.1097/MD.0000000000018225

Huang, Y., Ananthakrishnan, T., & Eid, J. E. (2003). Hydroxyurea-induced splenic regrowth in an adult patient with severe hemoglobin SC disease. American Journal of Hematology, 74(2), 125–126. https://doi.org/10.1002/ajh.10388

Lagunju, I., Brown, B. J., & Sodeinde, O. (2015). Hydroxyurea lowers transcranial Doppler flow velocities in children with sickle cell anaemia in a Nigerian cohort. Pediatric Blood & Cancer, 62(9), 1587–1591. https://doi.org/10.1002/pbc.25529

Lefèvre, N., Dufour, D., Gulbis, B., Lê, P.-Q., Heijmans, C., & Ferster, A. (2008). Use of hydroxyurea in prevention of stroke in children with sickle cell disease. Blood, 111(2), 963–964; author reply 964. https://doi.org/10.1182/blood-2007-08-102244

McGann, P. T., & Ware, R. E. (2015). Hydroxyurea therapy for sickle cell anemia. Expert Opinion on Drug Safety, 14(11), 1749–1758. https://doi.org/10.1517/14740338.2015.1088827

Naffaa, L. N., Tandon, Y. K., & Irani, N. (2015). Transcranial Doppler screening in sickle cell disease: The implications of using peak systolic criteria. World Journal of Radiology, 7(2), 52–56. https://doi.org/10.4329/wjr.v7.i2.52

Nottage, K. A., Ware, R. E., Winter, B., Smeltzer, M., Wang, W. C., Hankins, J. S., Dertinger, S. D., Shulkin, B., & Aygun, B. (2014). Predictors of splenic function preservation in children with sickle cell anemia treated with hydroxyurea. European Journal of Haematology, 93(5), 377–383. https://doi.org/10.1111/ejh.12361

Ogu, U. O., Badamosi, N. U., Camacho, P. E., Freire, A. X., & Adams-Graves, P. (2021). Management of sickle cell disease complications beyond acute chest syndrome. Journal of Blood Medicine, 12, 101–114. https://doi.org/10.2147/JBM.S291394

Ohene-Frempong, K., Weiner, S. J., Sleeper, L. A., Miller, S. T., Embury, S., Moohr, J. W., Wethers, D. L., Pegelow, C. H., Gill, F. M., & The C.S. of Sickle Cell Disease (1998). Cerebrovascular accidents in sickle cell disease: Rates and risk factors. Blood, 91(1), 288–294. https://pubmed.ncbi.nlm.nih.gov/9414296/

Olujohungbe, A., & Burnett, A. L. (2013). How I manage priapism due to sickle cell disease. British Journal of Haematology, 160(6), 754–765. https://doi.org/10.1111/bjh.12199

Osunkwo, I., O'Connor, H. F., & Saah, E. (2020). Optimizing the management of chronic pain in sickle cell disease. Hematology, 2020(1), 562–569. https://doi.org/10.1182/hematology.2020000143

Sarnaik, S., Slovis, T. L., Corbett, D. P., Emami, A., & Whitten, C. F. (1980). Incidence of cholelithiasis in sickle cell anemia using the ultrasonic gray-scale technique. The Journal of Pediatrics, 96(6), 1005–1008. https://doi.org/10.1016/s0022-3476(80)80626-3

Sundd, P., Gladwin, M. T., & Novelli, E. M. (2019). Pathophysiology of sickle cell disease. Annual Review of Pathology, 14, 263–292. https://doi.org/10.1146/annurev-pathmechdis-012418-012838

Switzer, J. A., Hess, D. C., Nichols, F. T., & Adams, R. J. (2006). Pathophysiology and treatment of stroke in sickle-cell disease: Present and future. The Lancet Neurology, 5(6), 501–512. https://doi.org/10.1016/S1474-4422(06)70469-0

Tshilolo, L., Tomlinson, G., Williams, T. N., Santos, B., Olupot-Olupot, P., Lane, A., Aygun, B., Stuber, S. E., Latham, T. S., McGann, P. T., Ware, R. E., & REACH Investigators. (2019). Hydroxyurea for children with sickle cell anemia in Sub-Saharan Africa. The New England Journal of Medicine, 380(2), 121–131. https://doi.org/10.1056/NEJMoa1813598

Verduzco, L. A., & Nathan, D. G. (2009). Sickle cell disease and stroke. Blood, 114(25), 5117–5125. https://doi.org/10.1182/blood-2009-05-220921

Verma, H. K., Lakkakula, S., & Lakkakula, B. V. K. S. (2018). Retrospection of the effect of hydroxyurea treatment in patients with sickle cell disease. Acta Haematologica Polonica, 49(1), Article 1. DOI: 10.2478/ahp-2018-0001

Ware, R. E. (2013). Hydroxycarbamide: Clinical aspects. Comptes Rendus Biologies, 336(3), 177–182. https://doi.org/10.1016/j.crvi.2012.09.006

Williams, T. N., Uyoga, S., Macharia, A., Ndila, C., McAuley, C. F., Opi, D. H., Mwarumba, S., Makani, J., Komba, A., Ndiritu, M. N., Sharif, S. K., Marsh, K., Berkley, J. A., & Scott, J. A. G. (2009). Bacteraemia in Kenyan children with sickle-cell anaemia: A retrospective cohort and case–control study. The Lancet, 374(9698), 1364–1370. https://doi.org/10.1016/S0140-6736(09)61374-X

Yawn, B., Buchanan, G., & Afenyi-Annan, A. (2014). Management of Sickle Cell Disease: Summary of the 2014 Evidence-Based Report by Expert Panel Members. JAMA, 312(10), 1033–1048. doi:10.1001/jama.2014.10517

6 Paediatric to Adult Transition Care for Patients with Sickle Cell Disorder

Tamunomieibi Wakama and Ekaete David

Goals

1 Adherence to therapy without supervision.
2 Independence to attend clinic visits and take decisions on their own.
3 Introduce advanced treatment modalities/new therapies as they become available.
4 Try to ensure the disease remains stable and does not progress.

Problems

1 No documented structure on how the transition should take place.
2 What parameters should be important to be looked out for?
3 What do the patients think is important for them to make the transition seamless?
4 Tracking process from the paediatric clinic so that follow-up can be carried out.
5 Stating those needed in the team and defining their job roles.

Scenario 1

Master Anayo is a 17-year-old boy, a known patient with sickle cell anaemia (SCA) diagnosed at the age of two years. He has been attending the paediatric sickle cell clinic mostly in the company of his mother in the last 15 years and has had several Emergency room (ER) and paediatric in-patient admissions. Shortly after his 16th birthday, he was brought to the children's emergency having developed features of vaso-occlusive crisis (VOC). The doctor in the ER directs them to the adult Emergency room, as 'he was no longer a child, and there is no suitable bed for his size in the children's emergency room'.

Anayo was seen by the casualty officer in the adult ER. Based on his medical history of SCA and the attendant pains, he was given parenteral Pentazocine, and a consult was sent to the adult Haematology team on call. The Haematology team reviewed him and subsequently admitted him to the adult Male medical ward for further management. After about five days of in-patient management, he was discharged to the adult sickle cell clinic for follow-up.

Master Anayo who is now a college student in a boarding school attended clinic appointments on two occasions with his mother and was later 'lost to follow up'.

DOI: 10.4324/9781003463931-7

After about a year he was brought to the adult ER with complaints of a three-day history of fever, chest pain and pain in the long bones which did not respond to treatment given at the school clinic. A review by the Haematology team revealed that he had gone back to the paediatric sickle cell clinic a couple of times when on holidays and defaults on his clinic appointments and his routine medications. He was also noticed to have developed severe pains in the right hip with some difficulty in movement. In view of this, the orthopedic team was invited to review him as a possible case of Avascular Necrosis of the right femoral head (AVN). He was discharged after a week of in-patient management in the adult male medical ward, to continue outpatient management at the adult sickle cell clinic and the orthopedic clinic on their respective clinic days.

Based on the above, the patient and the parents (who hitherto were not aware of the existence of 'another' sickle cell clinic in the hospital) were invited to have a session with the counselling team, the managing adult haematology team and his paediatric consultant paediatrician for counselling on his further management to transit seamlessly to adult care.

Introduction

Health care transition is defined as 'the purposeful, planned movement of adolescents and young adults (AYA) with chronic physical and medical conditions from child-centred to adult-oriented health care systems' (Blum et al., 1993). This definition was given by Blum and colleagues and covers all chronic diseases that patients need to live with throughout life (Blum et al., 1993).

The sickle cell disease spectrum is a disease that has over time evolved from being a childhood killer disease to one that is now a chronic illness with most people living into adulthood due to improved access to vaccinations, well-trained physicians, access to healthcare facilities, improved nutrition, better screening techniques, and more drug treatment options. Sickle cell disease is one of the oldest genetic diseases reported in the literature. Research is ongoing involving new drugs for the treatment of symptoms of the disease and complications that arise from the disease. The role of stem cell transplantation and gene therapy is also being explored as curative treatment methods.

Sickle cell disease is of global importance because of its prevalence rate in different parts of the world. The new born screening programme has given the following prevalence values: Sub-Saharan Africa 500–2,000/100,000 live births, South America and Caribbean Islands (20–1,000/100,000), and <500/100,000 live births in Europe. Colombatti et al. (2022) noted hotspots in Sub-Saharan Africa, India, North East Africa and the Middle East. Regional studies have tried to postulate the prevalence of sickle cell disease in Nigeria. A study done by Nwogoh et al. (2012) in Benin city south-south Nigeria gave a prevalence rate of 2.39% (Nwogoh et al., 2012).

The data presented above on prevalence rate and also data from high-income countries show that the mortality rate is highest in the 20–24-year age group with the increased frequency of presentation at emergency rooms. These facts highlight the need for a smooth transition process.

The transition process involves the process of change of caregivers due to age, social development, emotional development and disease management knowledge and skills. As people grow older there is a need to change caregivers. The children begin the process of transition from childhood to adolescence to adulthood. In each of these phases in life, there are peculiarities which need to be properly attended to. The use of age is the main criterion for transfer from paediatric to adult care. The age for transfer depends on the country or region. For example, it ranges from 12 years in the Middle East, 12–15 years in many African countries, to 16–18 years in the United Kingdom, 18–21 years in the United States of America and 17–19 years in Canada. There are arguments that only age should not be the main criterion for the transfer of patients as is commonly the case in the Middle East and some African countries (Inusa et al., 2020; Sobota et al., 2015; Treadwell et al., 2023). The age of commencement of the transition process and conversations also vary with the different regions of the world. It is noted to commence between the ages of 13–14 years in the United Kingdom and 15 years in the United States of America.

The transition period is critical because this also coincides with the period of adolescence. With so much going on at the same time for this age group, it can get overwhelming for them. This is the period also where complications of the disease begin to appear; these include iron overload, renal disease, neurosensory impairments, etc. This period has been linked to the period with an increase in morbidity and mortality.

A study by de Montalembert and Guitton (2013) of the French reference centre for sickle cell disease noted that clinical features of adolescents with sickle cell disease included chronic pain episodes, mental health challenges (depression, post-traumatic stress disorder, abuse of pain killers, etc.), academic difficulties (due to frequent school absences, stokes, brain infarcts, neurocognitive impairment, etc.), social difficulties (stigmatisation, transition to self-care, inability to play sports, etc.) (de Montalembert & Guitton, 2013). These features lead to the need for long-term care and frequent visits to the hospital. Complications of sickle cell disease have been noted to increase mortality in this group.

There are different suggestions as to the criteria for seamless transition. In Nigeria, there are currently no documented national guidelines on the seamless transition process/management. A guideline is needed for uniform provision of care and also allows for seamless care when patient relocates within the country.

The Transition Process

This is the process involved in ensuring a seamless transition from paediatric based care to adult based care. This will require the co-operation of the patients and their care givers to minimise or slow down development of complications of the disease.

In the transitioning process, the association of maternal and child health programmes of the United States of America states that for improved health outcomes and quality of life there are four standards for paediatric care settings and four standards for adult care settings (Saulsberry et al., 2019; Treadwell et al., 2023). See Table 6.1.

Table 6.1 Standards of care for the transition process

Peadiatric care standards	Adult care standards
Transition policy	Adolescent and young adult transition and care policy
Transition readiness	Orientation and integration to adult practice
Transfer of care	Initial visit plan
Transfer completion	Ongoing care

The important standards in paediatric settings are:

- **Transition policy**
  It is advocated that a transition policy is developed in every facility where this is to happen. The policy should clearly state what is to happen and have the input of caregivers of the paediatric patients and the patients themselves. This may include combined consultations with adult and paediatric physicians, a separate clinic location for the adolescents and staff trained to handle adolescents.
- **Transition readiness**
  A tool is used to assess the child's readiness to transition based on the ability to independently seek medical attention and self-care. This tool should help the assessment.
- **Transfer of care**
  This will be a document written by the paediatric physician detailing the full history of the patient, previous care plans, current care plan and transition care assessments.
- **Transfer completion**
  Ensure correspondence with the adult physician to confirm that the patient has registered and is attending the clinic.

On the other hand, the important standards in adult settings are:

- **Adolescent and young adult transition and care policy**
  Each institution where the transition process will occur should have a policy in the adult clinic setting stating how this transition will take place. The policy drafted should have input from the end users.
- **Orientation and integration to adult practice**
  This document should state the facilities that will carry out this important step. Also, there should be laid out steps on what is to be done at the first few visits to ensure proper integration. There must be documentation of receipt of documents from the paediatric facility. Ideally, such transfer may occur in the same facility.
- **Initial visit plan**
  This should comprise discussing the concerns of the patient about the transfer, reviewing the current care plan, making updates to the current plan as well as drawing up plans for the care of the patient. The initial visit can assess the patient's ability to

independently seek care when needed, assess understanding/knowledge of the disease and the role of the patient in ensuring good health. The plan can also document the concerns of the patient and what will be done to address such concerns.

• **Ongoing care**
  At this stage, the paediatric team is contacted to inform them that the patient has reported to the adult clinic, there are reviews with the patients to get feedback on services received and changes they wish to see. There will be a need to provide knowledge about the expectations on health-seeking behaviours and also personnel self-care. There will be a need to ensure that their mental health needs are adequately provided for through the transition period as this also coincides with puberty.

Another institution that has done a lot of work on the transition process is the Got transition/Centre for Health Care Transition Improvement. This was created by the National Alliance to Advance Adolescent Health, in partnership with the Maternal and Child Health Bureau. The GOT transition centre spelt out the six core elements of the sickle cell transition process and they include:

1 creating a transition policy,
2 tracking and monitoring progress,
3 assessing transition readiness,
4 planning for adult care,
5 transferring to adult care, and
6 integrating into adult care

Barriers to Effective Transition

Hobart and Phan in their article tried to itemise the factors that affect/hinder smooth healthcare transition (HCT) from paediatric to adult care (Hobart & Phan, 2019). These transitions have been categorised into modifiable and non-modifiable factors. These two main groups are seen to affect patients, caregivers as well as the healthcare system. The non-modifiable factors include ethnicity, sex, socioeconomic factors and age. Ethnicity would encompass factors like religious and cultural norms. This plays a very important role in health-seeking behaviours and will greatly affect the uptake of the service to be provided. Health facilities need to put this into consideration and ensure that the cultures and the norms of the environment they operate in are considered.

Socioeconomic factors are very important non-modifiable factors. The transition is the age where most people go off the insurance of their parents and have a dilemma on which insurance package they subscribe to. This extra cost of insurance is an extra burden on the caregivers and the patient. In many countries in the Sub-Saharan region, payment is out of pocket. This is a huge burden on the finances of the family.

The modifiable factors that are barriers to effective transition have been summarised in Table 6.2.

Table 6.2 Factors affecting paediatric to adult transition (Hobart & Phan, 2019).

Patient/caregiver factors	Healthcare system factors
Language proficiency	Lack of policies for structured HCT
Health literacy proficiency	Lack of training/insufficient training for teams involved in HCT
Perceived lack of support from clinicians	Lack of engagement between the HCT team and patients/caregivers
Fear of the unknown	Communication gaps between adult/ paediatric team

Global Practice on Transition

There are varying practices on transition in different parts of the globe. What is clear is that other than age, other factors such as the capabilities of the adolescents, their needs and their future aspirations play significant roles. Each country must write national policies on transition care for sickle cell disease patients. These national policies will act as templates for institutions to draw up their local policies.

Transition care is said to be a shared responsibility between paediatric care doctors and adult care doctors. The two sets of doctors must keep communicating with themselves and the patient throughout the transition process to ensure a seamless transfer process (Inusa et al., 2020; Saulsberry et al., 2019). It has been noticed that transition is more difficult and requires more human, educational and material resources when the patients need to be moved to a different facility for adult care. Certain factors need to be addressed as they have been noted to be of major concern to the patients these include:

  i Distance to the new facility from their residence
 ii The process for review by the physician in the new facility
iii The cost of care at the new facility
 iv Ease of referral to other specialist in the facility
  v Access to emergency care at the new site

A recent study done in Tanzania by Masamu et al. (2020) notes that there was a relationship between health status and loss of follow-up. However, this study also notes that phone follow-ups were not sufficient to ensure patient compliance with clinic visits and positive health-seeking behaviours.

They suggest the use of patient engagement groups to ensure continuous education of the patient. The second was the training and retraining of the staff to detect possible patterns of defaulters and how to stop them.

Successful Transition

To date, there are no metrics to measure successful transitions. The important benefit to be attained from a successful transition is having disease-specific knowledge as well as developing a positive mindset on disease management.

There are however other indicators for a successful transition in other chronic diseases which may be applicable to sickle cell.

These indicators are:

i Disease status at the point of transition: mild, moderate or severe
ii Health-care utilisation: use of clinics, day care centres as well as emergency room presentations. The aim is to minimise emergency room visits to the barest minimum
iii Patient-centred outcomes: independence in disease management and decision-making

Nigerian National Transition Plan

There is a need for the country to develop a national transition plan that will be used as a template for all health facilities to set up their transition plan for adolescents and young adults that have to transition from paediatric to adult care.

A laid down plan ensures that care is continuous, emergency care is reduced to the barest minimum and complications are picked and sorted out early.

Furthermore, the plan that is developed must be holistic to cover the education of all parties concerned, identification of gaps in the system, closure of such gaps and development of sickle cell disease registries as well as sickle cell transition registries.

The other important component of a national plan is the development of models to analyse outcome measures from the services provided and various intervention methods put in place.

The outcome measures need to cover quality of life, ease of transition, cost of care, the effect of cost of care-on-caregiver and patients, mental health, education of healthcare providers and patients/family members, and use of navigators.

The plan should also include ways the outcome measures will be effectively utilised to improve the present model of transition care with the ultimate goal of having excellent transition care. The ultimate goal is to develop excellent transition care that is suitable and acceptable by the patients, caregivers, healthcare facilities and healthcare providers.

A review of the literature reveals that though a large percentage of children with sickle cell disease are born and reside in Sub-Saharan Africa, there are no laid down transition plans. There are an increasing number of children with sickle cell disease living into adulthood (Inusa et al., 2020).

There are important points that must be captured in the national transition plan and they should be based on the SICKLE recommendations which are recommendations that have been developed for transition based on reviews, WHO standard recommendations and literature searches (Asnani et al., 2017; Inusa et al., 2020; WHO, 2015). Table 6.3 details the global standards for health as produced by the WHO (2015). The WHO global standards for quality healthcare services for adolescents have eight standards which must be attained.

Table 6.3 Global standards for quality healthcare services for adolescents (WHO, 2015).

Adolescents' health literacy
Community support
Appropriate package of services
Providers' competencies
Facility characteristics
Equity and non-discrimination
Data and quality improvement
Adolescents' participation

The components of the global standards for quality healthcare services for adolescents are listed in the table. The goal of the transition period is to move these patients from supervised care to independent care.

These international recommendations listed above were taken by experts and tailored specifically to sickle cell disease. This is known as the sickle recommendations which are discussed below.

- **The SICKLE recommendation** (Inusa et al., 2020).
  - **Skills transfer**
  Patients are taught how to recognise their symptoms particularly pain, and how to manage the onset of the pain. They are also taught to recognise when they need professional help for relief and how to book appointments. There is no recommended age, but it is thought that the caregivers and medical personnel decide this.
- **Increasing self-efficacy**
  The adolescents and young adults are encouraged to be actively involved in developing their care plan. This needs to be reviewed at each visit. The parents and caregivers are also counselled as they make up their support system. Changes to care plan should be made to suit the young patients' goals, aims and aspirations.
- **Coordination of transition**
  The transition process needs a lot of support so as to ensure the process is successful. In high-income countries, the young person is attached to a community nurse or health worker. The person provides information on the disease, medication adherence and other questions that the person has.

  The community health worker acts as a liaison with the doctors or nurses in the hospital.

  In low-income countries, community health extension workers (CHEW), medical officers and village liaison can be trained to perform this function. These personnel have to be supervised by a specific secondary or tertiary health facility that they report progress of the individuals and their families.

  They will also be valuable in following up patients when they default from the health facilities.
- **Knowledge transfer**
  All patients should have a good understanding of sickle cell disease, including its cause, signs and symptoms, potential complications, management, risks of

non-adherence to medication (hydroxyurea and penicillin), and prognosis before the transfer of care.

We recommend that multidisciplinary (including young people with sickle cell disease and their families) task forces develop a curriculum and handbook for the transition from paediatric to adult care.

- **Linking to adult services**

It is expected that young people should know when their care will be transferred and who the adult provider is or could be. They are also expected to have either a joint first consultation or a period of overlap whereby their first consultation with their adult care provider occurs before their last paediatric appointment. They should also be introduced to other services that they would need to access in the course of their adult care.

We recommend a mapping of all facilities offering specialist sickle cell care in the lower and middle-income countries for easy referral and identification of the nearest adult centred service for patients in care at paediatrics-only centres. Joint paediatric and adult care clinics should be established where resources are available. A minimum requirement is to offer such a clinic before care transfer.

- **Evaluating readiness**

Before the transfer of care, transition readiness should be assessed to ensure every young person is developmentally ready to assume complete responsibility for their healthcare and adequately prepared for doing so. Tracking the progress of the young adult for several years will enhance the evaluation of the success of the adolescent transition programme.

The aim of the standards as shown above is to ensure that adolescents and young adults get satisfactory services in both public and private health facilities. There also have to be measures put in place to assess the standards that have been suggested to be used for global use.

Mental health access must be included in their transition care plan as studies have shown that there is a high rate of depression among adolescents and young adults with sickle cell disease. Sehlo and Kamfar (2015) note that 46% of the children studied had depression (Allemang et al., 2019; Sehlo & Kamfar, 2015). Their quality of life was also noted to be altered due to emotional disturbances, social functioning and school functioning deficits and other criteria measured in the Paediatric Quality of Life Inventory, Version 4.0 Generic Core Scales (PedsQL 4.0).

Patient navigators are members of staff employed to act as a bridge between patients and the healthcare services providing information/education to patients and others, they must have excellent communication skills, practice professionally, give feedback to health facilities and generally ensure that patients' visits to the hospital are seamless. They follow up with patients to ensure they are compliant with treatment plans and follow up with phone calls and home visits if necessary. These patient navigators are very important especially in ensuring mental health access without delay for the patients.

There have also been studies done to show that the use of patient navigators in health facilities improved patient transition, appointment visits and drug use

(Allemang et al., 2019). It will be important to incorporate patient navigators into a national transition plan as studies have shown they positively affect the outcome.

Survivorship

As in medium and high-income countries, low-income countries have noticed that life expectancy has improved with the statistics showing that 50 percent of children born with sickle cell disease will live beyond ten years of age in Sub-Saharan Africa (Inusa, 2020). This recent data is in contrast to a study done in Northern Nigeria in the 1970s that showed that more than 90% of children with sickle cell disease born in rural communities did not see their fifth birthday. This great improvement in life has been attributed to several factors such as better health education and health awareness campaigns, improved nutrition, easier access to vaccination and health facilities, adequate support systems and new and emerging treatment options. These numbers still lag behind the figures in the United States of America and the United Kingdom where greater than 95% of children born with haemoglobinopathies are expected to survive into adulthood. There has been an improvement in survival but the fact remains that this group of people is expected to die between 10 and 20 years earlier than their age, sex and race-matched peers. The peak age for mortality is between the mid-20s and mid-40s. There are several postulations as to why this still exists which include the development of complications of the disease, poor compliance to outlined treatment protocols and financial constraints among others (Fleming et al., 1979; Grosse et al., 2011; Inusa et al., 2020; Treadwell et al., 2023

The countries of the Sub-Saharan Africa are striving to improve the age expectancy of those with sickle cell disease so that it matches those of middle- and high-income countries.

Conclusion

The sickle cell disease first discovered in 1910 has come a long way since its discovery. Recent advances in science and research have caused the disease to move from that disease with high infant mortality to a chronic disease. Many of the sufferers of the disease now live into adulthood in all parts of the world including low- and middle-income countries.

This new situation has brought up new challenges which need to be tackled to build on the gains of an improved life span. The proper framework for paediatric to adult transition is the bedrock of achieving an excellent quality of life in this group of people.

There is a need to develop guidelines that define the multidisciplinary team required to care for this group of people, their roles and ultimately a seamless transition from paediatric to adult care. Such teams have to be culturally sensitive and acceptable to all (patients, careers, clinicians and other health personnel).

The aim is to have adults with sickle cell disease with no or minimal complications of the disease that are debilitating and leave them hospital-bound or moribund. This chapter aims to drive conversations that will ensure that the sickle cell population in Nigeria and the world at large get excellent care at all stages of their lives.

References

Allemang, B., Allan, K., Johnson, C., Cheong, M., Cheung, P., Odame, I., Ward, R., Williams, S., Mukerji, G., & Kuo, K. H. (2019). Impact of a transition program with navigator on loss to follow-up, medication adherence, and appointment attendance in hemoglobinopathies. *Pediatric Blood & Cancer*, *66*(8), e27781. https://doi.org/10.1002/pbc.27781

Asnani, M. R., Barton-Gooden, A., Grindley, M., & Knight-Madden, J. (2017). Disease knowledge, illness perceptions, and quality of life in adolescents with sickle cell disease: Is there a link? *Global Pediatric Health*, *4*, 2333794X1773919. https://doi.org/10.1177/2333794x17739194

Blum, R. W., Garell, D., Hodgman, C. H., Jorissen, T. W., Okinow, N. A., Orr, D. P., & Slap, G. B. (1993). Transition from child-centered to adult health-care systems for adolescents with chronic conditions. *Journal of Adolescent Health*, *14*(7), 570–576. https://doi.org/10.1016/1054-139x(93)90143-d

Colombatti, R., Birkegård, C., & Medici, M. (2022). PB2215: Global epidemiology of sickle cell disease: A systematic literature review. *HemaSphere*, *6*, 2085–2086. https://doi.org/10.1097/01.hs9.0000851688.00394.f4

de Montalembert, M., & Guitton, C. (2013). Transition from paediatric to adult care for patients with sickle cell disease. *British Journal of Haematology*, *164*(5), 630–635. https://doi.org/10.1111/bjh.12700

Fleming, A. F., Storey, J., Molineaux, L., Iroko, E. A., & Attai, E. D. E. (1979, April). Abnormal haemoglobins in the Sudan savanna of Nigeria. *Annals of Tropical Medicine & Parasitology*, *73*(2), 161–172. https://doi.org/10.1080/00034983.1979.11687243

Grosse, S. D., Odame, I., Atrash, H. K., Amendah, D. D., Piel, F. B., & Williams, T. N. (2011). Sickle cell disease in Africa. *American Journal of Preventive Medicine*, *41*(6), S398–S405. https://doi.org/10.1016/j.amepre.2011.09.013

Hobart, C. B., & Phan, H. (2019). Pediatric-to-adult healthcare transitions: Current challenges and recommended practices. *American Journal of Health-System Pharmacy*, *76*(19), 1544–1554. https://doi.org/10.1093/ajhp/zxz165

Inusa, B. P. D., Stewart, C. E., Mathurin-Charles, S., Porter, J., Hsu, L. L. Y., Atoyebi, W., De Montalembert, M., Diaku-Akinwumi, I., Akinola, N. O., Andemariam, B., Abboud, M. R., & Treadwell, M. (2020, April). Paediatric to adult transition care for patients with sickle cell disease: A global perspective. *The Lancet Haematology*, *7*(4), e329–e341. https://doi.org/10.1016/s2352-3026(20)30036-3

Masamu, U., Sangeda, R. Z., Kandonga, D., Ondengo, J., Ndobho, F., Mmbando, B., Nkya, S., Msami, K., & Makani, J. (2020). Patterns and patient factors associated with loss to follow-up in the Muhimbili sickle cell cohort, Tanzania. *BMC Health Services Research*, *20*(1). https://doi.org/10.1186/s12913-020-05998-6

Nwogoh, B., Adewowoyin, A., Iheanacho, O. E., & Bazuaye, G. N. (2012). Prevalence of haemoglobin variants in Benin City, Nigeria. *Annals of Biomedical Sciences*, *11*(2), 60–64.

Saulsberry, A. C., Porter, J. S., & Hankins, J. S. (2019). A program of transition to adult care for sickle cell disease. *Hematology*, *2019*(1), 496–504. https://doi.org/10.1182/hematology.2019000054

Sehlo, M. G., & Kamfar, H. Z. (2015, April 11). Depression and quality of life in children with sickle cell disease: The effect of social support. *BMC Psychiatry*, *15*(1). https://doi.org/10.1186/s12888-015-0461-6

Sobota, A. E., Umeh, E., & Mack, J. W. (2015). Young adult perspectives on a successful transition from pediatric to adult care in sickle cell disease. *Journal of Hematology Research*, *2*(1), 17–24. https://doi.org/10.12974/2312-5411.2015.02.01.3

The National alliance to Advance Adolescent Health/Got Transition. (2020). The Six Core Elements of Health Care Transition. https://www.gottransition.org

Treadwell, M., Hankins, J. S., & King, A. (2023). Sickle cell disease (SCD) in adolescents and young adults (AYA): Transition from pediatric to adult care. https://www.medilib.ir/uptodate/show/112919

WHO (2015). *Global standards for quality health-care services for adolescents: a guide to implement a standards-driven approach to improve the quality of health care services for adolescents*. https://apps.who.int/iris/handle/10665/183935

Appendix to the chapter

The appendix document is found below which shows samples of transition documents.

got transition

Sample Transition Readiness Assessment for Parents/Caregivers
Six Core Elements of Health Care Transition 2.0

Please fill out this form to help us see what your child already knows about his or her health and the areas that you think he/she needs to learn more about. After you complete the form, compare your answers with the form your child has complete. Your answers may be different. We will help you work on some steps to increase your child's health care skills.

Date:

Name: Date of Birth:

Transition Importance and Confidence   On a scale of 0 to 10, please circle the number that best
describes how you feel right now.

How important is it for your child to prepare for/change to an adult doctor before age 22?

0 (not)	1	2	3	4	5	6	7	8	9	10 (very)

How confide   it do you feel about your child's ability to prepare for/change to an idult doctor?

0 (not)	1	2	3	4	5	6	7	8	9	10 (very)

My Health Please check the box that applies to your child right now.	Yes, he/she knows this	He/she needs to learn	Someone needs to do this... Who?
My child knows his/her medical needs.	☐	☐	☐
My child can explain his/her medical needs to others.	☐	☐	☐
My child knows his/her symptoms including ones that he/she quickly needs to see a doctor for.	☐	☐	☐
My child knows what to do in case he/she has a medical emergency.	☐	☐	☐
My child knows his/her own medicines, what they are for, and when he/she needs to take them.	☐	☐	☐
My child knows his/her allergies to medicines and medicines he/she should not take.	☐	☐	☐
My child carries important health information with him/her every day (e.g. insurance card, allergies, medications, emergency contact information, medical summary).	☐	☐	☐
My child knows he/she can see a doctor alone as I wait in the waiting room.	☐	☐	☐
My child understands how health care privacy changes at age 18.	☐	☐	☐
My child can explain to others how his/her customs and beliefs affect health care decisions and medical treatment.	☐	☐	☐
Using Health Care			
My child knows or can find his/her doctor's phone number.	☐	☐	☐
My child makes his/her own doctor appointments.	☐	☐	☐
Before a visit, my child thinks about questions to ask.	☐	☐	☐
My child has a way to get to his/her doctor's office.	☐	☐	☐
My child knows to show up 15 minutes before the visit to check in.	☐	☐	☐
My child knows where to go to get medical care when the doctor's office is closed.	☐	☐	☐
My child has a file at home for his/her medical information.	☐	☐	☐
My child has a copy of his/her current plan of care.	☐	☐	☐
My child knows how to fill out medical forms.	☐	☐	☐
My child knows how to get referrals to other providers.	☐	☐	☐
My child knows where his/her pharmacy is and how to refill his/her medicines.	☐	☐	☐
My child knows where to get blood work or x-rays if his/her doctor orders them.	☐	☐	☐
My child has a plan to keep his/her health insurance after ages 18 or older.	☐	☐	☐
My child and I have discussed his/her ability to make his/her own health care decisions at age 18.	☐	☐	☐
My child and I have discussed a plan for supported decision-making, if needed.	☐	☐	☐

Source: The Six Core Elements of Health Care Transition™ are the copyright of Got Transition. This version of the Six Core Elements has been modified and is used with permission.[1]

American Society of Hematology

Sickle Cell Disease Transition Readiness Assessment Template

Please fill out this form to help us see what you already know about your health and how to use health care and the areas that you want to learn more about. If you need help completing this form, please ask your parent/caregiver.

Date: Name: Date of Birth:

Transition and Self-Care Importance and Confidence   *On a scale of 0 to 10, please circle the number that best describes how you feel now.*

How important is it to you to manage your own health care?

0 (not)	1	2	3	4	5	6	7	8	9	10 (very)

How confident do you feel about your ability to manage your own health care?

0 (not)	1	2	3	4	5	6	7	8	9	10 (very)

How confident do you feel about preparing for/changing to an adult doctor before the age of 22?   Not Applicable ☐

0 (not)	1	2	3	4	5	6	7	8	9	10 (very)

My Health *Please check the box that applies to you right now.*	No, I do not know	No, but I am learning to do this	Yes, I have started doing this	Yes, I always do this when I need to
Disease Knowledge				
I know what type of sickle cell disease I have.				
I know my medical needs and can explain them to someone.				
I know what a hematologist is and why I go to one.				
I know what to do in case of a medical emergency.				
I understand what causes a pain episode.				
I understand how drugs, alcohol and tobacco affect sickle cell disease.				
I have friends that I can talk to about sickle cell disease.				
I know about necessary screening exams (echo annually, kidney function annually, retinal exams, etc.).				
I know how to get blood work and x-rays.				
Medication Management				
I know what my medications are for.				
I know the names and doses of my medications.				
I remember to take my medications without my parent reminding me.				
I fill prescriptions before I run out of medications.				
I am aware of what hydroxyurea is and how it prevents sickling of my red blood cells.				
I know how to prevent a pain episode and what to do if I have pain.				
Appointments				
I make my own doctors' appointments.				
I know how to get medical care when the doctor's office is closed.				
I fill out my own medical history form				
I keep track of my own medical information.				
I keep track of my doctors' and other appointments.				
I make a list of questions before my visit with my doctors.				
I answer questions on my own during medical visits.				
I arrange my own transportation to medical appointments.				
Insurance				
I carry my own insurance card.				
I understand my insurance plan.				
Privacy Information				
I understand how health care privacy changes at age 18, when I am legally an adult.				

Source: The Six Core Elements of Health Care Transition™ are the copyright of Got Transition. This version of the Six Core Elements has been modified and is used with permission.[2]

Notes

1 The National alliance to Advance Adolescent Health/Got Transition (2020). The Six Core Elements of Health Care Transition. https://www.gottransition.org
2 American Society of Hematology (2020). Sickle Cell disease Transition Readiness assessment Template. https://.www.hematology.org

7   Neurocognitive Complications of Sickle Cell Disease in Africa

Fenella Kirkham, Mary Ampomah, Mboka Jacob, Maryam Shehu, Dawn E. Saunders, Richard Idro and IkeOluwa Lagunju

Introduction

The sickle gene mutation is most common in equatorial Africa, related to the relative protection from severe malaria of heterozygosity (Piel et al., 2010). Stroke is a well-recognised complication of sickle cell disease (SCD) (Noubiap, Mengnjo, Nicastro, & Kamtchum-Tatuene, 2017), particularly in those with homozygous sickle cell anaemia (HbSS). Stroke also occurs, albeit less commonly, in compound heterozygotes, e.g. those with haemoglobin SC (HbSC) disease which is common in West Africa, or those with haemoglobin Sβ-thalassaemia, seen along the coast of East Africa. There is a wide variety of stroke syndromes, including arterial ischaemic stroke secondary to vasculopathy and/or thromboembolism, venous sinus thrombosis which may be associated with ischaemia or haemorrhage, posterior reversible encephalopathy syndrome (PRES) and haemorrhagic stroke. Cognitive difficulties are common in people with and without infarction on neuroimaging.

Acute Neurological Presentations

Definitions

Acute neurological symptoms and signs are common in SCD (Noubiap et al., 2017), and the underlying pathologies, particularly haemorrhage with intracranial hypertension, may be an important cause of rapid death (Lagunju, Brown, & Famosaya, 2011). There is a wide differential diagnosis (Noubiap et al., 2017; Stotesbury, Adams, & Kirkham, 2021) but published definitions have not been standardised until recently (Noubiap et al., 2017). However, more recent studies have used the World Health Organisation definition of clinical stroke, a focal neurological deficit lasting more than 24 hours, and transient ischaemic attack, a focal neurological deficit lasting less than 24 hours. Neuroimaging may be available (Green et al., 2019; Idro et al., 2022; Kija et al., 2019) and may distinguish ischaemic stroke in an arterial territory (Figure 7.1A) from alternative diagnoses associated with risk of ischaemia, such as PRES (Figure 7.1B). However, because of the cost, neuroimaging is rarely undertaken in the acute phase (Landoure et al., 2017; Ogwang, Odongo, Namusisi, Okello, & Acan, 2022) when haemorrhagic stroke could be

DOI: 10.4324/9781003463931-8

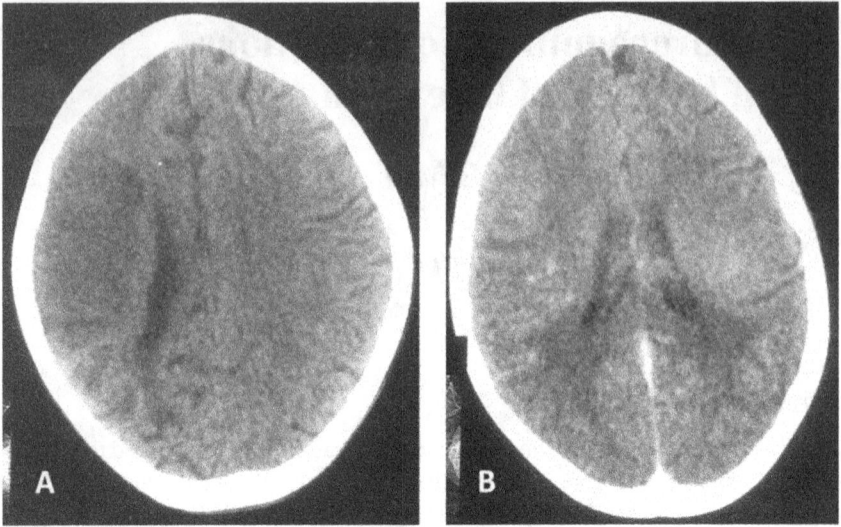

Figure 7.1 Acute CT head scans of children with (A) right middle cerebral artery territory infarct and (B) bilateral and symmetrical oedema of the parietal white matter and patchy cortical abnormality which has the appearance of PRES.

diagnosed in time for emergency treatment (Fatunde, Adamson, Ogunseyinde, Sodeinde, & Familusi, 2005; Njamnshi et al., 2006). Clinical presentations include headaches (Kehinde, Temiye, & Danesi, 2008; Lagunju & Brown, 2012), seizures (Adamolekun, Durosinmi, Olowu, & Adediran, 1993; Lagunju & Brown, 2012) and coma (Akpede & Airede, 1993) as well as stroke and transient ischaemic attack (TIA) (Lagunju & Brown, 2012). Previous asymptomatic cerebral infarction (silent or covert infarct) (Green et al., 2019; Houwing et al., 2020; Idro et al., 2022; Kija et al., 2019) or atrophy (Njamnshi et al., 2006) may be diagnosed if neuro-imaging is available, and should ideally be distinguished, in patients presenting acutely. Young children presenting with acute seizures/status epilepticus may have ischaemia, infarction or infection, including tuberculous (Figure 7.2A) and bacterial meningitis (Figure 7.2B) (Lagunju & Brown, 2012), which may be associated with arterial (Figure 7.2A) and venous (Figure 7.2B) strokes or bacterial abscess (Figure 7.2C).

Epidemiology

Stroke

Without screening and prophylactic treatment, between 5% and 17% of SCD patients living in Africa will suffer a first stroke during childhood or adolescence (Fatunde et al., 2005; Green et al., 2019; Lagunju et al., 2011; Njamnshi et al., 2006; Saidi et al., 2016). In Africa, SCD is typically the most common cause of stroke in childhood (Fatunde et al., 2005; Macharia et al., 2018; Obama, Dongmo,

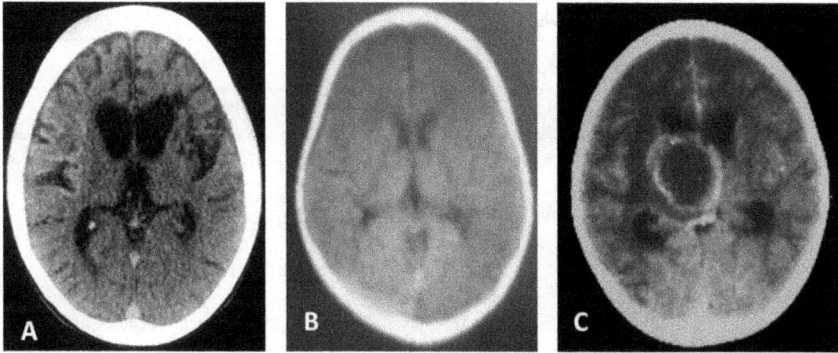

Figure 7.2 CT scans of central nervous system infections in sickle cell disease. (A) Tuberculous meningitis with acute hydrocephalus and cerebral ischaemia and cortical
contrast enhancement. (B) Pneumococcal meningitis with acute cerebral ischaemia with some cerebral swelling of the anterior and middle cerebral circula-
tions and left posterior circulation secondary to venous sinus thrombosis with
an empty delta sign posteriorly. (C) Enhanced scan showing a cerebral abscess.

Nkemayim, Mbede, & Hagbe, 1994) with a recent estimated prevalence of 7.4 per
1,000 patients (Jude et al., 2014). Adults are also affected, with a prevalence of
17.7 per 1,000 patients in the same Nigerian study (Jude et al., 2014). As intracranial bleeding may be a cause of sudden death (Lagunju et al., 2011), the incidence
of haemorrhagic stroke is almost certainly underestimated. However, although
haemorrhagic stroke does occur in children with SCD living in Africa (Lagunju
& Brown, 2012), the available data suggests a greater proportion in adulthood
(Njamnshi et al., 2006) as in the Co-operative study of SCD (CSSCD) in the USA
(Ohene-Frempong et al., 1998).

Small series have reported a wide range of prevalences of stroke from a number
of African countries (Table 7.1), at least in part because the ages reported have been
different. In an initial study in Ibadan between 2004 and 2008 Lagunju et al. found
a prevalence of 6.8% (24/351) (Lagunju et al., 2011) while with CT scan for all
patients and using the WHO criteria for stroke and TIA, the prevalence increased
to 8.4% (Lagunju & Brown, 2012). A meta-analysis of 30 studies in Africa, including all age groups, reported an overall prevalence for stroke of 4.2%, with a higher
prevalence of 6.4% in those using the WHO definition with neuroimaging compared with 2.2% of those not clearly described (Noubiap et al., 2017). In another
systematic review and meta-analysis of ten cross-sectional clinic-based studies,
prevalence ranged from 2.9% to 16.9%, leading to an estimate of 30,000–60,000
children affected (Marks et al., 2018). In a case-control study in Nigeria, paraplegia and stroke were both more common in children, adolescents and adults than in
healthy controls (Kehinde et al., 2008); it is not clear whether the paraplegias were
related to prematurity, spinal stroke or acquired disease of the white matter secondary to status epilepticus.

Table 7.1 Prevalence of all stroke presenting clinically.

	Stroke prevalence	
	Population	Number stroke (%)
Algeria	87	1 (1) (de Montalembert, Beauvais, Bachir, Galacteros & Girot, 1993).
Egypt	100	5 (5) (Bakr, Khorshied, Talha, Jaffer, Soliman, Eid, El-Ghamrawy & 2019)
	60	4 (7) Abou-Elew, Youssry, Hefny, Hashem, Fouad, & Zayed, 2018)
Nigeria	5,721	71 (1) Jude, Aliyu, Nalado, Garba, Florence, Hassan, A. et al. (2014)
Enugu	3,195	23 (0.7) Izuora, Kaine & Emodi (1989)
Lagos	322	17 (5) Kehinde, Temiye, & Danesi. (2008)
Ibadan	500	27 (5) Fatunde, Adamson, Ogunseyinde, Sodeinde, & Familusi, (2005)
Ibadan	351	24 (7) Lagunju, Brown & Famosaya. (2011)
Ibadan	214	7 (3) Akingbola, Tayo, Salako, Layden, Hsu, Cooper, Gordeuk, & Saraf (2014)
Kano	60	7 (12) Tabari & Ismail 2013
Port Harcourt	256	11 (4) George & Frank-Briggs. (2011)
South West	240	7 (3) Adegoke, Adeodu & Adekile. (2015)
Senegal	438	7 (2) Diagne, Diagne-Guèye, Fall, Ndiaye, Camara, Diouf, Signate-Sy & Kuakuvi. (2001)
Angola	200	6 (3) [106] Santos, Delgadinho, Ferreira, Germano, Miranda, Arez, Faustino & Brito. (2020)
Cameroon	113	8 (7) Rumaney, Ngo Bitoungui, Vorster, Ramesar, Kengne, Ngogang, Wonkam. (2014)
	120	8 (7) Njamnshi, Mbong, Wonkam, Ongolo-Zogo, Djientcheu, Sunjoh, et al. (2006)
	96	7 (7) Ruffieux N, Njamnshi, Wonkam, Hauert, Chanal, Verdon. et al. (2013)
DR Congo	500	14 (3) [Djunga & Clarysse. (1977)
Congo	1,422	14 (1) [111] Babela, Nzingoula & Senga. (2005)
Kenya		
Nairobi	360	12 (3) Amayo, Owade, Aluoch & Njeru. (1992)
Kilifi	105	1 (1) Makani, Kirkham, Komba, Ajala-Agbo, Otieno, Fegan et al. (2009).
Uganda	2,870	147 (7) Munube, Katabira, Ndeezi, Joloba, Lhatoo, Sajatovic & Tumwine. (2016)
	256	15 (6) [Green, N, Munube, Bangirana, Buluma, Kebirungi, Opoka. et al. (2019).
Tanzania		
NorthWest	124	21 (17) Saidi, Smart, Kamugisha, Ambrose, Soka, Peck et al. (2016).
Dar es Salaam	200	15 (8) [86] Kija, Saunders, Munubhi, Darekar, Barker, Cox et al. (2019).
Malawi	117	10 (9%) [114] Heimlich, Chipoka, Kamthunzi, Krysiak, Majawa, Mafunga, Fedoriw, Phiri, Key, Ataga, & Gopal. (2016)

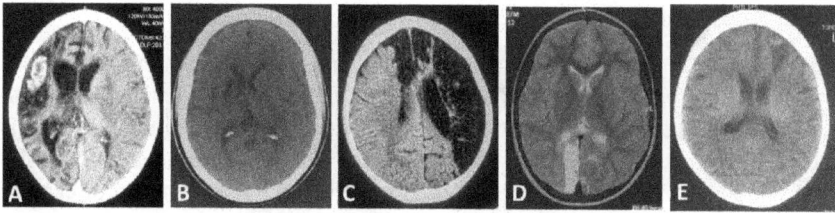

Figure 7.3 CT/MRI head scans of children with mature infarcts of differing type and distribution. (A) Right middle cerebral artery territory infarcts with atrophy, calcification and enlargement of the lateral ventricles. (B) Right striatocapsular (basal ganglia) infarct. (C) Left anterior and middle and right anterior territory infarction with volume loss. (D) MRI scan showing a posterior cerebral artery territory infarct. (E) Left superficial watershed territory infarct between left anterior and middle cerebral artery territory with marginal cortical calcification.

Overt ischaemic stroke is common in mid-childhood, between 2 and 10 years of age (Ohene-Frempong et al., 1998) and presents with motor difficulties, typically hemiparesis, secondary to unilateral or bilateral focal infarction (Lagunju et al., 2011; Njamnshi et al., 2006). Stroke syndromes reported from Africa include symptoms and signs secondary to infarction in the middle (typically hemiparesis; Figure 7.3A,B,C), anterior (cognitive and behvioural difficulties or apparently asymptomatic; Figure 7.3C) and posterior (visual loss, ataxia; Figure 7.3D) cerebral artery territories, equally distributed across both hemispheres but with more subcortical than cortical infarcts (Idro et al., 2022). Infarction in the watershed regions between the main cerebral arteries is not uncommon (Figure 7.3E), sometimes if blood pressure has been reduced rapidly in PRES (Figure 7.1B). Venous sinus thrombosis may be diagnosed as the empty delta sign on CT scan (Figure 7.2B).

Without secondary prevention, the annual recurrence rate is around 25% (Lagunju et al., 2011; Njamnshi et al., 2006) but may be as high as 78% (Noubiap et al., 2017). In one study of children, the nine recurrences occurred from 3 to 48 months after the initial stroke (Lagunju et al., 2019); one had a third stroke eight months after the second.

Incidence of Ischaemic Stroke

The few available data (Noubiap et al., 2017) suggests that overall, the incidence of stroke in children with SCD residing in Africa is at least 0.88 per 100 PYO (Abdullahi, DeBaun, Jordan, Rodeghier, & Galadanci, 2019). The incidence may be even higher, for example, 1.7 per 100 PYO in Ibadan from 2004 to -2008 (12.5% recurrences) and 3 per 100 PYO in another study from Ibadan of 66 children aged 37–197 months and followed for 12 months (Noubiap et al., 2017). The incidence of recurrent stroke in untreated patients appears to be as high as 17–28 recurrent strokes per 100 PYO (Abdullahi et al., 2019; Lagunju, Brown, & Sodeinde, 2013).

Acute Treatment of Ischaemic Stroke

Diagnosis and management of acute seizures and status epilepticus along local guidelines (see below) is crucial to prevent further brain injury, adequate hydration is important, particularly if there is evidence of venous sinus thrombosis, and blood pressure should be stabilised to prevent hypotension and extension of any infarction. Partial exchange blood transfusion is the standard of care for acute treatment of stroke, and it is rated by expert consensus to be superior to simple transfusion, with evidence for a reduction in risk of recurrence (Hulbert et al., 2006). It is safe and well tolerated and was associated with complete resolution of symptoms and signs in one series (Faye et al., 2017), but it carries the same risk as top up (simple) transfusions for other indications. In Africa, where resources are limited and facilities for automated red cell exchange are not readily available, the exchange is done manually and therefore requires skill and expertise. The donor blood must be of the haemoglobin A phenotype and packed cells are preferred over whole blood transfusion in order to achieve significant reduction in %HbS concentration. Despite increased exposure to donors with red cell exchange compared to simple transfusions, several studies have shown no increase in the rates of allo-immunisation (Venkateswaran, Teruya, Bustillos, Mahoney, Jr., & Mueller, 2011).

Rehabilitation in the acute phase should also be considered and may be economically feasible using smartphone technology with trained therapists (Boma, Panda, Ngoy Mande, & Bonnechere, 2023).

Secondary Prevention of Ischaemic Stroke in Patients with SCD Living in Africa

Chronic Blood Transfusion

Although the evidence is of low quality (Estcourt, Kohli, Hopewell, Trivella, & Wang, 2020), in the USA and Europe, if tolerated, chronic transfusion is the mainstay of the prevention of recurrent ischaemic stroke (Stotesbury et al., 2021a). Although this is relatively costly and the risk of infection may be greater, many centres in Africa offer this option to patients who have had an ischaemic stroke (Boma et al., 2017; Dokekias & Basseila, 2010; Duru et al., 2021). Partial manual exchange is offered in some centres (Dokekias & Basseila, 2010; Boma et al., 2017). Alloimmunisation may occur, particularly to E, D, C and K antigens, with a risk of 7.4 (95% confidence interval: 5.1–10.0) per 100 transfused patients in a systematic review of African studies (Boateng, Ngoma, Bates, & Schonewille, 2019); the risk increases with age and number of transfusions. Chelation increases the annual cost – from US$3,345 without iron chelation and >US $5,000 with chelation (Boma et al., 2017). For secondary prevention where the benefit:risk ratio has been established in the USA in comparison with switching to hydroxyurea (Ware et al., 2011), families may refuse chronic transfusion for a number of reasons. High economic costs with out-of-pocket payment, unavailability of blood, need to regularly seek for blood donors, cultural beliefs and high frequency of transfusion reactions are major challenges to a successful chronic blood transfusion programme in African countries such as Nigeria (Lagunju & Brown, 2012).

Hydroxyurea

In a study from Ibadan, 13 children who had had an ischaemic stroke received hydroxyurea to maximum tolerated dose (20–25 mg/kg/day) while 18 declined. The secondary stroke incidence of 7/100 person years in the hydroxyurea group was significantly lower than the 28/100 person years in the non-HU group (P = 0.001, OR 3.808, 95% confidence intervals 1.556, 9.317) (Lagunju et al., 2013). A randomised trial of hydroxyurea at low (10 mg/kg) and moderate (20 mg/kg) dose conducted in northern Nigeria showed no difference between the groups for the incidence of recurrent stroke (7.1 and 6.0 per 100 PYO, respectively) (Abdullahi et al., 2023) compared with 17.4 per 100 PYO in the feasibility study (Abdullahi et al., 2019). The authors concluded that 10 mg/kg was the minimum efficacious dose of hydroxyurea for secondary stroke prevention (Abdullahi et al., 2023).

Primary Prevention of Stroke in Patients with SCD Living in Africa

Newborn Screening and Prevention of Infection

The later the diagnosis, the higher the stroke incidence in children (Lagunju et al., 2011); so newborn screening and prevention of complications, including acute anemia and infection, might prevent stroke. Meningitis secondary to *Streptococcus pneumoniae* and *Haemophilus influenzae* may be associated with cerebrovascular disease and contemporaneous or later stroke, but whether or not this has been an important cause in SCD is controversial (Kehinde et al., 2008).

Transcranial Doppler Ultrasound (TCD)

Screening for stroke risk using transcranial Doppler (TCD) and appropriate management for those at high risk does appear to have successfully achieved primary stroke prevention (Kirkham & Lagunju, 2021). Non-imaging pulsed TCD has been used to measure the time-averaged maximum of the mean velocities (TAMMV) along the length of the intracranial arteries (distal internal carotid (ICA), middle cerebral (MCA), anterior cerebral (ACA) and posterior cerebral (PCA) arteries) which are typically affected in SCD (Nichols, Jones, & Adams, 2001). Increased TCD velocities may be associated with increased cerebral blood flow (CBF) in the presence of anaemia (Prohovnik, Hurlet-Jensen, Adams, De, & Pavlakis, 2009) or narrowing of the artery diameter (Adams, Aaslid, el, Nichols, & McKie, 1988; Adams, Nichols, Figueroa, McKie, & Lott, 1992). ICA/MCA TAMMV equal or greater than 200 cm/sec (defined as Abnormal; Figure 7.4A) are associated with a 40% risk of stroke over a three year-period, while there is a 7% risk over the same period for Conditional TAMMV (Figure 7.4B) (170–199 cm/sec) (Adams et al., 1997). There are no longitudinal data on stroke risk using

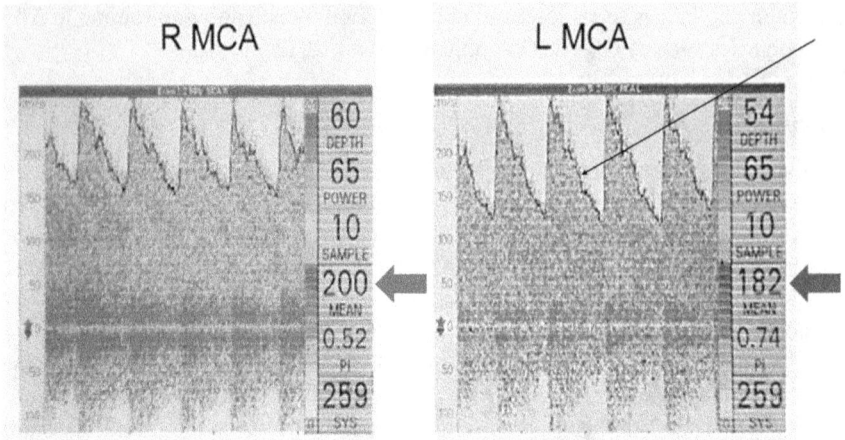

Figure 7.4 Spectrograms from a transcranial Doppler study showing (A) abnormal time-averaged mean of the maximum velocity (TAMMV; black line; 40% stroke risk over three years) of 200 cm/sec. (B) Conditional TAMMV of 182 cm/sec (black line with arrow; 7% stroke risk over three years) when normal (low stroke risk) is <170 cm/sec.

peak systolic velocity (PSV) (Modebe et al., 2023) but for trials of treatment, cutoffs of >250 cm/sec for Abnormal and of 200–249 cm/sec for Conditional TCD appear appropriate.

Imaging TCD (TCDi) in SCD has been undertaken using Duplex Doppler on available ultrasound machines purchased for cardiac, foetal or peripheral vascular work (Malouf, Jr. et al., 2001; Mohammed-Nafi'u, Oniyangi, Akano, Aikhionbare, & Okon, 2021; Neish, Blews, Simms, Merritt, & Spinks, 2002; Salama, Rady, Hashem, & El-Ghamrawy, 2020), although there is a lack of data on the cutoff for prediction of stroke risk. An Egyptian study using TCDi routinely operated by radiologists found only five (6%) patients had Conditional TAMMV, 4 with HbSS, while one (1%) with HbSβ-thalassaemia had Abnormal TCD velocities in the right MCA (Salama et al., 2020). Studies have shown that TCDi velocity values for stroke prevention in sickle cell anaemia children and adults yield lower values compared to the STOP criteria (Jones et al., 2001; McCarville, Li, Xiong, & Wang, 2004). Angle corrected TCDi, on the other hand, can give lower or higher TAMMV values in some vessels which may lead to over- or under-estimation of abnormal TCD (Krejza et al., 2007). Currently, if there has been angle correction, ICA/MCA TAMMV >185 cm/sec should be considered Abnormal. However, studies where TCDi without angle correction was compared with non-imaging TCD yielded comparable velocities in the MCA and tICA (Padayachee, Thomas, Arnold, & Inusa, 2012). If TCDi is used, there should be no angle correction, in which case the criteria for Abnormal and Conditional TCD are the same as for non-imaging TCD.

Prevalence of Abnormal and Conditional Transcranial Doppler in Africa

The prevalence of abnormal TCD varies across studies conducted in Africa (Table 7.2). The rate was nearly 5% in Nigeria (Lagunju, Sodeinde, & Telfer, 2012) and 7% in Tanzania (Cox et al., 2014) but has been reported to be lower in other African countries, including Kenya (Makani et al., 2009) and Uganda (Green et al., 2019). In the African meta-analysis, the prevalence of abnormal and conditional TCD was 10.6% and 6.1%, respectively (Noubiap et al., 2017).

The STOP study demonstrated that TCD is a useful tool for screening and detection of patients at risk of stroke in the sickle population with a 92%

Table 7.2 TCD screening and chronic transfusion for primary prevention of stroke in children with SCD in Africa.

	n Studied	Conditional	Abnormal	Conditional + abnormal
		Transcranial Doppler prevalence conditional/abnormal		
Egypt	52			14 (30) Abou-Elew, Youssry, Hefny, Hashem, Fouad, & Zayed. (2018).
	78	5 (6) [92]	0	5 (6) Salama, Rady, Hashem, & El-Ghamrawy. (2020).
	60	10	0	10 Tantawy, Andrawes, Adly, El Kady & Shalash. (2013)
Sudan	119	0	0	0 Ismail, Elnour & Mustafa (2019)
Mali	572	68 (12)	30 (5)	98 (17) Dorie, Guindo, Saro, Touré, Fané, Dembelé & Diallo
Nigeria Ibadan	145	29 (20)	6 (4)	35 (24) Lagunju, Sodeinde & Telfer. (2012).
	265	45 (17)	19 (7)	64 (18) [99] Lagunju, Brown & Sodeinde (2015)
	396	74 (19)	28 (7)	102 (26) Lagunju, Labaeka, Ibeh, Orimadegun, Brown & Sodeinde. (2021).
Cameroon	32			12 (38) Ruffieux, Njamnshi, Wonkam, Hauert, Chanal, Verdon et al. (2013)
Kenya	105	0 (0)	3 (3)	3 (3) Makani, Kirkham, Komba, Ajala-Agbo, Otieno, Fegan. et al. (2009)
Uganda	256	38 (15)	5 (2)	43 (17) Green, Munube, Bangirana, Buluma, Kebirungi, Opoka et al. (2019)
Tanzania Dar es Salaam	601	25 (4)	42 (7)	67 (11) [Cox, Makani, Soka, L'Esperence, Kija, Dominguez-Salas, et al. (2014)
	200	1 (0.5)	11 (5.5)	12 (6) Kija, Saunders, Munubhi, Darekar, Barker, Cox, et al. (2019)
	224	3 (1)	1 (0.5)	4 (2) Jacob, Saunders, Sangeda, Ahmed, Tutuba, Kussaga, et al. (2020a).

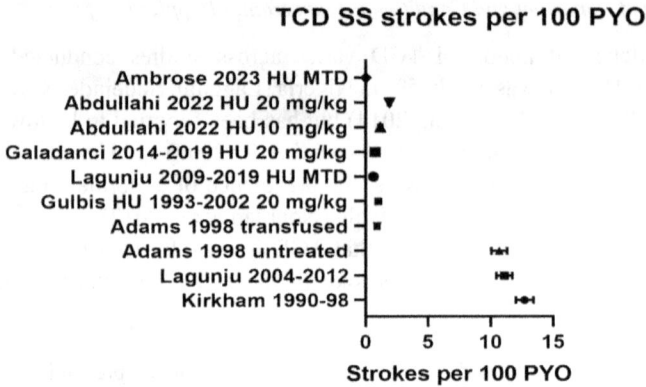

Figure 7.5 The effect in reducing the incidence of stroke in children with sickle cell disease of screening with transcranial Doppler and treating those with abnormal TAMMV (>200 cm/sec) with chronic blood transfusion or hydroxyurea.

reduction in stroke risk for those who were transfused (Kirkham & Lagunju, 2021) (Figure 7.5). Epidemiological evidence suggests that has been a parallel fall in the overall incidence of stroke in SCD in the USA since TCD screening/chronic transfusions began from around 0.88 to 0.17–0.24 per 100 patient years (Kirkham & Lagunju, 2021); this strategy appears to be cost effective (Mazumdar, Heeney, Sox, & Lieu, 2007). However, as for secondary prevention as discussed above, chronic transfusion programmes may not be feasible in Africa.

Effect of Hydroxyurea on Risk of Stroke in Children with SCD and Abnormal TCD

The available data shows that hydroxyurea reduces TAMMV in those with abnormal and conditional velocities (Ambrose et al., 2023; DeBaun et al., 2020) and reduces the incidence of first strokes in children with SCD living in Africa (Figure 7.5). In a cohort study of 34 patients with abnormal TCD in Belgium treated with hydroxyurea 20 mg/kg/day, the incidence of stroke was 1 per 100 PYO and in a feasibility single arm trial of fixed-dose 20 mg/kg hydroxyurea in northern Nigeria, the rate was 0.76 per 100 PYO (Galadanci et al., 2020), both less than the expected rate of 10.7 strokes per 100 PYO in the untreated arm of the STOP study (Galadanci et al., 2020). In the randomised SPRING trial comparing 10 and 20 mg/kg fixed dose hydroxyurea for patients with abnormal TCD velocities (>200 cm/sec) with a primary stroke endpoint, the incidence rates were 1.19 and 1.92 per 100 person-years, respectively, suggesting that an affordable dose as low at 10 mg/kg is effective in reducing stroke risk and requires minimal monitoring on sites only able to perform haematocrit. If monitoring of white cell count is available, escalation to maximum tolerated dose of hydroxyuea is feasible and may further reduce stroke risk. A study in Ibadan using maximum tolerated dose hydroxyurea for 396 children with conditional or abnormal TCD velocities (≥170 cm/sec) with follow-up over 5–10 (median 7.2) years found that velocities reduced significantly over 5–35 (median 10) months with doses of 15–31 mg/kg; two children had a stroke with an incidence of 0.08 per 100 PYO (Lagunju et al., 2021). In an open label Phase II study of maximum tolerated dose of hydroxyurea in children with conditional or abnormal velocities in Mwanza, Tanzania with a primary endpoint of change of TCD velocity after 12 months, 86% reverted to normal velocities and there were no clinical strokes (Ambrose et al., 2023). An open label, single arm clinical trial is being conducted over three years in Uganda (https://www.clinicaltrials.gov/study/ NCT04750707) to test the impact of hydroxyurea treatment at a dose of 20 mg/kg/ day on neurological and cognitive tests and TAMMV in 270 children with SCA starting at ages 3–9 years; a random 90 will also be offered MRI at baseline and three years (R Idro, personal communication).

Intracranial Haemorrhage

CLINICAL PRESENTATION AND EPIDEMIOLOGY

People with SCD may suffer spontaneous intracranial haemorrhage into the extra-dural (Figure 7.6A), subdural (Figure 7.6B) and subarachnoid (Figure 7.6C) spaces as well as intracerebrally (Figure 7.6D). In the USA CSSCD, the risk of haemor-rhagic stroke was highest during early adulthood when the risk of ischaemic stroke was lowest, potentially indicating different underlying mechanisms or progressive vasculopathy (Ohene-Frempong et al., 1998). It is not yet clear whether the inci-dence of haemorrhagic stroke has been altered by interventions for children with SCD (Fox et al., 2022).

There is a paucity of case series of haemorrhagic stroke in SCD from African countries, probably related to the difficulty in making a provisional diagnosis and obtaining immediate imaging as well as the high early mortality (Matuja, Mun-seri, & Khanbhai, 2020; Njamnshi et al., 2006). Even with neuroimaging it may be difficult to diagnose subtle intracranial haemorrhage, e.g. in the subarachnoid space, without specialist MRI sequences such as gradient echo or susceptibility

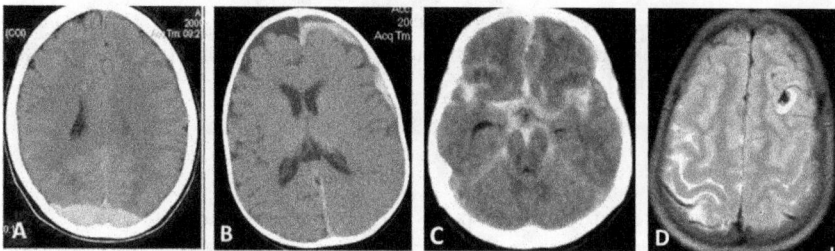

Figure 7.6 CT scans showing haemorrhage in children with sickle cell disease. (A) Extra-dural haemorrhage. (B) Left convexity and interhemispheric subdural haema-toma and left cerebral swelling. (C) Left frontal subarachnoid haemorrhage in a child with bilateral posterior frontal/parietal cortical iatrophy. (D) Intraparen-chymal haemorrhage

(Stotesbury et al., 2021a). A CT study of 14 children with stroke in the context of SCD from Ibadan found that 21% had intracranial haemorrhage (Ogunseyinde, Obajimi, & Fatunde, 2005). The two patients with suspected haemorrhagic stroke, one with a parieto-occipital haematoma on CT, in a study from Cameroon were both on their 20s (Njamnshi et al., 2006). In a study of adults with intracranial haemorrhage from Burkina Faso (mean age 56 years), there appeared to be an apparent excess of people with HbAS and HbAC, as well as 3 of 74 patients homozygous for haemoglobin C (Napon et al., 2012), but no patients with SCD, perhaps because haemorrhage in this condition has the highest incidence in young adults (20–30 years) and mortality is high (Matuja et al., 2020; Ohene-Frempong et al., 1998; Ohene-Frempong et al., 1998).

Subarachnoid (Figure 7.6C) and intracerebral (Figure 7.6D) haemorrhage occur in the context of acute hypertension and may be associated with corticosteroid use, recent transfusion or bone marrow transplantation (Strouse, Hulbert, DeBaun, Jordan, & Casella, 2006). Intracranial haemorrhage in older patients is commonly related to aneurysm formation (Preul, Cendes, Just, & Mohr, 1998). The aneurysms which rupture are typically located at the bifurcations of major vessels, particularly in the vertebrobasilar circulation. Intraparenchymal bleeding may be associated with large-vessel vasculopathy, especially if moyamoya formation is present (Dobson et al., 2002). Venous sinus thrombosis (Sebire et al., 2005) and reversible posterior leukencephalopathy (Henderson et al., 2003) may also be associated with haemorrhage. Extradural (Figure 7.6A) (Iversen et al., 2019; Saha & Saha, 2019) and subdural (Figure 7.6B) (Obajimi, Jumah, & Iddrisu, 2002) haematomata occur in the absence of significant head trauma in SCD, probably related to hypervascular areas of bone.

MANAGEMENT OF HAEMORRHAGIC STROKE

Careful nursing of a comatose patient to avoid secondary complications, such as aspiration pneumonia and skin breakdown, is important. If blood pressure is high, it should be monitored very closely and brought down slowly, over at least 48–72 hours, as the autoregulatory range may be higher than normal and secondary ischaemia may supervene. Space-occupying intracranial haematomas (intracerebral, subdural, extradural) and clipping of any aneurysm require neurosurgical intervention if available.

PREVENTION OF HAEMORRHAGIC STROKE

Although blood pressure may be lower in the population of people with SCD, the available evidence suggests that relative (Benneh-Akwasi et al., 2018), and perhaps progressive, hypertension is an important risk factor for haemorrhagic stroke (Nguweneza et al., 2022a, 2022b). Hypertension may also be associated with other presentations, e.g. with acute visual loss (Lagunju & Brown, 2012) and/ or seizures in the context of PRES (Figure 7.1B), which may lead to ischaemic or haemorrhagic stroke (Stotesbury et al., 2021a). Regular measurement of systolic, diastolic and pulse pressure (Benneh-Akwasi et al., 2018) and plotting on an appropriate centile chart for people with SCD could allow the development of management strategies to decrease the risk of PRES and haemorrhagic stroke risk and increase life expectancy.

Seizures

Epidemiology

Patients with SCD may also have single and recurrent seizures (Kehinde et al., 2008; Lagunju & Brown, 2012). ICA/MCA TAMMV on TCD is higher in children with SCD and recent seizures, while regional cerebral blood flow is lower ipsilateral to the electroencephalographic abnormality (Prengler, Boyd, Lane, & Kirkham, 2001). Most of the cohort data comes from low-middle income countries where neuroimaging is unaffordable, making the distinction between febrile and acute symptomatic seizures in young children very difficult. Between 7% and 10% of individuals with SCD will experience at least one seizure (Lagunju & Brown, 2012). A case-control study from Lagos, Nigeria, found that 10% of children with SCD had febrile seizures compared with 2% of controls (Kehinde et al., 2008). Febrile seizures (HbSS; n = 6, HbSC; n = 1), acute symptomatic seizures (n = 5), single unprovoked seizures (n = 2) and epilepsy (separate occurrence of two or more unprovoked seizures; n = 6) were all diagnosed in Lagunju's description of adverse neurological outcomes in 214 Nigerian children with SCD (Lagunju & Brown, 2012). In a meta-analysis of studies from Africa, the prevalence of seizures was 4.4% (Noubiap et al., 2017) and was higher in studies with a smaller sample size and in more recent studies.

Treatment

A single seizure does not mandate anticonvulsant treatment but if available TCD should be performed and treatment with hydroxyurea should be considered for Conditional or Abnormal TAMMV in view of the evidence that the drug reduces TAMMV. Treatment of seizures in SCD should follow the standard protocol for management of seizures, including febrile, acute symptomatic and epileptic seizures. Children with SCD and epilepsy have been shown to respond to first-line anti-epileptic drugs, with five of six children attaining seizure remission on carbamazepine monotherapy, the drug of choice for focal seizures(Lagunju & Brown, 2012). If there is more than one seizure, local guidelines for management of epilepsy should be followed using available drugs including Phenobarbitone and Carbamazepine. After a period of seizure freedom of 1–2 years withdrawal of anticonvulsants should be considered, typically during long school holidays when the child can be monitored for recurrence of seizures by the family.

Headache

Epidemiology

Headache affects between 20% and 45% of patients with SCD and may occur at any age, including in young children (Noubiap et al., 2017). A case-control study from Lagos, Nigeria, found that 25% of children with SCD aged 4–14 years had headaches compared with 7.3% of healthy controls with HbAA recruited from a local school (Kehinde et al., 2008); the proportion in the SCD population stayed the same in adolescents and adults, while that in controls recruited from the university increased in adolescence, although the difference remained statistically significant at all ages. Severe headache can also be a symptom of intracranial haemorrhage: subdural, intraparenchymal, subarachnoid, or intraventricular (Adams, 1994) and neuroimaging (Figure 7.5D) should be performed as an emergency at initial presentation. Venous sinus thrombosis and pseudotumor cerebri have also been reported and should be excluded in those presenting with acute headache (Stotesbury et al., 2021a).

Treatment

Acute presentation with headache in SCD can present a diagnostic challenge and a thorough evaluation is indicated to exclude severe and potentially devastating conditions like stroke, intracranial haemorrhage, venous sinus thrombosis, moyamoya, PRES, facial and orbital bone infarcts, dental pain and osteomyelitis (Vgontzas, Charleston, & Robbins, 2016). Headache is not a typical symptom in an acute painful crisis. Once serious disease has been excluded, benign headaches, including migraine, in children with SCD, have been found to respond to simple analgesics taken at onset and lifestyle modifications (Lagunju & Brown, 2012). Headache frequency in some patients with migraine is reduced by cutting out food triggers, including chocolate, cheese and orange juice, which can be helpful at times of additional stress, e.g. with school examinations.

Central Nervous System Infections

Children with SCD can present with central nervous system infections such as meningitis (Figure 7.2A,B) (Lagunju & Brown, 2012), bacterial abscess (Figure 7.2C), malaria and parasitic diseases, including neurocysticercosis and Hydatid cyst. The incidence of pneumococcal disease has decreased with penicillin prophylaxis and immunisation in the USA, but these preventative strategies are not widely available in Africa (Chen et al., 2019), where bacterial infections are still prevalent alongside malaria. Anaemia is a risk factor for meningitis (Pelkonen, Roine, Kallio, Jahnukainen, & Peltola, 2022) and SCD was found in 10% of children with meningitis in Angola, fivefold more than in the general population (Pelkonen, Roine, Bernardino, Jahnukainen, & Peltola, 2022). The same study reported a higher prevalence of pneumococcal meningitis, a higher risk of death and a significantly longer period of hospitalisation in children with meningitis and SCD compared with those without SCD (Pelkonen et al., 2022).

Other Neurological Presentations

There are clinical descriptions of paraplegia (Lagunju & Brown, 2012; Kehinde et al., 2008), myopathy (Landoure et al., 2017), myelopathy and neuropathy (Prengler, Pavlakis, Prohovnik, & Adams, 2002) but access to a neurological opinion and investigation with electromyography and nerve conduction and/or muscle biopsy may not be available. There are few population-based studies of prevalence but one case-control study in Nigeria found a high prevalence of sensory neuropathy (Kehinde et al., 2008). This study also found a trend for an excess of tremor (Kehinde et al., 2008), which might be related to basal ganglia ischaemia.

Cognitive Impairment

Cognitive difficulties are common in SCD and may be particularly debilitating due to potential adverse effects on educational achievement, employment opportunities, social and economic mobility, disease self-management, healthcare use, mental health and quality of life. Cognitive impairment may manifest in infancy, during the preschool years affecting school readiness, with academic difficulties during childhood through adolescence, and employment difficulties during adulthood. Throughout childhood, adolescence and adulthood, patients continue to be at risk of impairment across a range of domains, including general intelligence, executive function, attention, visuo-spatial abilities, verbal abilities, processing speed, working memory and visual and verbal short-term memory (Stotesbury et al., 2021a). Adaptive and behavioural difficulties increase with age, but it is not yet clear whether this is related to a difference in developmental trajectory (Hamdule et al., 2023; Jacob et al., 2022; Koelbel et al., 2023) or a decline in performance through childhood (Wang et al., 2001) and/or adulthood (Ampomah et al., 2022).

Where resources allow, brief neuropsychological screening ought to feature as part of routine care from early childhood. Tests undertaken in African settings include the Mullen Scales of Early Learning (Green et al., 2019; Bangirana, Boehme, Birabwa, Opoka, Munube, Mupere, Kasirye, Ru, Idro & Green (2023)), the Kaufman Assessment Battery for Children (Green et al., 2019), Raven's progressive matrices (Jacob et al., 2022), measures of processing speed (coding, symbol search, cancellation), working memory (letter-number sequencing and digit span) (Jacob et al., 2022; Ruffieux et al., 2013) and perceptual reasoning (block design, picture concept, matrix reasoning) (Jacob et al., 2022) from the Wechsler scales and tests of motor speed (Purdue pegboard) and executive function (e.g. Trails) (Ampomah et al., 2022; Ruffieux et al., 2013). Computerised tests and executive function questionnaires have also been used effectively (Bangirana et al., 2023).

Studies rarely report formal diagnoses of cognitive impairment, which makes meaningful comment on the prevalence challenging. The overwhelming majority of studies also report sample-level mean performance on cognitive tests, rather than the proportion of patients with scores that fall into established clinical categories. A study from Cameroon found that 37.5% of children had mild to severe cognitive difficulties (Ruffieux et al., 2013). In a study in Tanzanian children, processing speed was lower than controls (mean difference 4.15 points; p = .002) and there was a trend for lower working memory index (mean difference 4.14 points; p = .089) (Jacob et al., 2022). For coding and cancellation, both measures of processing speed and attention improvement in performance with age was slower in the children with SCD (Jacob et al., 2022). Using the Rey-Osterrieth Complex figure and a block design test to test memory, visuo-spatial skills and executive function, Matondo et al. found impaired IQ on block design (mental age <80% chronological age) in 73% of 80 Tanzanian sibling controls and in 85% of 233 children with SCD aged 9–15 years, most of whom had had access to primary education (Matondo, Kija, & Manji, 2020). Ability to copy the Rey-Osterrieth Complex figure was impaired in 68% of those with SCD and 45% of siblings (Matondo et al., 2020). For all tests, the proportion of impaired children with SCD increased with increasing age and school absence, while low body mass index had an effect on copying only (Matondo et al., 2020). A study of Ghanian adults found that those with SCD performed worse than controls in all cognitive test domains and showed declines in visuospatial abilities, processing speed and executive functioning (Ampomah et al., 2022). Although there is significant variability within SCD populations, patients are at greater risk of clinically significant cognitive impairment. Neurodevelopmental screening using questionnaires and relatively simple tools with minimal cultural and educational biases, such as cancellation, is recommended in the recent guidelines, particularly in early childhood (DeBaun et al., 2020) and will allow urgently needed trials of treatment (https://www.clinicaltrials.gov/study/NCT04750707). There may be opportunities for trials of disease-modifying strategies, but caregiver education and nutrition are also very important in cognitive development (Bangirana et al., 2023).

Abnormalities Detectable on Cross-Sectional Neuroimaging in Asymptomatic Patients

Covert (Silent) Cerebral Infarction

Magnetic resonance imaging, when available, can show the distribution of infarction in overt (clinical) and covert (silent) stroke (Figure 7.7). Silent cerebral infarction (SCI) infarction is found in up to 40% of patients with SCD without clinical symptoms overall, with a steady rate of accumulation (Houwing et al., 2020). Prevalence estimates may vary not only with age, but also with scanner magnet strength and voxel size (Stotesbury, Kawadler, Saunders, & Kirkham, 2021). Using a 1.5T MRI scanner, studies in Tanzania found that 27% of children aged 5–19 years with no neurological history had SCI (Jacob et al., 2020a), while in Uganda, >50% of children had SCI and or MRA abnormality despite having no history of stroke,

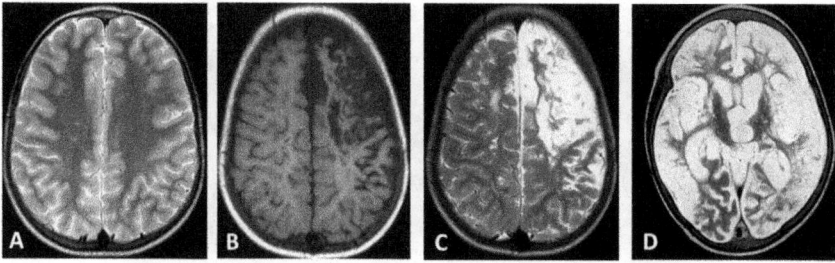

Figure 7.7 Axial MRI scans of mature infarction in children with sickle cell disease. (A) T2-weighted images showing silent deep white matter infarcts in the centrum semiovale. (B) Axial T1- and (C) T2-weighted showing a mature left anterior and middle cerebral artery territory infarcts. (D) Axial T2-weighted images showing almost complete cerebral cortical infarction (some sparing of the right occipital lobe) and external capsular infarction with atrophy of the basal ganglia in a child with cerebral vasculopathy.

normal TCD and normal cognition (Idro et al., 2022). Patients with SCD and overt or silent infarction may be more likely to have abnormal psychometric testing (Idro et al., 2022; Kawadler, Clayden, Clark, & Kirkham, 2016; Prussien, Jordan, De-Baun, & Compas, 2019). In the Ugandan study two-thirds of those with abnormal cognition on screening had SCI on MRI compared with one-third of those with normal cognition (Idro et al., 2022) while only processing speed performance was worse in those with SCI compared with those without SCI and sibling controls in a Tanzanian study (Jacob et al., 2022). However, studies at higher field strength have been less likely to find an association between cognitive function and SCI (Stotesbury et al., 2022). Quantitative MRI may clarify some of these issues (Jacob et al., 2020b, 2023; Stotesbury et al., 2021b) as well as providing information of clinical use in addition to an experienced radiologist's reading of the conventional MRI study. In the CSSCD, SCI was also associated with cognitive decline (Wang et al., 2001), but this is controversial (Hogan et al., 2008).

Cerebrovascular Disease on Magnetic Resonance Angiography

In SCD, magnetic resonance angiography (MRA) can be up to 85% accurate when compared with conventional angiography (Kandeel, Zimmerman, & Ohene-Frempong, 1996). Turbulence or signal dropout on MRA may be graded as mild, moderate and severe (Dlamini et al., 2017; Jacob et al., 2020a) (Figure 7.8). Alternatively the degree of apparent stenosis can be estimated using the criteria from the SWiTCH trial (Helton et al., 2014; Idro et al., 2022) although there are few data looking at the relationship with the degree of arterial stenosis on conventional angiography and MRA may overestimate.

In a Tanzanian study of children with SCD, 48/200 with either low (<50 cm/sec), absent or elevated (>150 cm/sec). MCA TAMMV underwent MRA of which 24 (50%) were abnormal, including all six with prior stroke (Kija et al., 2019).

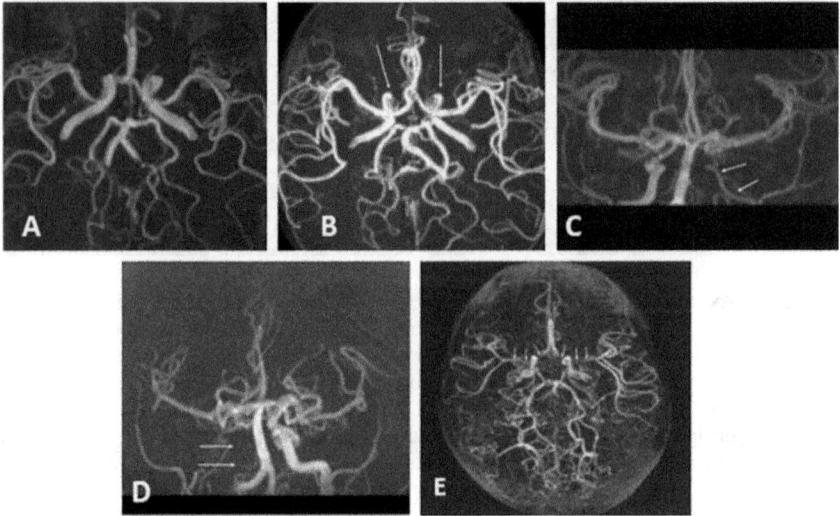

Figure 7.8 Magnetic resonance angiography in Tanzanian children with sickle cell disease. (A) Normal middle cerebral artery (MCA; Grade 0). (B) Turbulent flow within the cavernous carotid arteries probably related to anaemia (Grade 1 vasculopathy.) (C) Marked narrowing of the left internal carotid artery (ICA) at the skull base (arrows; Grade 2 vasculopathy). The right terminal ICA is also narrowed and much of the supply will be coming through the posterior circulation. (D) Occluded right ICA with good flow through the left ICA and posterior circulation (Grade 3 vasculopathy). (E) Moyamoya syndrome; bilateral narrowing of the terminal ICA and branches with moyamoya and posterior cerebral artery collaterals (Grade 4 vasculopathy).

A study of 81 children with SCD in Uganda, 52 of whom had either had a stroke, a conditional (TAMMV>170 cm/sec) or abnormal (TAMMV>200 cm/sec) TCD or cognitive difficulties, found MRA abnormalities in 22 (31%) (Idro et al., 2022). Another study of 224 Tanzanian children with no previous neurological presentations found stenosis and occlusion in 16 (7%) and 2 (1%), respectively (Jacob et al., 2020a). Cognitive difficulties were not worse in those with MRA abnormalities (Jacob et al., 2022). Occlusion or severe stenosis, typically of the distal internal carotid, with collaterals, or moyamoya (Figure 7.8), was reported in one patient in Tanzania and four patients in Uganda (Idro et al., 2022; Kija et al., 2019). In Sudan (Khartoum) moyamoya angiographic features were also reported in 48 of the 50 patients with SCD who had a Brain MRA (Elmahdi et al., 2022).

Extracranial ICA stenosis and occlusion in children with SCD have been reported in Europe and the USA (Telfer et al., 2011); pathogenesis is unclear but some may be secondary to extracranial dissection (Telfer et al., 2011), while others appear to be associated with intracranial stenosis (Schlotman et al., 2021). There is controversy over whether extracranial stenosis is associated with SCI (Bernaudin et al., 2015; Schlotman et al., 2021). There are few data from Africa but extracranial carotid artery occlusion or dissection should be considered in children with SCDpresenting with symptoms of stroke and, if available, imaging of the neck vessels should be part of the investigation of these patients in the acute phase (Telfer et al., 2011).

Quantitative MRI: Compromise of White Matter Integrity and Brain Volume

Quantitative MRI measures for investigation of brain structure and function in SCD have been developed over the last few years (Stotesbury et al., 2021a; Stotesbury et al., 2021b). Diffusion tensor imaging has been used to investigate white matter integrity (Gonzalez-Zacarias et al., 2022; Jacob et al., 2020b; Kawadler et al., 2015; Stotesbury et al., 2018). In a study from Tanzania (Jacob et al., 2020b) radial diffusivity was higher in patients with SCD and SCI, while mean diffusivity and axial diffusivity were negatively correlated with haemoglobin and fractional anisotropy was lower in those with MRA abnormality in a number of white matter regions. Measurement of total, cortical and subcortical brain volumes has shown differences from controls (Choi et al., 2019; Darbari et al., 2018; Hamdule et al., 2023; Jacob et al., 2023; Kawadler et al., 2013). In her Tanzanian cohort, Jacob et al. (2023)found reduced grey matter volumes in the patients with SCD, but some white matter areas appeared to be spared.

Risk Factors for Neurological, Cognitive and Neuroradiological Abnormalities

The various neurological and cognitive complications of SCD share some risk factors but not others (Hirtz & Kirkham, 2019). The phenotype may be influenced by the different β-haplotypes (the nucleotide 5′ and 3′ sickle cell gene sequence). There are three major African and African American haplotypes: Senegal, Benin and Bantu (or Central African Republic) (Serjeant, 1997). In addition, there is an independent haplotype in India and Saudi Arabia (Ballas, 1998). However, the majority of the available data suggests that the β-haplotypes are not associated with stroke (Abou-Elew et al., 2018; Belisario et al., 2010; Domingos et al., 2014; Hatzlhofer et al., 2021; Rodrigues et al., 2016) and, although there have been few studies in Africa, there is currently no evidence that there are large difference in prevalence of stroke between populations (Marks et al., 2018; Noubiap et al., 2017). Stroke risk is reduced in the presence of co-inherited alpha-thalassemia (Cox et al., 2014; Hatzlhofer et al., 2021; Neonato et al., 2000). The effect of co-inherited Glucose-6-phosphate dehydrogenase deficiency remains controversial (Cox et al., 2014; Belisario et al., 2016; Bernaudin et al., 2008; Joly et al., 2016; Miller, Milton, & Steinberg, 2011; Rees et al., 2009; Thangarajh et al., 2012).

In addition to abnormal TCD in cohort studies (Hirtz & Kirkham, 2019), the biggest risk factor for stroke in population studies of children and adults with SCD is hypertension (Pegelow et al., 1997; Strouse, Jordan, Lanzkron, & Casella, 2009), with diabetes mellitus, hyperlipidemia, atrial fibrillation, and renal disease also risk factors in adults (Strouse et al., 2009). Predictors of ICA/MCA velocity and/ or abnormal TCD (Hirtz & Kirkham, 2019) include low haemoglobin (Lagunju, Sodeinde, Brown, Akinbami, & Adedokun, 2014; Rankine-Mullings et al., 2018; Rees et al., 2008), haematocrit (Brass, Pavlakis, DeVivo, Piomelli, & Mohr, 1988), haemoglobin oxygen saturation (Lagunju et al., 2014; Makani et al., 2009; Quinn, Variste, & Dowling, 2009; Rankine-Mullings et al., 2018), and markers of hae-molysis including reticulocyte count (Rankine-Mullings et al., 2018), aspartate transaminase (Rees et al., 2008) and lactate dehydrogenase (O'Driscoll, Height, Dick, & Rees, 2008).

Conclusion

Although in SCD the incidence of first clinical stroke has fallen over the past 3–4 decades in the USA and Europe, this is still a highly prevalent problem in Africa, where the majority of the people with this condition live and where resources for screening and preventative treatment remain scarce. Evidence-based prevention of haemorrhagic stroke at any age and ischaemic stroke in adults is not yet feasible. Further epidemiological studies may allow cost-effective prevention of stroke and other neurological problems across the World.

References

Abdullahi, S. U., DeBaun, M. R., Jordan, L. C., Rodeghier, M., & Galadanci, N. A. (2019). Stroke recurrence in Nigerian children with sickle cell disease: Evidence for a secondary stroke prevention trial. *Pediatr. Neurol., 95*, 73–78.

Abdullahi, S. U., Sunusi, S., Abba, M. S., Sani, S., Inuwa, H. A., Gambo, S. et al. (2023). Hydroxyurea for secondary stroke prevention in children with sickle cell anemia in Nigeria: A randomized controlled trial. *Blood, 141*, 825–834.

Abou-Elew, H. H., Youssry, I., Hefny, S., Hashem, R. H., Fouad, N., & Zayed, R. A. (2018). Beta(S) globin gene haplotype and the stroke risk among Egyptian children with sickle cell disease. *Hematology, 23*, 362–367.

Adamolekun, B., Durosinmi, M. A., Olowu, W., & Adediran, I. (1993). The prevalence and classification of epileptic seizures in Nigerians with sickle-cell anaemia. *J. Trop. Med. Hyg., 96*, 288–290.

Adams, R. J. (1994). Neurological complications. In S. Embury, R. P. Hebbel, N. Mohandas, & M. H. Steinberg (Eds.), *Sickle cell disease: Basic principles and clinical practice.* (1 ed., pp. 599–621). New York: Raven Press Ltd.

Adams, R. J., Aaslid, R., el Gammal, T., Nichols, F. T., & McKie, V. (1988). Detection of cerebral vasculopathy in sickle cell disease using transcranial Doppler ultrasonography and magnetic resonance imaging. Case report. *Stroke, 19*, 518–520.

Adams, R. J., McKie, V. C., Carl, E. M., Nichols, F. T., Perry, R., Brock, K. et al. (1997). Long-term stroke risk in children with sickle cell disease screened with transcranial Doppler. *Ann. Neurol., 42*, 699–704.

Adams, R. J., Nichols, F. T., Figueroa, R., McKie, V., & Lott, T. (1992). Transcranial Doppler correlation with cerebral angiography in sickle cell disease. *Stroke, 23*, 1073–1077.

Adegoke, S. A., Adeodu, O. O., & Adekile, A. D. (2015). Sickle cell disease clinical pheno-types in children from South-Western, Nigeria. *Niger. J. Clin. Pract., 18*, 95–101.

Akingbola, T. S., Tayo, B. O., Salako, B., Layden, J. E., Hsu, L. L., Cooper, R. S., Gordeuk, V. R., & Saraf, S. L. (2014). Comparison of patients from Nigeria and the USA highlights modifiable risk factors for sickle cell anemia complications. *Hemoglobin, 38*, 236–243.

Akpede, G. O. & Airede, A. I. (1993). Acute encephalopathy, hypertension and gram negative sepsis in sickle cell disease. *West Afr. J. Med., 12*, 180–184.

Amayo, E. O., Owade, J. N., Aluoch, J. R., & Njeru, E. K. (1992). Neurological complications of sickle cell anaemia at KNH: A five-year retrospective study. *East Afr. Med. J., 69*, 660–662.

Ambrose, E. E., Latham, T. S., Songoro, P., Charles, M., Lane, A. C., Stuber, S. E. et al. (2023). Hydroxyurea with dose escalation for primary stroke risk reduction in children with sickle cell anaemia in Tanzania (SPHERE): An open-label, phase 2 trial. *Lancet Haematol., 10*, e261–e271.

Ampomah, M. A., Drake, J. A., Anum, A., Amponsah, B., Dei-Adomakoh, Y., Anie, K. et al. (2022). A case-control and seven-year longitudinal neurocognitive study of adults with sickle cell disease in Ghana. *Br. J. Haematol., 199*, 411–426.

Babela, J. R., Nzingoula, S., & Senga, P. (2005). Les crises vaso-occlusives drépanocytaires chez l'enfant et l'adolescent a Brazzaville, Congo. Etude rétrospective de 587 cas [Sickle-cell crisis in the child and teenager in Brazzaville, Congo. A retrospective study of 587 cases]. *Bull. Soc. Pathol. Exot., 98*, 365–370.

Bakr S., Khorshied M., Talha N., Jaffer K. Y., Soliman N., Eid K., & El-Ghamrawy M. (2019). Implication of HMOX1 and CCR5 genotypes on clinical phenotype of Egyptian patients with sickle cell anemia. *Ann. Hematol., 98*, 1805–1812.

Ballas, S. K. (1998). Sickle cell disease: Clinical management. *Baillieres Clin. Haematol., 11*, 185–214.

Bangirana, P., Boehme, A. K., Birabwa, A., Opoka, R. O., Munube, D., Mupere, E., Kasirye, P., Ru, G., Idro, R., & Green, N. S. (2023). Neurocognitive impairment in Ugandan children with sickle cell disease compared to sibling controls: A cross-sectional study. *medRxiv* [Preprint].

Belisario, A. R., Martins, M. L., Brito, A. M., Rodrigues, C. V., Silva, C. M., & Viana, M. B. (2010). Beta-globin gene cluster haplotypes in a cohort of 221 children with sickle cell anemia or Sbeta(0)-thalassemia and their association with clinical and hematological features. *Acta Haematol., 124*, 162–170.

Belisario, A. R., Rodrigues, S. R., Evelin, T. N., Velloso-Rodrigues, C., Maria, S. C., & Borato, V. M. (2016). Glucose-6-phosphate dehydrogenase deficiency in Brazilian children with sickle cell anemia is not associated with clinical ischemic stroke or high-risk transcranial Doppler. *Pediatr. Blood Cancer, 63*, 1046–1049.

Benneh-Akwasi, K. A., Owusu-Ansah, A. T., Ampomah, M. A., Sey, F., Olayemi, E., Nouraie, M. et al. (2018). Prevalence of relative systemic hypertension in adults with sickle cell disease in Ghana. *PLoS One, 13*, e0190347.

Bernaudin, F., Verlhac, S., Arnaud, C., Kamdem, A., Vasile, M., Kasbi, F. et al. (2015). Chronic and acute anemia and extracranial internal carotid stenosis are risk factors for silent cerebral infarcts in sickle cell anemia. *Blood, 125*, 1653–1661.

Bernaudin, F., Verlhac, S., Chevret, S., Torres, M., Coic, L., Arnaud, C. et al. (2008). G6PD deficiency, absence of alpha-thalassemia, and hemolytic rate at baseline are significant independent risk factors for abnormally high cerebral velocities in patients with sickle cell anemia. *Blood, 112*, 4314–4317.

Boateng, L. A., Ngoma, A. M., Bates, I., & Schonewille, H. (2019). Red blood cell alloimmunization in transfused patients with sickle cell disease in Sub-Saharan Africa; A systematic review and meta-analysis. *Transfus. Med Rev., 33*, 162–169.

Boma, M. P., Kaluila Mamba, J. F. J., Muhau, P. P., Bilo, V., Panda Mulefu, J. D., & Diallo, D. A. (2017). Effectiveness, safety, and cost of partial exchange transfusions in patients with sickle-cell anemia at a sickle cell disease center in sub-Saharan Africa. *Med Sante Trop., 27*, 387–391.

Boma, P. M., Panda, J., Ngoy Mande, J. P., & Bonnechere, B. (2023). Rehabilitation: A key service, yet highly underused, in the management of young patients with sickle cell disease after stroke in DR of Congo. *Front. Neurol., 14*, 1104101.

Brass, L. M., Pavlakis, S. G., DeVivo, D., Piomelli, S., & Mohr, J. P. (1988). Transcranial Doppler measurements of the middle cerebral artery. Effect of hematocrit. *Stroke, 19*, 1466–1469.

Chen, C. J., Bakeera-Kitaka, S., Mupere, E., Kasirye, P., Munube, D., Idro, R. et al. (2019). Paediatric immunisation and chemoprophylaxis in a Ugandan sickle cell disease clinic. *J Paediatr. Child Health, 55*, 795–801.

Choi, S., O'Neil, S. H., Joshi, A. A., Li, J., Bush, A. M., Coates, T. D. et al. (2019). Anemia predicts lower white matter volume and cognitive performance in sickle and non-sickle cell anemia syndrome. *Am. J. Hematol., 94*, 1055–1065.

Cox, S. E., Makani, J., Soka, D., L'Esperence, V. S., Kija, E., Dominguez-Salas, P. et al. (2014). Haptoglobin, alpha-thalassaemia and glucose-6-phosphate dehydrogenase poly-morphisms and risk of abnormal transcranial Doppler among patients with sickle cell anaemia in Tanzania. *Br. J. Haematol., 165*, 699–706.

Darbari, D. S., Eigbire-Molen, O., Ponisio, M. R., Milchenko, M. V., Rodeghier, M. J., Casella, J. F. et al. (2018). Progressive loss of brain volume in children with sickle cell anemia and silent cerebral infarct: A report from the silent cerebral infarct transfusion trial. *Am. J. Hematol., 93*, E406–E408.

DeBaun, M. R., Jordan, L. C., King, A. A., Schatz, J., Vichinsky, E., Fox, C. K. et al. (2020). American Society of Hematology 2020 guidelines for sickle cell disease: Prevention, diagnosis, and treatment of cerebrovascular disease in children and adults. *Blood Adv., 4*, 1554–1588.

de Montalembert, M., Beauvais, P., Bachir, D., Galacteros, F., & Girot, R. (1993). Cerebro-vascular accidents in sickle cell disease. Risk factors and blood transfusion influence. French Study Group on Sickle Cell Disease. *Eur. J. Pediatr., 52*, 201–204.

Diagne, I., Diagne-Guèye, N. R., Fall, L., Ndiaye, O., Camara, B., Diouf, S., Signate-Sy, H., & Kuakuvi, N. (2001). Manifestations encéphaliques aiguës chez l'enfant drépano-cytaire sénégalais [Acute encephalic manifestations in Senegalese children with sickle cell disease]. *Dakar Med., 46*, 116–120.

Djunga, S. & Clarysse, J. (1977). L'hémoglobinopathie S. et complications neurologiques [Neurological complications in sickle cell disease (author's transl)]. *Acta. Neurol. Belg., 77*, 105–114.

Dlamini, N., Saunders, D. E., Bynevelt, M., Trompeter, S., Cox, T. C., Bucks, R. S. et al. (2017). Nocturnal oxyhemoglobin desaturation and arteriopathy in a pediatric sickle cell disease cohort. *Neurology, 89*, 2406–2412.

Dobson, S. R., Holden, K. R., Nietert, P. J., Cure, J. K., Laver, J. H., Disco, D. et al. (2002). Moyamoya syndrome in childhood sickle cell disease: A predictive factor for recurrent cerebrovascular events. *Blood, 99*, 3144–3150.

Dokekias, A. E. & Basseila, G. B. (2010). [Results of partial transfusion exchange in 42 homozygous sickle cell patients at university hospital of Brazzaville]. *Transfus. Clin. Biol., 17*, 232–241.

Domingos, I. F., Falcao, D. A., Hatzlhofer, B. L., Cunha, A. F., Santos, M. N., Albuquerque, D. M. et al. (2014). Influence of the betas haplotype and alpha-thalassemia on stroke development in a Brazilian population with sickle cell anaemia. *Ann. Hematol.*, *93*, 1123–1129.

Dorie, A., Guindo, A., Saro, Y. S., Touré, A., Fané, B., Dembelé, A. K., & Diallo, D. A. (2015). Dépistage de la vasculopathie cérébrale drépanocytaire par doppler transcrânien au Mali [Screening of cerebral vasculopathy in sickle cell anemia children using transcranial Doppler]. *Arch. Pediatr.*, *22*, 260–266.

Duru, A., Madu, A. J., Okoye, H., Nonyelu, C., Obodo, O., Okereke, K. et al. (2021). Variations and characteristics of the various clinical phenotypes in a cohort of Nigerian sickle cell patients. *Hematology*, *26*, 684–690.

Elmahdi, M., Fadalla, T., Suliman, M., Elsayed, M., Awad Elhaj, A. M., & Hussein, H. (2022). Moyamoya syndrome and stroke among pediatric sickle cell disease patients in Sudan: A cross-sectional study. *Ann. Med. Surg. (Lond.)*, *78*, 103815.

Estcourt, L. J., Kohli, R., Hopewell, S., Trivella, M., & Wang, W. C. (2020). Blood transfusion for preventing primary and secondary stroke in people with sickle cell disease. *Cochrane Database Syst. Rev.*, *7*, CD003146.

Fatunde, O. J., Adamson, F. G., Ogunseyinde, O., Sodeinde, O., & Familusi, J. B. (2005). Stroke in Nigerian children with sickle cell disease. *Afr. J. Med. Med. Sci.*, *34*, 157–160.

Faye, B. F., Sow, D., Seck, M., Dieng, N., Toure, S. A., Gadji, M. et al. (2017). Efficacy and safety of manual partial red cell exchange in the management of severe complications of sickle cell disease in a developing country. *Adv. Hematol.*, *2017*, 3518402.

Fox, C. K., Leykina, L., Hills, N. K., Kwiatkowski, J. L., Kanter, J., Strouse, J. J. et al. (2022). Hemorrhagic stroke in children and adults with sickle cell anemia: The post-STOP cohort. *Stroke*, *53*, e463–e466.

Galadanci, N. A., Abdullahi, S. U., Ali, A. S., Wudil, J. B., Aminu, H., Tijjani, A. et al. (2020). Moderate fixed-dose hydroxyurea for primary prevention of strokes in Nigerian children with sickle cell disease: Final results of the SPIN trial. *Am. J. Hematol.*, *95*, E247–E250.

George, I. O. & Frank-Briggs, A. I. (2011). Stroke in Nigerian children with sickle cell anaemia. *J. Public Health Epidemiol.*, *3*, 407–409.

Gonzalez-Zacarias, C., Choi, S., Vu, C., Xu, B., Shen, J., Joshi, A. A. et al. (2022). Chronic anemia: The effects on the connectivity of white matter. *Front. Neurol.*, *13*, 894742.

Green, N. S., Munube, D., Bangirana, P., Buluma, L. R., Kebirungi, B., Opoka, R. et al. (2019). Burden of neurological and neurocognitive impairment in pediatric sickle cell anemia in Uganda (BRAIN SAFE): A cross-sectional study. *BMC Pediatr.*, *19*, 381.

Hamdule, S., Kolbel, M., Stotesbury, H., Murdoch, R., Clayden, J. D., Sahota, S. et al. (2023). Effects of regional brain volumes on cognition in sickle cell anemia: A developmental perspective. *Front. Neurol.*, *14*, 1101223.

Hatzlhofer, B. L. D., Pereira-Martins, D. A., de Farias Domingos, I., Arcanjo, G. D. S., Weinhauser, I., Falcao, D. A. et al. (2021). Alpha thalassemia, but not beta(S)-globin haplotypes, influence sickle cell anemia clinical outcome in a large, single-center Brazilian cohort. *Ann. Hematol.*, *100*, 921–931.

Heimlich, J. B., Chipoka, G., Kamthunzi, P., Krysiak, R., Majawa, Y., Mafunga, P., Fedoriw, Y., Phiri, A., Key, N. S., Ataga, K. I., & Gopal, S. (2016). Establishing sickle cell diagnostics and characterizing a paediatric sickle cell disease cohort in Malawi. *Br. J. Haematol.*, *174*, 325–329.

Helton, K. J., Adams, R. J., Kesler, K. L., Lockhart, A., Aygun, B., Driscoll, C. et al. (2014). Magnetic resonance imaging/angiography and transcranial Doppler velocities in sickle cell anemia: Results from the SWiTCH trial. *Blood*, *124*, 891–898.

Henderson, J. N., Noetzel, M. J., McKinstry, R. C., White, D. A., Armstrong, M., & DeBaun, M. R. (2003). Reversible posterior leukoencephalopathy syndrome and silent cerebral infarcts are associated with severe acute chest syndrome in children with sickle cell disease. *Blood, 101*, 415–419.

Hirtz, D. & Kirkham, F. J. (2019). Sickle cell disease and stroke. *Pediatr. Neurol., 95*, 34–41.

Hogan, A., Telfer, P., Prengler, M., Saunders, D., Wade, A. M., Vargha-Khadem, F. et al. (2008). Intellectual function in children with sickle cell anemia: Longitudinal data from the East London cohort. *Br. J. Haematol., 141*, 111.

Houwing, M. E., Grohssteiner, R. L., Dremmen, M. H. G., Atiq, F., Bramer, W. M., de Pagter, A. P. J. et al. (2020). Silent cerebral infarcts in patients with sickle cell disease: A systematic review and meta-analysis. *BMC Med., 18*, 393.

Hulbert, M. L., Scothorn, D. J., Panepinto, J. A., Scott, J. P., Buchanan, G. R., Sarnaik, S. et al. (2006). Exchange blood transfusion compared with simple transfusion for first overt stroke is associated with a lower risk of subsequent stroke: A retrospective cohort study of 137 children with sickle cell anemia. *J. Pediatr., 149*, 710–712.

Idro, R., Boehme, A. K., Kawooya, M., Lubowa, S. K., Munube, D., Bangirana, P. et al. (2022). Brain magnetic resonance imaging and angiography in children with sickle cell anaemia in Uganda in a cross-sectional sample. *J. Stroke Cerebrovasc. Dis., 31*, 106343.

Ismail, W. I. M., Elnour, M., & Mustafa, A. E. M. (2019). Evaluation of transcranial Doppler abnormalities in children with sickle cell disease in El-Obeid Specialized Children's Hospital. *J. Family Med. Prim. Care, 8*, 1176–1181.

Iversen, P. O., Jacob, M., Makame, J., Abisay, M., Yonazi, M., Schuh, A. et al. (2019). A massive extradural hematoma in sickle cell disease and the importance of rapid neuroimaging. *Case Rep. Hematol.*, 1742472.

Izuora, G. I., Kaine, W. N., & Emodi, I. (1989). Neurological disorders in Nigerian children with homozygous sickle cell anaemia. *East Afr. Med. J., 66*, 653–657.

Jacob, M., Kawadler, J. M., Murdoch, R., Ahmed, M., Tutuba, H., Masamu, U. et al. (2023). Brain volume in Tanzanian children with sickle cell anaemia: A neuroimaging study. *Br. J. Haematol., 201*, 114–124.

Jacob, M., Saunders, D. E., Sangeda, R. Z., Ahmed, M., Tutuba, H., Kussaga, F. et al. (2020a). Cerebral infarcts and vasculopathy in Tanzanian children with sickle cell anemia. *Pediatr. Neurol., 107*, 64–70.

Jacob, M., Stotesbury, H., Kawadler, J. M., Lapadaire, W., Saunders, D. E., Sangeda, R. Z. et al. (2020b). White matter integrity in Tanzanian children with sickle cell anemia: A diffusion tensor imaging study. *Stroke, 51*, 1166–1173.

Jacob, M., Stotesbury, H., Kija, E., Saunders, D., Mtei, R. J., Tutuba, H. et al. (2022). Effect of age, cerebral infarcts, vasculopathy and haemoglobin on cognitive function, in Tanzanian children with sickle cell anaemia. *Eur. J. Paediatr. Neurol., 37*, 105–113.

Joly, P., Garnier, N., Kebaili, K., Renoux, C., Dony, A., Cheikh, N. et al. (2016). G6PD deficiency and absence of alpha-thalassemia increase the risk for cerebral vasculopathy in children with sickle cell anemia. *Eur. J. Haematol., 96*, 404–408.

Jones, A. M., Seibert, J. J., Nichols, F. T., Kinder, D. L., Cox, K., Luden, J. et al. (2001). Comparison of transcranial color Doppler imaging (TCDI) and transcranial Doppler (TCD) in children with sickle-cell anemia. *Pediatr. Radiol., 31*, 461–469.

Jude, M. A., Aliyu, G. N., Nalado, A. M., Garba, K. U., Florence, F. O., Hassan, A. et al. (2014). Stroke prevalence amongst sickle cell disease patients in Nigeria: A multi-centre study. *Afr. Health Sci., 14*, 446–452.

Kandeel, A. Y., Zimmerman, R. A., & Ohene-Frempong, K. (1996). Comparison of magnetic resonance angiography and conventional angiography in sickle cell disease: Clinical significance and reliability. *Neuroradiology, 38*, 409–416.

Kawadler, J. M., Clayden, J. D., Clark, C. A., & Kirkham, F. J. (2016). Intelligence quotient in paediatric sickle cell disease: A systematic review and meta-analysis. *Dev. Med. Child Neurol.*, *58*, 672–679.

Kawadler, J. M., Clayden, J. D., Kirkham, F. J., Cox, T. C., Saunders, D. E., & Clark, C. A. (2013). Subcortical and cerebellar volumetric deficits in paediatric sickle cell anaemia. *Br. J. Haematol.*, *163*, 373–376.

Kawadler, J. M., Kirkham, F. J., Clayden, J. D., Hollocks, M. J., Seymour, E. L., Edey, R. et al. (2015). White matter damage relates to oxygen saturation in children with sickle cell anemia without silent cerebral infarcts. *Stroke*, *46*, 1793–1799.

Kehinde, M. O., Temiye, E. O., & Danesi, M. A. (2008). Neurological complications of sickle cell anemia in Nigerian Africans – a case-control study. *J. Natl. Med. Assoc.*, *100*, 394–399.

Kija, E. N., Saunders, D. E., Munubhi, E., Darekar, A., Barker, S., Cox, T. C. S. et al. (2019). Transcranial Doppler and magnetic resonance in Tanzanian children with sickle cell disease. *Stroke*, *50*, 1719–1726.

Kirkham, F. J. & Lagunju, I. A. (2021). Epidemiology of stroke in sickle cell disease. *J. Clin. Med.*, *10*, 4232.

Koelbel, M., Hamdule, S., Kirkham, F. J., Stotesbury, H., Hood, A. M., & Dimitriou, D. (2023). Mind the gap: Trajectory of cognitive development in young individuals with sickle cell disease: A cross-sectional study. *Front. Neurol.*, *14*, 1087054.

Krejza, J., Rudzinski, W., Pawlak, M. A., Tomaszewski, M., Ichord, R., Kwiatkowski, J. et al. (2007). Angle-corrected imaging transcranial Doppler sonography versus imaging and nonimaging transcranial Doppler sonography in children with sickle cell disease. *AJNR Am. J. Neuroradiol.*, *28*, 1613–1618.

Lagunju, I., Brown, B. J., Oyinlade, A. O., Asinobi, A., Ibeh, J., Esione, A. et al. (2019). Annual stroke incidence in Nigerian children with sickle cell disease and elevated TCD velocities treated with hydroxyurea. *Pediatr. Blood Cancer*, *66*, e27252.

Lagunju, I., Sodeinde, O., Brown, B., Akinbami, F., & Adedokun, B. (2014). Transcranial Doppler ultrasonography in children with sickle cell anemia: Clinical and laboratory correlates for elevated blood flow velocities. *J. Clin. Ultrasound*, *42*, 89–95.

Lagunju, I., Sodeinde, O., & Telfer, P. (2012). Prevalence of transcranial Doppler abnormalities in Nigerian children with sickle cell disease. *Am. J. Hematol.*, *87*, 544–547.

Lagunju, I. A. & Brown, B. J. (2012). Adverse neurological outcomes in Nigerian children with sickle cell disease. *Int. J. Hematol.*, *96*, 710–718.

Lagunju, I. A., Brown, B. J., & Famosaya, A. A. (2011). Childhood stroke in sickle cell disease in Nigeria. *J. Pediatr. Neurol.*, 9(1), 49–53.

Lagunju, I. A., Brown, B. J., & Sodeinde, O. O. (2013). Stroke recurrence in Nigerian children with sickle cell disease treated with hydroxyurea. *Niger. Postgrad. Med. J.*, *20*, 181–187.

Lagunju, I., Brown, B. J., & Sodeinde, O. (2015). Hydroxyurea lowers transcranial Doppler flow velocities in children with sickle cell anaemia in a Nigerian cohort. *Pediatr. Blood Cancer*, *62*, 1587–1591.

Lagunju, I. A., Labaeka, A., Ibeh, J. N., Orimadegun, A. E., Brown, B. J., & Sodeinde, O. O. (2021). Transcranial Doppler screening in Nigerian children with sickle cell disease: A 10-year longitudinal study on the SPPIBA cohort. *Pediatr. Blood Cancer*, *68*, e28906.

Landoure, G., Cisse, L., Toure, B. A., Yalcouye, A., Coulibaly, T., Karambe, M. et al. (2017). Neurological complications in subjects with sickle cell disease or trait: Genetic results from Mali. *Glob. Heart*, *12*, 77–80.

Macharia, A. W., Mochamah, G., Uyoga, S., Ndila, C. M., Nyutu, G., Makale, J. et al. (2018). The clinical epidemiology of sickle cell anemia in Africa. *Am. J. Hematol.*, *93*, 363–370.

Makani, J., Kirkham, F. J., Komba, A., Ajala-Agbo, T., Otieno, G., Fegan, G. et al. (2009). Risk factors for high cerebral blood flow velocity and death in Kenyan children with sickle cell anaemia: Role of haemoglobin oxygen saturation and febrile illness. *Br. J. Haematol.*, *145*, 529–532.

Malouf, A. J., Jr., Hamrick-Turner, J. E., Doherty, M. C., Dhillon, G. S., Iyer, R. V., & Smith, M. G. (2001). Implementation of the STOP protocol for stroke prevention in sickle cell anemia by using duplex power Doppler imaging. *Radiology*, *219*, 359–365.

Marks, L. J., Munube, D., Kasirye, P., Mupere, E., Jin, Z., LaRussa, P. et al. (2018). Stroke prevalence in children with sickle cell disease in Sub-Saharan Africa: A systematic review and meta-analysis. *Glob. Pediatr. Health*, *5*, 2333794X18774970.

Matondo, L. O., Kija, E., & Manji, K. P. (2020). Neurocognitive functioning among children with sickle cell anemia attending SCA clinic at MNH, Dar es Salaam, Tanzania. *Neurol. Res. Int.*, *2020*, 3636547.

Matuja, S. S., Munseri, P., & Khanbhai, K. (2020). The burden and outcomes of stroke in young adults at a tertiary hospital in Tanzania: A comparison with older adults. *BMC. Neurol.*, *20*, 206.

Mazumdar, M., Heeney, M. M., Sox, C. M., & Lieu, T. A. (2007). Preventing stroke among children with sickle cell anemia: An analysis of strategies that involve transcranial Doppler testing and chronic transfusion. *Pediatrics*, *120*, e1107–e1116.

McCarville, M. B., Li, C., Xiong, X., & Wang, W. (2004). Comparison of transcranial Doppler sonography with and without imaging in the evaluation of children with sickle cell anemia. *AJR Am. J. Roentgenol.*, *183*, 1117–1122.

Miller, S. T., Milton, J., & Steinberg, M. H. (2011). G6PD deficiency and stroke in the CSSCD. *Am. J. Hematol.*, *86*, 331.

Modebe, E., Nonyelu, C., Duru, A., Ezenwosu, O., Chukwu, B., Madu, A. et al. (2023). Cerebral artery conditional blood velocity in sickle cell disease: A multicentre study and evidence for active treatment. *Arch. Dis. Child*, *108*, 440–444.

Mohammed-Nafi'u, R., Oniyangi, O., Akano, A. O., Aikhionbare, H. A., & Okon, E. J. (2021). Transcranial Doppler ultrasonography imaging studies in children with sickle cell anaemia in a tertiary Hospital, Abuja, Nigeria. *West Afr. J. Med.*, *38*, 460–464.

Munube, D., Katabira, E., Ndeezi, G., Joloba, M., Lhatoo, S., Sajatovic, M., & Tumwine, J. K. (2016). Prevalence of stroke in children admitted with sickle cell anaemia to Mulago Hospital. *BMC Neurol.*, *16*, 175.

Napon, C., Kabore, A., Ouedraogo, M., Drave, A., Lompo, L., & Kabore, J. (2012). [Strokes and hemoglobinopathies in Burkina Faso]. *Med Sante Trop.*, *22*, 390–393.

Neish, A. S., Blews, D. E., Simms, C. A., Merritt, R. K., & Spinks, A. J. (2002). Screening for stroke in sickle cell anemia: Comparison of transcranial Doppler imaging and nonimaging US techniques. *Radiology*, *222*, 709–714.

Neonato, M. G., Guilloud-Bataille, M., Beauvais, P., Begue, P., Belloy, M., Benkerrou, M. et al. (2000). Acute clinical events in 299 homozygous sickle cell patients living in France. French Study Group on Sickle Cell Disease. *Eur. J. Haematol.*, *65*, 155–164.

Nguweneza, A., Ngo Bitoungui, V. J., Mnika, K., Mazandu, G., Nembaware, V., Kengne, A. P. et al. (2022a). Clinical characteristics and risk factors of relative systemic hypertension and hypertension among sickle cell patients in Cameroon. *Front. Med. (Lausanne)*, *9*, 924722.

Nguweneza, A., Oosterwyk, C., Banda, K., Nembaware, V., Mazandu, G., Kengne, A. P. et al. (2022b). Factors associated with blood pressure variation in sickle cell disease patients: A systematic review and meta-analyses. *Expert. Rev. Hematol.*, *15*, 359–368.

Nichols, F. T., Jones, A. M., & Adams, R. J. (2001). Stroke prevention in sickle cell disease (STOP) study guidelines for transcranial Doppler testing. *J. Neuroimag.*, *11*, 354–362.

Njamnshi, A. K., Mbong, E. N., Wonkam, A., Ongolo-Zogo, P., Djientcheu, V. D., Sunjoh, F. L. et al. (2006). The epidemiology of stroke in sickle cell patients in Yaounde, Cameroon. *J. Neurol. Sci.*, *250*, 79–84.

Noubiap, J. J., Mengnjo, M. K., Nicastro, N., & Kamtchum-Tatuene, J. (2017). Neurologic complications of sickle cell disease in Africa: A systematic review and meta-analysis. *Neurology*, *89*, 1516–1524.

O'Driscoll, S., Height, S. E., Dick, M. C., & Rees, D. C. (2008). Serum lactate dehydrogenase activity as a biomarker in children with sickle cell disease. *Br. J. Haematol.*, *140*, 206–209.

Obajimi, M. O., Jumah, K. B., & Iddrisu, M. (2002). CT evaluation of intracranial subdural haematoma: An Accra experience. *Afr. J. Med. Med. Sci.*, *31*, 321–324.

Obama, M. T., Dongmo, L., Nkemayim, C., Mbede, J., & Hagbe, P. (1994). Stroke in children in Yaounde, Cameroon. *Indian Pediatr.*, *31*, 791–795.

Ogunseyinde, A. O., Obajimi, M. O., & Fatunde, O. J. (2005). Computed tomographic pattern of stroke in children with sickle cell anaemia in Ibadan. *Afr. J. Med. Med. Sci.*, *34*, 115–118.

Ogwang, E., Odongo, C. N., Namusisi, J., Okello, P. A., & Acan, M. (2022). Hair-on-end sign in a 9-year-old girl presenting with acute stroke in sickle cell disease. *Int. Med. Case Rep. J.*, *15*, 69–73.

Ohene-Frempong, K., Weiner, S. J., Sleeper, L. A., Miller, S. T., Embury, S., Moohr, J. W. et al. (1998). Cerebrovascular accidents in sickle cell disease: Rates and risk factors. *Blood*, *91*, 288–294.

Padayachee, S. T., Thomas, N., Arnold, A. J., & Inusa, B. (2012). Problems with implementing a standardised transcranial Doppler screening programme: Impact of instrumentation variation on STOP classification. *Pediatr. Radiol.*, *42*, 470–474.

Pegelow, C. H., Colangelo, L., Steinberg, M., Wright, E. C., Smith, J., Phillips, G. et al. (1997). Natural history of blood pressure in sickle cell disease: Risks for stroke and death associated with relative hypertension in sickle cell anemia. *Am. J. Med.*, *102*, 171–177.

Pelkonen, T., Roine, I., Bernardino, L., Jahnukainen, K., & Peltola, H. (2022). Bacterial meningitis in children with sickle cell disease in Angola. *Pediatr. Infect. Dis. J.*, *41*, e335–e338.

Pelkonen, T., Roine, I., Kallio, M., Jahnukainen, K., & Peltola, H. (2022). Prevalence and significance of anaemia in childhood bacterial meningitis: A secondary analysis of prospectively collected data from clinical trials in Finland, Latin America and Angola. *BMJ Open*, *12*, e057285.

Piel, F. B., Patil, A. P., Howes, R. E., Nyangiri, O. A., Gething, P. W., Williams, T. N. et al. (2010). Global distribution of the sickle cell gene and geographical confirmation of the malaria hypothesis. *Nat. Commun.*, *1*, 104.

Prengler, M., Boyd, S., Lane, R., & Kirkham, F. J. (2001). Seizures in sickle cell disease. *Eur. J. Paediatr. Neurol.*, *5*, 143.

Prengler, M., Pavlakis, S. G., Prohovnik, I., & Adams, R. J. (2002). Sickle cell disease: The neurological complications. *Ann. Neurol.*, *51*, 543–552.

Preul, M. C., Cendes, F., Just, N., & Mohr, G. (1998). Intracranial aneurysms and sickle cell anemia: Multiplicity and propensity for the vertebrobasilar territory. *Neurosurgery*, *42*, 971–977.

Prohovnik, I., Hurlet-Jensen, A., Adams, R., De Vivo, D., & Pavlakis, S. G. (2009). Hemodynamic etiology of elevated flow velocity and stroke in sickle-cell disease. *J. Cereb. Blood Flow Metab.*, *29*, 803–810.

Prussien, K. V., Jordan, L. C., DeBaun, M. R., & Compas, B. E. (2019). Cognitive function in sickle cell disease across domains, cerebral infarct status, and the lifespan: A meta-analysis. *J. Pediatr. Psychol.*, *44*, 948–958.

Quinn, C. T., Variste, J., & Dowling, M. M. (2009). Haemoglobin oxygen saturation is a determinant of cerebral artery blood flow velocity in children with sickle cell anaemia. *Br. J. Haematol., 145,* 500–505.

Rankine-Mullings, A. E., Morrison-Levy, N., Soares, D., Aldred, K., King, L., Ali, S. et al. (2018). Transcranial Doppler velocity among Jamaican children with sickle cell anaemia: Determining the significance of haematological values and nutrition. *Br. J. Haematol., 181,* 242–251.

Rees, D. C., Dick, M. C., Height, S. E., O'Driscoll, S., Pohl, K. R., Goss, D. E. et al. (2008). A simple index using age, hemoglobin, and aspartate transaminase predicts increased intracerebral blood velocity as measured by transcranial Doppler scanning in children with sickle cell anemia. *Pediatrics, 121,* e1628–e1632.

Rees, D. C., Lambert, C., Cooper, E., Bartram, J., Goss, D., Deane, C. et al. (2009). Glucose 6 phosphate dehydrogenase deficiency is not associated with cerebrovascular disease in children with sickle cell anemia. *Blood, 114,* 742–743.

Rodrigues, D. O., Ribeiro, L. C., Sudario, L. C., Teixeira, M. T., Martins, M. L., Pittella, A. M. et al. (2016). Genetic determinants and stroke in children with sickle cell disease. *J. Pediatr. (Rio J.), 92,* 602–608.

Ruffieux, N., Njamnshi, A. K., Wonkam, A., Hauert, C. A., Chanal, J., Verdon, V. et al. (2013). Association between biological markers of sickle cell disease and cognitive functioning amongst Cameroonian children. *Child Neuropsychol., 19,* 143–160.

Rumaney, M. B., Ngo Bitoungui, V. J., Vorster, A. A., Ramesar, R., Kengne, A. P., Ngogang, J., & Wonkam. A. (2014). The co-inheritance of alpha-thalassemia and sickle cell anemia is associated with better hematological indices and lower consultations rate in Cameroonian patients and could improve their survival. *PLoS One, 9,* e100516.

Saha, B. & Saha, A. (2019). Spontaneous epidural hemorrhage in sickle cell disease, are they all the Same? A case report and comprehensive review of the literature. *Case Rep. Hematol., 2019,* 8974580.

Saidi, H., Smart, L. R., Kamugisha, E., Ambrose, E. E., Soka, D., Peck, R. N. et al. (2016). Complications of sickle cell anaemia in children in Northwestern Tanzania. *Hematology, 21,* 248–256.

Salama, K., Rady, R., Hashem, R. H., & El-Ghamrawy, M. (2020). Transcranial Doppler velocities among sickle cell disease patients in steady state. *Hemoglobin, 44,* 418–422.

Santos, B., Delgadinho, M., Ferreira, J., Germano, I., Miranda, A., Arez, A. P., Faustino P., & Brito, M. (2020). Co-inheritance of alpha-thalassemia and sickle cell disease in a cohort of Angolan pediatric patients. *Mol. Biol. Rep., 47,* 5397–5402.

Schlotman, A. A., Donahue, M. J., Kassim, A. A., Lee, C. A., Waddle, S. L., Pruthi, S. et al. (2021). Intracranial and extracranial vascular stenosis as risk factors for stroke in sickle cell disease. *Pediatr. Neurol., 114,* 29–34.

Sebire, G., Tabarki, B., Saunders, D. E., Leroy, I., Liesner, R., Saint-Martin, C. et al. (2005). Cerebral venous sinus thrombosis in children: Risk factors, presentation, diagnosis and outcome. *Brain, 128,* 477–489.

Serjeant, G. R. (1997). Sickle-cell disease. *Lancet, 350,* 725–730.

Stotesbury, H., Adams, R. J., & Kirkham, F. J. (2021a). Stroke and cognitive dysfunction. In M. T. Gladwin, G. J. Kato, & E. M. Novelli (Eds.), *Sickle cell disease* (1st ed.). New York: McGraw Hill.

Stotesbury, H., Kawadler, J. M., Clayden, J. D., Saunders, D. E., Hood, A. M., Koelbel, M. et al. (2022). Quantification of silent cerebral infarction on high-Resolution FLAIR and cognition in sickle cell anemia. *Front. Neurol., 13,* 867329.

Stotesbury, H., Kawadler, J. M., Saunders, D. E., & Kirkham, F. J. (2021b). MRI detection of brain abnormality in sickle cell disease. *Expert Rev. Hematol.*, 14, 473–491.

Stotesbury, H., Kirkham, F. J., Kolbel, M., Balfour, P., Clayden, J. D., Sahota, S. et al. (2018). White matter integrity and processing speed in sickle cell anemia. *Neurology*, 90, e2042–e2050.

Strouse, J. J., Hulbert, M. L., DeBaun, M. R., Jordan, L. C., & Casella, J. F. (2006). Primary hemorrhagic stroke in children with sickle cell disease is associated with recent transfusion and use of corticosteroids. *Pediatrics*, 118, 1916–1924.

Strouse, J. J., Jordan, L. C., Lanzkron, S., & Casella, J. F. (2009). The excess burden of stroke in hospitalized adults with sickle cell disease. *Am. J. Hematol.*, 84, 548–552.

Tabari, A. M. & Ismail A. (2013). Doppler ultrasound velocimetry of middle cerebral arteries of patients with sickle cell disease at Aminu Kano Teaching Hospital: A preliminary report. *Ultrasound Q.*, 29, 61–65.

Tantawy, A. A., Andrawes, N. G., Adly, A. A., El Kady, B. A., & Shalash, A. S. (2013). Retinal changes in children and adolescents with sickle cell disease attending a paediatric hospital in Cairo, Egypt: Risk factors and relation to ophthalmic and cerebral blood flow. *Trans. R. Soc. Trop. Med. Hyg.*, 107, 205–211.

Telfer, P. T., Evanson, J., Butler, P., Hemmaway, C., Abdulla, C., Gadong, N. et al. (2011). Cervical carotid artery disease in sickle cell anemia: Clinical and radiological features. *Blood*, 118, 6192–6199.

Thangarajh, M., Yang, G., Fuchs, D., Ponisio, M. R., McKinstry, R. C., Jaju, A. et al. (2012). Magnetic resonance angiography-defined intracranial vasculopathy is associated with silent cerebral infarcts and glucose-6-phosphate dehydrogenase mutation in children with sickle cell anaemia. *Br. J. Haematol.*, 159, 352–359.

Venkateswaran, L., Teruya, J., Bustillos, C., Mahoney, D., Jr., & Mueller, B. U. (2011). Red cell exchange does not appear to increase the rate of allo- and auto-immunization in chronically transfused children with sickle cell disease. *Pediatr. Blood Cancer*, 57, 294–296.

Vgontzas, A., Charleston, L., & Robbins, M. S. (2016). Headache and facial pain in sickle cell disease. *Curr. Pain Headache Rep.*, 20, 20.

Wang, W., Enos, L., Gallagher, D., Thompson, R., Guarini, L., Vichinsky, E. et al. (2001). Neuropsychologic performance in school-aged children with sickle cell disease: A report from the cooperative study of sickle cell disease. *J. Pediatr.*, 139, 391–397.

Ware, R. E., Schultz, W. H., Yovetich, N., Mortier, N. A., Alvarez, O., Hilliard, L. et al. (2011). Stroke with transfusions changing to hydroxyurea (SWiTCH): A phase III randomized clinical trial for treatment of children with sickle cell anemia, stroke, and iron overload. *Pediatr. Blood Cancer*, 57, 1011–1017.

8 Overview of Organ Dysfunction in Sickle Cell Disease

*Ruth Namazzi, Catherine Nabaggala, Annet Nakirulu,
Philip Kasirye and Deogratais Munube*

Introduction

Globally, sickle cell disease (SCD) is the most common inherited haemoglobinopathy affecting approximately 300,000 new births annually. The condition is caused by a single-point mutation that leads to the production of haemoglobin S, instead of the normal adult haemoglobin A. The hallmark of the disease is recurrent polymerisation of the haemoglobin S molecule under conditions of low oxygen tension and this causes chronic haemolysis and recurrent vaso-occlusion. Chronic haemolysis (Kato, Gladwin, & Steinberg, 2007) and recurrent vaso-occlusion damage blood vessels, block microvasculature and causing tissue hypoxia that damage multiple body organs and cause organ dysfunction including kidney injury, pulmonary hypertension and brain injury.

Over the past decades, survival among patients with SCD has improved, with median survival age increasing up to 55 years. However, these improved survival rates imply that persons with SCD live long enough to experience SCD-related organ damage and its effects on quality of life.

Organ dysfunction and the resultant end organ failure contributes up to 50% of mortality among adults with SCD and also causes poor quality of life among survivors. In less developed countries where childhood mortality from SCD remains high, organ dysfunction and the associated morbidity and mortality in adults are is poorly described.

Organ dysfunction in SCD can occur irrespective of severity of clinical symptoms and may remain asymptomatic but progress to end organ damage unless detected by systematic screening. For example, routine screening for cerebral vascular velocities in children and young adults can detect those at increases risk of stroke.

Pathophysiology of SCD-Associated Organ Dysfunction

Organ dysfunction in SCD is an insidious but progressive process. Clinical presentation of the organ dysfunction usually manifests from early to mid-adulthood. The onset and frequency of organ dysfunction are not necessarily correlated with severity of SCD and may occur among patients with seemingly milder phenotypes

DOI: 10.4324/9781003463931-9

Mechanical Vascular Damage

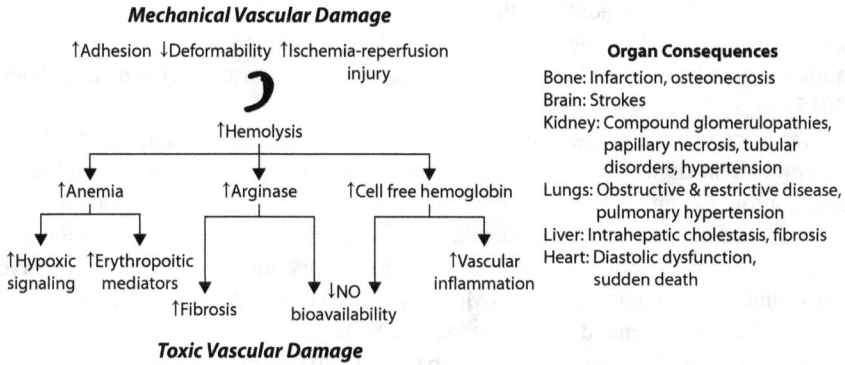

Figure 8.1 Mechanical and toxic vascular damage.

(van Beers et al., 2008). Single or multiple organs can be affected (Thein, Igbineweka, & Thein, 2017), the most affected being highly vascularised organs such as the kidneys, brain and lungs, but bone as well as eye complications have also been described. The organs damaged or affected by SCD vary with age, and SCD genotype as well as environmental factors.

Haemoglobin polymerisation with the resultant chronic haemolysis, anaemia, vaso-occlusion and systemic inflammation is the central mechanism underlying organ damage in SCD (Figure 8.1). Vaso-occlusion causes blockage in the small microvasculature leading to tissue ischaemia related injury and necrosis in various body organs. Subsequent reperfusion allowing re-entry of oxygen causes local ischaemia/reperfusion tissue injury (Hebbel, Belcher, & Vercellotti, 2020; Kalogeris, Baines, Krenz, & Korthuis, 2016). Further, the ischaemia/perfusion injury invokes systemic inflammation through activation of leucocytes and cytokines (Solovey et al., 2017), endothelial activation through up regulation of P selectin and vascular cell adhesion molecule VCAM (Belcher et al., 2005; Takano et al., 2002). Additionally, chronic haemolysis releases heme and free haemoglobin which induce oxidative stress, systemic inflammation, hypercoagulability, nitric oxide deficiency and endothelial activation (Belcher et al., 2014).

Spectrum of Organ Dysfunction in SCD

Kidney Dysfunction

The kidneys are among the most frequently affected organs in SCD (Powars, Chan, Hiti, Ramicone, & Johnson, 2005). Patients with SCD face a number of kidney complications that include acute kidney injury (AKI), chronic kidney disease (CKD), hyperfiltration (Ware et al., 2010), microalbuminuria, haematuria and hyposthenia. The types of kidney complications vary with age: children develop hyposthenuria, hyperfiltration, impaired potassium secretion and acidification and papillary necrosis, while adults have CKD.

Nearly 30–50% of adults with SCD are affected by one or more kidney complications. Kidney complications develop in later childhood and progress well into adulthood and are associated with increased risk of mortality (Nath & Hebbel, 2015).

Vaso-occlusion and haemolysis (Van Avondt, Nur, & Zeerleder, 2019) play a central role in tissue damage in the kidneys. Because of low oxygen partial pressures, a low PH and high osmolality, the renal medulla provides an ideal environment for red cells to sickle. Ischaemia reperfusion injury from vaso-occlusion and free heme from haemolysis contribute to kidney injury and CKD through oxidative stress and complement activation (Merle et al., 2018; Van Avondt et al., 2019).

Risk factors for renal dysfunction include SCD genotypes (more common in the HBSS and HBS/β^0,) severe anaemia (Aban et al., 2017) and hypertension (Lebensburger, Cutter, Howard, Muntner, & Feig, 2017).

Types of Kidney Dysfunction in SCD

Hyposthenuria

Hyposthenia, the inability of the kidney to concentrate urine beyond 450 mOS/kg in conditions of water deprivation, is common and starts from early childhood. It manifests as nocturnal enuresis and polyuria. Repeated sickling causes eventual ischaemia in the vas recta, formation of collaterals, and loss of the long loops of Henle, which reduces the reabsorption of free water.

No definitive treatments are known, but hydroxyurea was shown to improve the concentrating capacity in children with SCD (Alvarez et al., 2012).

Glomerular Hyperfiltration

Defined as glomerualar filteration rate (GFR) > 130 ml/min//1.73 m^2 in women, 140 ml/min//1.73 m^2 in men and >180 ml/min/1.73 m^2 in children, glomerular hyperfiltration starts early in childhood (Ware et al., 2010). Hyperfiltration typically precedes the occurrence of albuminuria (Lebensburger et al., 2019). Increased GFRs result from increased renal blood flow from increased cardiac output from chronic anaemia and release of vasodilator/tors due to vaso-occlusion.

Tubular Dysfunction

Glomerular hyperfiltration causes a reactionary increased reabsorption of sodium and water in the proximal tubules. This also drives up the reabsorption of solutes such as phosphate and β_2 microglobulin and secretion of uric acid and creatinine (Nath & Hebbel, 2015).

Further, there is decreased secretion of hydrogen ions and potassium in the distal tubules causes an incomplete type IV renal tubular acidosis. However, hyperkalaemia is rare unless there are additional exacerbating factors which compromise renal compensatory mechanism – such acute illness or use of renin angiotensin converting enzyme inhibitor drugs.

Haematuria

Haematuria occurs commonly in SCD, and it is due micro infracts in the renal papillae (Naik & Derebail, 2017). Although usually painless, and self-limiting, occasionally, an extensive micro infarct can cause renal papillary necrosis and cause pain. Painless haematuria is usually self-limiting, requiring good hydration and pain killers for resolution.

Acute Kidney Injury

AKI occurs in 10–20% of adults and 17–48.7% of children (Baddam et al., 2017, 2022) admitted with SCD-associated complications such as acute chest syndrome and acute pain crises.(AKI is associated with a reversible reduction of up to 15% in creatinine clearance during acute vaso-occlusioncrises. Infections (Batte et al., 2022), dehydration, use of renal toxic drugs as well as worsening anaemia (Baddam et al., 2017) are associated with increased risk of AKI.

Chronic Kidney Disease

CKD incidence increases with age, occurring in up to 25% of patients above 50 years. CKD usually develops insidiously, starting as glomerular hyperfiltration in early childhood, and micro albuminuria in late childhood and adolescence, which progresses slowly to unselective proteinuria and CKD (Sharpe & Thein, 2014). Although not all patients progress to CKD, for those who are diagnosed, they have an increased risk of death with an estimated overall five- year survival of only 55% (Nielsen et al., 2016).

Treatment Approach for SCD-Associated Renal Dysfunction

Screening for renal disease, monitoring of renal function and early treatment are recommended treatment approaches for patients with SCD, especially as they age. Screening for microalbuminuria, haematuria and changes in GFR should be part of the routine care especially for older patients with SCD (Vichinsky, 2017). Importantly, changes in creatinine and or GFR are more meaningful given the limitations of using creatinine as marker of renal disease in patients with SCD. Monitoring for renal disease using surrogate markers of kidney function for example serum Cystatin C, urine N-acetyl-β-D-glycosaminidase might be of value. Treatment of known risk factors such as hypertension helps to abate the progression of kidney dysfunction. The American Society of Haematology guidelines suggests a target blood pressure of 130/90 mmHg (Liem et al., 2019)

Hydroxyurea therapy has been shown to reduce GFR (Aygun et al., 2013) and improve urine concentrating capacity in children (Alvarez et al., 2012). In adults, it reduces proteinuria (Laurin, Nachman, Desai, Ataga, & Derebail, 2014) and therefore should be considered for all patients with SCD-associated kidney disease. Angiotensin-converting enzyme inhibitors (ACEis) or angiotensin receptor blockers have been shown to reduce proteinuria and are recommend for use in patients with SCD glomerulopathy (Falk et al., 1992).

The effectiveness of regular blood transfusions on the onset and progression of proteinuria in children needs further supporting evidence. One study suggested that regular and early initiation blood transfusions delayed the onset of proteinuria in children (Alvarez, Montane, Lopez, Wilkinson, & Miller, 2006), while two other studies failed to see a proactive effect (Becton et al., 2010; Lebensburger et al., 2011). Blood transfusion is however useful in slowing progression of CKD, especially when hydroxyurea is not effective (Sharpe & Thein, 2014).

Erythropoiesis stimulating agents are useful in patients with worsening anaemia and CKD because of a reduced synthesis of erythropoietin. Erythropoietin analogues should be used in combination with hydroxyurea with the aim of raising haemoglobin levels. Target haemoglobin levels are about 10 g/dL to reduce on the risk of vaso-occlusion crises (Liem et al., 2019).

Renal Replacement Therapy (RRT)

Renal replacement therapy is necessary when GFR falls below 40 mL/min/1.73 m^2. Early referral to nephology for planning is important since SCD patients may face unique risks associated with RRT. Both haemodialysis and peritoneal dialysis have been successfully performed in patients with SCD end stage renal disease (ESRD) (Liem et al., 2019).

Renal Transplant

Kidney transplant should be considered for patients with ESKD. Regular blood transfusion (preferably exchange transfusion) should be started months before the transplant and until the graft is taken.

Brain Dysfunction

Neurological complications are common in persons with SCD and range from silent cerebral infracts to overt ischaemic and haemorrhagic strokes, and neurocognitive impairment. The pathophysiology of brain dysfunction remains poorly understood. Risk factors for stroke and cerebral infarcts include chronic anaemia, acute drops in haemoglobin levels, low oxygen saturation and presence of infections.

Spectrum of Brain Dysfunction

Overt Stroke

Stroke is the most devastating neurological complication of SCD that can cause permanent motor sequelae and poor quality of life. Overt stroke occurs in up to 11% of children by age 20 years with SCD (HBSS) (Ohene-Frempong et al., 1998) in the absence of a preventive strategy. Without secondary preventive measures, strokes have a high recurrence rate of up to 50% and 66% within the first two and nine years of initial stroke, respectively (Powars, Wilson, Imbus, Pegelow, & Allen, 1978). Overt strokes in SCD are ischaemic in 75% of cases and haemorrhagic in 25% (Strouse, Lanzkron, & Urrutia, 2011).

Ischaemic strokes occur commonly in childhood, and older adults while haemorrhagic strokes occur most commonly in the 20–30 age group (Powars et al., 1978).

Stroke is associated with cerebral vascular vasculopathy in large vessels in the circle of Willis, that compromises cerebral blood flow. Furthermore, the presence of a previous cerebral infarct increases the risk of recurrent stroke, especially in the first 2–3 years. Other risk factors for stroke include low oxygen saturation (Quinn & Sargent, 2008), acute drops in haemoglobin levels (Dowling et al., 2012), acute infections (Dowling et al., 2012), hypertension, diabetics mellitus and renal disease (Strouse et al., 2011).

Magnetic resonance imaging is preferred over computed tomography for diagnosis of stroke (Lansberg, Albers, Beaulieu, & Marks, 2000). Additionally, use of diffusion weighted MRI helps to differentiate acute infarcts from sub-acute infracts.

The management of stroke encompasses treatment of the acute ischaemic episodes and secondary prevention of recurrent stroke. Data from prospective randomised trials are lacking to guide management of acute ischaemic episodes in SCD. Management of acute stroke should be multidisciplinary involving haematologists, neurologists, neuroradiologists and blood transfusion specialists if available. The American Society of Haematology guidelines recommend that children and adults showing signs of stroke should receive blood transfusion within 2 hours of presentation. Further, exchange blood transfusion is preferred over simple blood transfusion with a target of reducing the haemoglobin S level to about 30% (DeBaun et al., 2020). In the absence of exchange transfusion, for example, in low-middle income countries (LMIC), simple transfusion should be given within 2 hours of presentation. Other measures such hydration, pain control and maintaining oxygen levels above 90% should be instituted.

Primary stroke prevention in persons with SCD involves routine screening with annual Trans Doppler Ultra Sound scans (TCD) to identify children at risk of stroke. Blood transfusion among children with TCD velocities of greater than 200 cm/sec reduces the risk of stroke by 92% (Adams et al., 1998).

Blood transfusion is also efficacious in reducing risk of stroke in children with abnormal TCD velocities and demonstrated vasculopathy on MRA.

In LMIC where blood transfusion capacity is limited, TCD screening and the use of hydroxyurea for primary stroke prevention are a reasonable approach compared to no therapy (Galadanci et al., 2020). The optimal dosing of hydroxyurea for stroke prevention, and frequency of monitoring remains undetermined for patients in LMIC. (Abdallahi et al,2022)

Secondary stroke prevention after a first stroke involves chronic blood transfusion although protection is not complete as some secondary cerebral infracts can still occur despite blood transfusion (Hulbert et al., 2011).

Silent Cerebral Infarcts

Silent cerebral infarcts (SCI) are defined as a neurological infarct (>3 mm lesion on T2 weighted images on two planes on fluid attenuated inversion recovery) (Kassim et al., 2016) on imaging but without associated history of or examination findings of overt neurological deficits. SCI are among the most common neurological complications of SCD. They occur early in life (Wang et al., 2008), most occurring by six years of age (Kinney et al., 1999; Wang et al., 1998). The incidence increases with age; 39% by age 18 (Bernaudin et al., 2015; Vichinsky, 2017) and 53% of adults by age 30 (Kassim et al., 2016) have infarcts. There is no age associated plateauing in the incidence of SCI among persons with SCD (Bernaudin et al., 2015). SCI are associated with overall decreased academic performance (King et al., 2014), cognitive impairment (Vichinsky et al., 2010) and future overt strokes (Miller et al., 2001).

Low base line haemoglobin (DeBaun et al., 2012) and rate of episodes of acute anaemia exacerbations have been associated with increased risk of SCI (Bernaudin et al., 2015). Most SCI lesions occur in the water shade areas in the deep white matter (Zimmerman, 2005). These areas are at highest risk of hypoxia during acute severe anaemia episodes. Additional risk factors include intra and extracranial carotid artery stenosis, age, history of seizures and high white cell count of above 11,000 per μl (Kinney et al., 1999; Kwiatkowski et al., 2009)

Because they are clinically silent, the onset of SCI is usually unknown. Diagnosis is made by magnetic resonance imaging with diffusion weighted imaging which can differentiate between acute and chronic events.

Management of SCI

There is no current for primary prevention of SCI among persons with SCD. Current treatment approaches include chronic blood transfusion and hydroxyurea.

From the Stroke Prevention in Sickle cell Disease STOP trial, chronic blood transfusion prevented the recurrence of both strokes and SCI in persons with SCA and abnormal TCD velocities (Adams et al., 1998). The Silent Cerebral Infract Transfusion SIT trial in children aged 5–15 years showed a 58% reduction in risk of recurrent infract (SCI and or overt stroke) in children who received blood transfusion when compared to those in the observation arm (DeBaun et al., 2014). Protection from recurrence by blood transfusion is however not complete, and some children may still get secondary SCI despite blood transfusion. The duration of the blood transfusion remains unclear. The SIT trial transfused children for 36 months. The risks of chronic blood transfusion such as alloimmunisation and iron overload must be considered and discussed with the patients or parents of patients, especially in LMIC where extended matching for red cell antigens is limited.

Neurocognitive Dysfunction

Neurocognitive dysfunction is one of the most common complications affecting persons with SCD. Neurocognitive derangement ranges from decreases in

IQ scores, attention and executive functioning. Adults with SCD show clinically significant differences in performances in language, memory, learning and attention compared to controls (Feliu et al., 2011). Similarly, children with SCD score up to seven full scale IQ points lower than controls (Armstrong et al., 1996) have attention and executive function deficits (Berkelhammer et al., 2007)

Risk factors for neurocognitive dysfunction include age, anaemia (Steen et al., 2003), prior stroke and SCI (Vichinsky et al., 2010). The association of anaemia with cognitive dysfunction suggests that chronic cerebral hypoxia may lead to cognitive dysfunction in SCD. Other risk factors include sleep apnoea, hypertension, smoking, renal and lung disease.

There are no recommendations to screen for neurocognitive deficits in neurologically asymptomatic patients. Early recognition of neurocognitive deficits enables remediation.

Hydroxyurea has been shown to improve cognition in adults (Puffer, Schatz, & Roberts, 2007). Other management strategies include treatment of modifiable risk factors like hypertension and nocturnal hypoxaemia. Furthermore, education and cognitive accommodation are helpful for persons with SCD-related neurocognitive dysfunction (Vichinsky, 2017).

Pulmonary Dysfunction

SCD-associated pulmonary complications are many and may be acute and chronic. Acute and chronic pulmonary complications in SCD are a major cause of morbidity and mortality (Hamideh & Alvarez, 2013).These complications usually begin in childhood and progress with age (Mehari & Klings, 2016). The disease manifestations can either be acute or chronic. SCD-associated pulmonary complications can involve the lung vascular, parenchyma and or airways.

The symptomatology of disease can be reflected in the following conditions:

- Pulmonary function abnormalities
- Asthma or recurrent wheezing without a diagnosis of asthma
- Sleep disordered breathing
- Pulmonary hypertension

Pulmonary Function Abnormalities

Pulmonary function abnormalities are common in children and adolescents with SCD and deteriorate with age (Lunt et al., 2016). Lung function abnormalities in SCD are characterised as obstructive restrictive lung pattern and mixed. A restrictive pattern is more evident among the older age group while an obstructive pattern is seen among younger children. *Cohen et al. reported* an abnormal lung function in 30% of children and adolescents with SCD, with the obstructive type being the most common (Cohen et al., 2016). In a longitudinal study for children aged 5–18 years, children had mainly obstructive lung abnormalities at baseline (Greenough & Inusa, 2016). Furthermore, longitudinal data among children with SCD show that a restrictive pattern increases with age, and adults tend to have a more restrictive type of lung disease.

The pathophysiology of abnormality of the lung function tests is not clear. Small airways may be compressed by congested peripheral pulmonary vessels (Wedder-burn et al., 2014). The restrictive pattern which is more common in adults with SCD may be, in part, due to increased circulation of activate fibrocytes, leading to lung fibrosis (Mehrad et al., 2017).

Asthma which is common in SCD could contribute to obstructive lung function abnormalities although obstructive pattern is not restricted to asthma patients with SCD. Data from studies suggest that methacholine sensitivity as well as eosino-philic inflammation are not associated with airway obstruction in SCD children (Arigliani & Gupta, 2020; Greenough & Inusa, 2016).

Strategies to reduce decline of pulmonary function with age may include use of hydroxyurea. A retrospective study among children >5 years and adoles-cents showed that the annual decline in Forced Expiratory Volume (FEV_1) was less in those on hydroxyurea therapy (McLaren et al., 2017). Although the prog-nostic implications of abnormal lung function tests in children are not clear, in adults, reduced FEV_1 is associated with increased risk of early mortality (Kassim et al., 2015). Although routine pulmonary function testing is not recommended for asymptomatic children and adults, persons with asthma, exercise intolerance, his-tory of recurrent acute chest syndrome among others need monitoring and testing and review by pulmonologists (Arigliani & Gupta, 2020; Liem et al., 2019; Mehari & Klings, 2016).

Sleep Disordered Breathing and Hypoxaemia

Sleep disordered breathing (SDB) including obstructive sleep apnoea (OSA) and nocturnal hypoxaemia is common in children and adolescents with SCD (Arigliani & Gupta, 2020). In a Sleep and Asthma prospective cohort study among children, it was noted that the prevalence of OSA was 41% and 25% using obstructive ap-noea hypopnea index cut points of >1 or > 5, respectively (Rosen et al., 2014). A prospective study among 20 adults with sickle cell anaemia found 50% had OSA (Whitesell et al., 2016). In this study, OSA was associated with a reduced health-related quality of life.

The aetiology of SDB is not clear. Children with SCD have reduced upper air-way diameters, increased adenoid and tonsillar size. Abnormalities with the lung parenchyma, airways and blood vessel changes may lead to reduced gas exchange and ventilation-perfusion mismatch. A study among adults and children showed that nocturnal hypoxemia was associated with reduced (Strunk et al., 2014). SDB and SCD potentiate each other clinical effects. In children with SCD, nocturnal hypoxae-mia is associated with anaemia (Halphen et al., 2014), increased risk of brain injury (Kirkham et al., 2001), cardiac abnormalities (Johnson et al., 2010), and pain crises and acute chest syndrome (Hargrave, Wade, Evans, Hewes, & Kirkham, 2003).

Screening for SDB in asymptomatic patients is not recommended. The American Society of Haematology guidelines recommends a formal polysomnography (sleep study) for symptomatic patients with SCD. This includes SCD patients with history of snoring, witnessed apnoea, nonrestorative sleep and or excessive daytime sleepiness, obesity, early morning headaches, unexplained desaturation or hypoxemia, carbon dioxide retention on arterial blood gas, history of poorly controlled hypertension or congestive heart failure, history of nocturnal enuresis in an older child, history of recurrent priapism or frequent daytime or nocturnal vaso-occlusion pain, PH as confirmed by right heart catheterisation, history of ischaemic stroke without evidence of vasculopathy, history of memory loss, difficulty with concentration or unexplained episodes of confusion and symptoms of attention deficit-hyperactivity disorder, poor academic achievement and performance or behaviour problems in children (Liem et al., 2019).

Treatment with hydroxyurea may reduce nocturnal hypoxaemia (van Geyzel et al., 2020). The management of OSA in the setting of SCD is similar to management in general population without SCD including use of corticosteroids and adenotonsillectomy.

Asthma and Wheezing

Asthma is a common condition in SCD especially among children and adolescents (Boyd, Macklin, Strunk, & DeBaun, 2006; Strunk et al., 2014) and is associated with a higher risk of vaso-occlusion pain episodes, acute chest syndrome (ACS) (Boyd et al., 2006). A retrospective case control study of children admitted with a vaso-occlussive crisisVOC reported that patients with asthma were four times more likely to develop ACS. Asthma-induced ventilation-perfusion mismatch subsequently causes local tissue hypoxia and increasing the sickling of the red cells, which causes a number of SCD-related clinical complications including ACS (Miller & Gladwin, 2012). Asthma in SCD can result from multiple mechanisms including SCD-associated chronic inflammation of the airway and airway remodelling (Strunk et al., 2014), increased air way responsiveness (Field et al., 2011), and obstructive lung disease (Cohen et al., 2016).

The diagnosis of asthma in SCD is confirmed by the presence of airflow obstruction relieved by bronchodilators, although making the diagnosis is complicated by the high prevalence of wheezing among patients with SCD who do not have asthma (Strunk et al., 2014).

There is limited data on the management of asthma in the context of SCD. Treatment is therefore according to national and international guidelines. Hypoxaemia should be corrected, and short acting β_2 agonists given (Arigliani & Gupta, 2020).

Caution should be excised when using oral corticosteroids in moderate and severe asthmatic exacerbations due to increased risk of vaso-occlusioncrisis.

Pulmonary Hypertension

In SCD, pulmonary hypertension (a mean pulmonary artery pressure of ≥25 mmHg determined by cardiac catherisation at rest, Badesch et al., 2009) occurs in about 6–10% adults with SCD (Mehari, Gladwin, Tian, Machado, & Kato, 2012; Parent et al., 2011). Pulmonary hypertension in SCD is classified as Group 5 indicating pulmonary hypertension with unclear or multiple aetiologies (Simonneau et al., 2013). Furthermore, pulmonary hypertension can be precapillary and postcapillary.

In SCD, recurrent intravascular haemolysis leads to the release of free heme: free heme inhibits nitric oxide and impairs vascular endothelial function (Gladwin et al., 2003; Rother, Bell, Hillmen, & Gladwin, 2005). Markers of haemolysis are associated with endothelial dysfunction and pulmonary hypertension (Mehari et al., 2012; Nouraie et al., 2013). Other potential mechanisms contributing to pulmonary hypertension in SCD include chronic thromboembolism (Anthi et al., 2007), chronic hypoxia (Shimoda & Semenza, 2011), and in the postcapillary type, left ventricular diastolic dysfunction (Gladwin & Sachdev, 2012).

Pulmonary hypertension is associated with increased risk of mortality (Mehari et al., 2012; Parent et al., 2011). The association with increased mortality underscores the need for screening for pulmonary hypertension. The American Thoracic Society Ad hoc committee on pulmonary hypertension in SCD recommends regular screening by measurement of the tricuspid regurgitation velocity (TRV) on doppler echocardiography. Elevated TRV correlates with pulmonary hypertension (Fonseca, Souza, Salemi, Jardim, & Gualandro, 2012; Parent et al., 2011). Patients with TRV between 2.5 and 2.8 m/sec with symptoms of pulmonary hypertension such as dyspnoea on exertion should have cardiac catheterisation for confirmatory diagnosis of pulmonary hypertension.

Management of pulmonary hypertension in SCD includes control of underlying SCD pathology by use of hydroxyurea at maximum tolerated dose if possible and or chronic blood transfusion. No large clinical trials have been successfully done to guide management of pulmonary hypertension. The American Society of Haematology guideline panel suggests the use of pulmonary hypertension-specific therapies under the care of a specialist given the lack of alternative treatment options and associated high morbidity and mortality (Liem et al., 2019). These targeted therapies include Prostacyclin agonists, endothelin receptor antagonists, soluble guanylate cyclase stimulators and phosphodiesterase-5 inhibitors (Hayes et al., 2014).

Cardiac Dysfunction

Cardiovascular complications are a common in SCD. They are an unrecognised cause of morbidity and premature mortality in SCD (Gladwin, 2016) and affect 20–32% SCD patients (Hammoudi, Lionnet, Redheuil, & Montalescot, 2020). Common manifestations of cardiac dysfunction in SCD include elevated pulmonary artery systolic pressure, cardiomyopathy (left ventricular diastolic) heart failure and myocardial infarction, dysrhythmia and sudden death

Pathophysiology

Chronic haemolytic anaemia results in reduced oxygen carrying capacity of blood thus inducing an increased cardiac output (compensatory mechanism) to deal with the body metabolic demand (Figure 8.2) (Hammoudi et al., 2020; Kaur, Aurif, Kittaneh,

Chronic anemia

High cardiac output
(high volume with mild
increase in heart rate)

Peripheral vascular dilation
(decreased systemic vascular
resistance)

Renin-angiotensin-aldosterone
system(RAAS) activation causing
water and salt retention

Volume overload causing
increased cardiac preload

Sickled RBC in blood vessel

Microvascular occlusion

Reduced perfusion

Myocardial fibrosis

Cardiac remodeling-LV cavity dilation associated with
compensatory eccentric myocardial hypertrophy

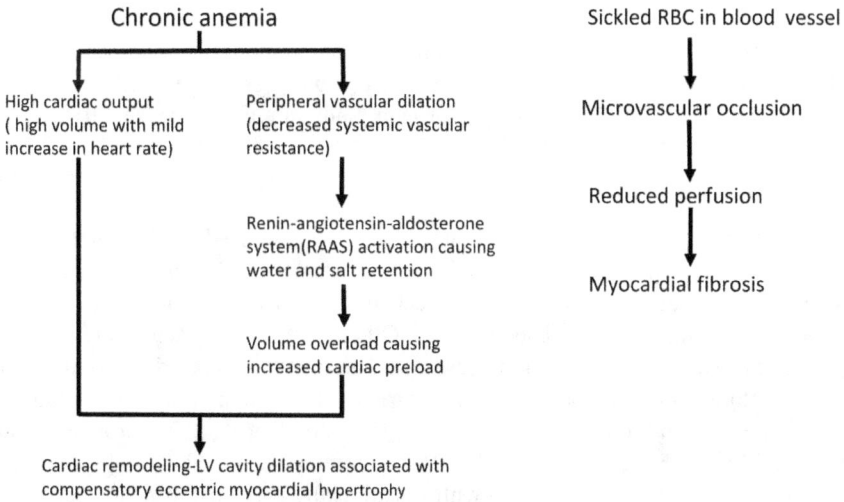

Figure 8.2 Sequential changes in pathophysiology of SCD-related cardiomyopathy.

Chio, & Malik, 2020). Anaemia also induces peripheral vascular dilation leading to decreased systemic resistance resulting in low blood pressure. This high-output state in SCD patients is related to a major increase in stroke volume associated with only a mild increase of heart rate (Hammoudi et al., 2014). This stimulates the renin–angiotensin–aldosterone system (RAAS) to increase plasma volume leading to left ventricular (LV) structure modification with compensatory myocardial hypertrophy (Kaur et al., 2020; Mushemi-Blake et al., 2015). This process usually begins early in childhood and advances with age (Harrington et al., 2017).

Chronic volume overload induces morphological cardiac remodelling that can be tolerated for a long time, however long-term severe anaemia will lead to cardiac fibrosis, LV dysfunction and congestion (Hammoudi et al., 2020).

Elevated Pulmonary Artery Systolic Pressure and Systemic Arterial Hypertension

Elevated pulmonary artery systolic pressure and systemic arterial hypertension occurs in 22.9% of persons with SCD (Sokunbi, Ekure, Temiye, Anyanwu, & Okoromah, 2017). Patients with SCD have generally lower blood pressure than reported normal values (Pegelow et al., 1997): A mild increase may reflect an alteration of systemic microcirculation (Hammoudi et al., 2020). Elevated pulmonary artery systolic pressure increases the risk of death (Lamina, Animasahun, Akinwumi, & Njokanma, 2019; Sokunbi et al., 2017).

Systemic arterial hypertension is associated with increased risk of stroke, left ventricular diastolic dysfunction (LVDD) and early mortality (Desai et al., 2014; Hammoudi et al., 2020; Kaur et al., 2020; Sokunbi et al., 2017). Kidney dysfunction is usually present because of shared underlying mechanisms. Further, the co-existent CKD may contribute to progressive vascular plus myocardial impairment thus further aggravating SCD-related cardiac remodelling and dysfunction (Hammoudi et al., 2020). Echocardiography usually shows elevated tricuspid regurgitant velocity (≥2.50 m/sec) (Noronha, Sadreameli, & Strouse, 2016).

Cardiomyopathy and Heart Failure

SCD-associated cardiomyopathy is associated with reduced quality of life and early mortality. Chronic anaemia leads to heart chamber dilation with a compensatory increase in left ventricular mass accompanied by left ventricular diastolic dysfunction (Gladwin & Sachdev, 2012). Other contributing factors include hypoxemia (Gladwin, 2016) with increased cardiac output, increased left ventricular stroke volume, and dilation of the left ventricle (Hammoudi et al., 2020), pulmonary hypertension (Fonseca & Souza, 2015; Hammoudi et al., 2020), iron overload (Chrifi, 2021; de Montalembert et al., 2017; Hammoudi et al., 2020) and alterations in intravascular volume associated with vasculopathy and renal insufficiency.

Left-sided diastolic dysfunction is increasingly being identified in patients with pulmonary hypertension and early cor-pulmonale (Niss et al., 2016) and increases with age.

A study among 134 patients with SCD who underwent screening echocardiography showed more than half had restrictive cardiomyopathy with diastolic dysfunction and left atrial enlargement (Niss et al., 2016). Progressive myocardial damages due to chronic volume overload lead to exercise intolerance and heart failure (Hammoudi et al., 2020). SCD mainly leads to right-sided heart failure with increased jugular venous pressure, tender hepatomegaly and peripheral oedema (Hammoudi et al., 2020; Thota et al., 2021).

Myocardial Infarction and Dysrhythmia

Myocardial Infarction

Myocardial injury is related to microvascular perfusion (Allali, Taylor, Brice, & de Montalembert, 2021); sickling in the coronary vasculature causes microvascular occlusion that results in chronic, indolent myocardial ischaemia (Di Maria et al., 2015).

Myocardial infarction is common in children and adolescents (Bode-Thomas, Hyacinth, Ogunkunle, & Omotoso, 2011). An autopsy study done on 72 hearts from patients with SCD between 1950 and 1982 showed about 10% had evidence of myocardial infarction, regardless of the lack of presence of obstructive or atherosclerotic lesions (Pannu et al., 2008). The commonly seen electrocardiogram (ECG) abnormality in these patients is prolonged corrected QT interval (QTc) (Indik et al., 2016).

Dysrhythmia

These are on the rise and a major indicator for worsening outcomes (Patel et al., 2020). A study done from 2010 to 2014 showed that the frequency of any arrhythmias and atrial fibrillation in hospitalised SCD patients relatively increased by

29.6% and 38.5%, respectively, with nearly a twofold increase in the frequency of arrhythmia among patients aged <18 years (Patel et al., 2020). Reported conduction abnormalities seen include QT prolongation, ventricular arrhythmias, first-degree AV block and nonspecific ST-T wave changes (Gladwin & Sachdev, 2012).

Management Approach

Management is multidisciplinary and is case based since disease severity varies widely among patients. The goals of treatment are to treat the congestion and underlying SCD and to manage comorbidities. Cardiovascular medications include low dose loop diuretics to reduce congestion (Hammoudi et al., 2020) and ACEis and angiotensin II receptor blockers which are cardiorenal protective and can reduce peak TRV (Haymann et al., 2017).

Hydroxyurea therapy is associated with better survival and may reverse cardiac remodelling. (Adjagba et al., 2017; Harrington et al., 2017; Sachdev et al., 2017). Chronic transfusion should be considered as an alternative therapy in patients at high mortality risk who are not responding to hydroxyurea (Klings et al., 2014). Comorbidities and risk management including weight loss, treatment of systemic arterial hypertension and renal failure improve cardiac function (Haymann et al., 2017).

Musculoskeletal Dysfunction: Osteonecrosis

Osteonecrosis affects about 30% of persons with SCD, with the femoral heads of the hip joints being the most affected joint. However multifocal joint involvement has also been reported (Adesina & Neumayr, 2019; Akinyoola, Adediran, & Asaleye, 2007).

Pathophysiology and Clinical Presentation

Ischaemic bone injury with infarction resulting from the occlusion of the microvasculature supplying the involved bones is the main underlying mechanism.

In the acute phases of infarction, compensatory bone marrow hyperplasia with osteolysis occurs before the eventual development of the degenerative bone changes with joint destruction. degenerative changes being a sequelae of irreversible bone destruction with repeated vaso-occlusion. The femoral bones are particularly vulnerable to microcirculation due to lack of collateral blood flow.

Symptoms range from no to mild pain to waxing and waning pain. Others include joint pains and stiffness on attempted movement.

Diagnosis

Diagnosis is often preceded by a thorough evaluation of the patient's history followed by a physical examination that confirms the presence of pain/tenderness, reduced range of motion of the affected limb or limb shortening,

However, imaging with MRI is the gold standard for diagnosis. MRI may also show diseased areas that are not yet causing any symptoms. A plain x-ray can also be performed on affected joints but largely useful in the later stages of the disease

Staging

Osteonecrosis can be categorised using four stages;

Stage 1 has a normal x-ray but MRI reveals the dead bone. Stage 2 can be seen on regular x-ray but there is no collapse of the femoral ball. Stage 3 shows signs of collapse (called a crescent sign) on x-ray. Stage 4 has collapse on x-ray and signs of cartilage damage (osteoarthritis).

Treatment

Beyond the pain management, several non-surgical as well as surgical interventions have been proposed. However, definitive treatment depends on the stage and severity of disease.

Non-operative treatments include hyperbaric oxygen therapy, shock wave therapy, electrical stimulation, pharmaceuticals (anticoagulants, bisphosphonates, vasodilators, lipid lowering agents), physiotherapy and muscle strengthening exercises. However, these non-operative treatments may be part of a wait-and-see approach based on the size of the area of dead bone.

Reduced weight bearing which is often recommended does not alter the course of the disease. Surgical treatments for osteonecrosis include: core decompression (Mukisi-Mukaza et al., 2009) which involves drilling a hole in the area of the affected bone to reduce pressure within the bone, works best in early stages of the disease.

Osteotomy which involves surgical reshaping of the bone to reduce stress on the affected area is most effective for patients with advanced osteonecrosis and those with a small area of affected bone.

Total hip arthroplasty is the definitive treatment and involves hip replacement. However, recent literature suggests maintenance of evidence-based perioperative SCD management for superior postoperative outcomes after cementless total hip arthroplasty in sickle cell–related osteonecrosis of the femoral head (Hernigou, Hernigou, & Scarlat, 2020).

In conclusion, organ dysfunction, which affects multiple body organs, is of growing significance among patients with SCD. It is progressive in nature, and it can start in childhood and peaks in early adulthood, culminating into end stage organ failure in late adulthood. Organ dysfunction is a predictor of early mortality in persons with SCD and is associated with poor quality of life in survivors. Early recognition through screening and monitoring of progression are important to reduce associated mortality.

Authorship

RN wrote the first draft, CN, PK, DM, made significant revisions and additions to the book chapter.

Conflict of Interest Disclosure

The authors declare no conflict of interest.

References

Aban, I., Baddam, S., Hilliard, L. M., Howard, T. H., Feig, D. I., & Lebensburger, J. D. (2017). Severe anemia early in life as a risk factor for sickle-cell kidney disease. *Blood, 129*(3), 385.

Adams, R. J., McKie, V. C., Hsu, L., Files, B., Vichinsky, E., Pegelow, C., ... Nichols, F. T. (1998). Prevention of a first stroke by transfusions in children with sickle cell anemia and abnormal results on transcranial Doppler ultrasonography. *New England Journal of Medicine, 339*(1), 5–11.

Adesina, O. O., & Neumayr, L. D. (2019). Osteonecrosis in sickle cell disease: An update on risk factors, diagnosis, and management. *Hematology 2014, the American Society of Hematology Education Program Book, 2019*(1), 351–358.

Adjagba, P. M., Habib, G., Robitaille, N., Pastore, Y., Raboisson, M.-J., Curnier, D., & Dahdah, N. (2017). Impact of sickle cell anaemia on cardiac chamber size in the paediatric population. *Cardiology in the Young, 27*(5), 918–924.

Akinyoola, A. L., Adediran, I. A., & Asaleye, C. M. (2007). Avascular necrosis of the femoral head in sickle cell disease in Nigeria: A retrospective study. *The Nigerian Postgraduate Medical Journal, 14*(3), 217–220.

Allali, S., Taylor, M., Brice, J., & de Montalembert, M. (2021). Chronic organ injuries in children with sickle cell disease. *Haematologica, 106*(6), 1535.

Alvarez, O., Miller, S. T., Wang, W. C., Luo, Z., McCarville, M. B., Schwartz, G. J., ... Rana, S. R. (2012). Effect of hydroxyurea treatment on renal function parameters: Results from the multi-center placebo-controlled BABY HUG clinical trial for infants with sickle cell anemia. *Pediatric Blood & Cancer, 59*(4), 668–674.

Alvarez, O., Montane, B., Lopez, G., Wilkinson, J., & Miller, T. (2006). Early blood transfusions protect against microalbuminuria in children with sickle cell disease. *Pediatric Blood & Cancer, 47*(1), 71–76.

Anthi, A., Machado, R. F., Jison, M. L., Taveira-DaSilva, A. M., Rubin, L. J., Hunter, L., ... Avila, N. A. (2007). Hemodynamic and functional assessment of patients with sickle cell disease and pulmonary hypertension. *American Journal of Respiratory and Critical Care Medicine, 175*(12), 1272–1279.

Arigliani, M., & Gupta, A. (2020). Management of chronic respiratory complications in children and adolescents with sickle cell disease. *European Respiratory Review, 29*(157), 200054.

Armstrong, F. D., Thompson Jr, R. J., Wang, W., Zimmerman, R., Pegelow, C. H., Miller, S., ... Vass, K. (1996). Cognitive functioning and brain magnetic resonance imaging in children with sickle cell disease. *Pediatrics, 97*(6), 864–870.

Aygun, B., Mortier, N. A., Smeltzer, M. P., Shulkin, B. L., Hankins, J. S., & Ware, R. E. (2013). Hydroxyurea treatment decreases glomerular hyperfiltration in children with sickle cell anemia. *American Journal of Hematology, 88*(2), 116–119.

Baddam, S., Aban, I., Hilliard, L., Howard, T., Askenazi, D., & Lebensburger, J. D. (2017). Acute kidney injury during a pediatric sickle cell vaso-occlusionpain crisis. *Pediatric Nephrology, 32*(8), 1451–1456.

Badesch, D. B., Champion, H. C., Gomez Sanchez, M. A., Hoeper, M. M., Loyd, J. E., Manes, A., ... Oudiz, R. J. (2009). Diagnosis and assessment of pulmonary arterial hypertension. *Journal of the American College of Cardiology, 54*(1_Supplement_S), S55–S66.

Batte, A., Menon, S., Ssenkusu, J., Kiguli, S., Kalyesubula, R., Lubega, J., … Starr, M. C. (2022). Acute kidney injury in hospitalized children with sickle cell anemia. *BMC Nephrology, 23*(1), 1–13.

Becton, L. J., Kalpatthi, R. V., Rackoff, E., Disco, D., Orak, J. K., Jackson, S. M., & Shatat, I. F. (2010). Prevalence and clinical correlates of microalbuminuria in children with sickle cell disease. *Pediatric Nephrology, 25*(8), 1505–1511.

Belcher, J. D., Chen, C., Nguyen, J., Milbauer, L., Abdulla, F., Alayash, A. I., … Vercellotti, G. M. (2014). Heme triggers TLR4 signaling leading to endothelial cell activation and vaso-occlusion in murine sickle cell disease. *Blood, The Journal of the American Society of Hematology, 123*(3), 377–390.

Belcher, J. D., Mahaseth, H., Welch, T. E., Vilback, A. E., Sonbol, K. M., Kalambur, V. S., … Vercellotti, G. M. (2005). Critical role of endothelial cell activation in hypoxia-induced vasoocclusion in transgenic sickle mice. *American Journal of Physiology-Heart and Circulatory Physiology, 288*(6), H2715–H2725.

Berkelhammer, L. D., Williamson, A. L., Sanford, S. D., Dirksen, C. L., Sharp, W. G., Margulies, A. S., & Prengler, R. A. (2007). Neurocognitive sequelae of pediatric sickle cell disease: A review of the literature. *Child Neuropsychology, 13*(2), 120–131.

Bernaudin, F., Verlhac, S., Arnaud, C., Kamdem, A., Vasile, M., Kasbi, F., … Biscardi, S. (2015). Chronic and acute anemia and extracranial internal carotid stenosis are risk factors for silent cerebral infarcts in sickle cell anemia. *Blood, The Journal of the American Society of Hematology, 125*(10), 1653–1661.

Bode-Thomas, F., Hyacinth, H., Ogunkunle, O., & Omotoso, A. (2011). Myocardial ischaemia in sickle cell anaemia: Evaluation using a new scoring system. *Annals of Tropical Paediatrics, 31*(1), 67–74.

Boyd, J. H., Macklin, E. A., Strunk, R. C., & DeBaun, M. R. (2006). Asthma is associated with acute chest syndrome and pain in children with sickle cell anemia. *Blood, 108*(9), 2923–2927.

Chrifi, F.-Z. (2021). La Readaptation Cardiaque Chez Les Patients En Insuffisance Cardiaque À Fevg Réduite (À Propos De 70 Cas).

Cohen, R. T., Strunk, R. C., Rodeghier, M., Rosen, C. L., Kirkham, F. J., Kirkby, J., & DeBaun, M. R. (2016). Pattern of lung function is not associated with prior or future morbidity in children with sickle cell anemia. *Annals of the American Thoracic Society, 13*(8), 1314–1323.

de Montalembert, M., Ribeil, J.-A., Brousse, V., Guerci-Bresler, A., Stamatoullas, A., Vannier, J.-P., … Bouabdallah, K. (2017). Cardiac iron overload in chronically transfused patients with thalassemia, sickle cell anemia, or myelodysplastic syndrome. *PLoS One, 12*(3), e0172147.

DeBaun, M. R., Gordon, M., McKinstry, R. C., Noetzel, M. J., White, D. A., Sarnaik, S. A., … Inusa, B. P. (2014). Controlled trial of transfusions for silent cerebral infarcts in sickle cell anemia. *New England Journal of Medicine, 371*(8), 699–710.

DeBaun, M., Jordan, L., King, A., Schatz, J., Vichinsky, E., Fox, C., … Daraz, L. (2020). American Society of Hematology 2020 guidelines for sickle cell disease: Prevention, diagnosis, and treatment of cerebrovascular disease in children and adults. *Blood Advances, 4*(8), 1554–1588.

DeBaun, M. R., Sarnaik, S. A., Rodeghier, M. J., Minniti, C. P., Howard, T. H., Iyer, R. V., … Quinn, C. T. (2012). Associated risk factors for silent cerebral infarcts in sickle cell anemia: Low baseline hemoglobin, sex, and relative high systolic blood pressure. *Blood, The Journal of the American Society of Hematology, 119*(16), 3684–3690.

Desai, A. A., Patel, A. R., Ahmad, H., Groth, J. V., Thiruvoipati, T., Turner, K., … Machado, R. F. (2014). Mechanistic insights and characterization of sickle cell disease–associated cardiomyopathy. *Circulation: Cardiovascular Imaging, 7*(3), 430–437.

Di Maria, M. V., Hsu, H. H., Al-Naami, G., Gruenwald, J., Kirby, K. S., Kirkham, F. J., … Younoszai, A. K. (2015). Left ventricular rotational mechanics in Tanzanian children with sickle cell disease. *Journal of the American Society of Echocardiography, 28*(3), 340–346.

Dowling, M. M., Quinn, C. T., Plumb, P., Rogers, Z. R., Rollins, N. K., Koral, K., & Buchanan, G. R. (2012). Acute silent cerebral ischemia and infarction during acute anemia in children with and without sickle cell disease. *Blood, The Journal of the American Society of Hematology, 120*(19), 3891–3897.

Falk, R. J., Scheinman, J., Phillips, G., Orringer, E., Johnson, A., & Jennette, J. C. (1992). Prevalence and pathologic features of sickle cell nephropathy and response to inhibition of angiotensin-converting enzyme. *New England Journal of Medicine, 326*(14), 910–915.

Feliu, M. H., Crawford, R. D., Edwards, L., Wellington, C., Wood, M., Whitfield, K. E., & Edwards, C. L. (2011). Neurocognitive testing and functioning in adults sickle cell disease. *Hemoglobin, 35*(5–6), 476–484.

Field, J. J., Stocks, J., Kirkham, F. J., Rosen, C. L., Dietzen, D. J., Semon, T., … DeBaun, M. R. (2011). Airway hyperresponsiveness in children with sickle cell anemia. *Chest, 139*(3), 563–568.

Fonseca, G., & Souza, R. (2015). Pulmonary hypertension in sickle cell disease. *Current Opinion in Pulmonary Medicine, 21*(5), 432–437.

Fonseca, G. H. H., Souza, R., Salemi, V., Jardim, C., & Gualandro, S. (2012). Pulmonary hypertension diagnosed by right heart catheterisation in sickle cell disease. *European Respiratory Journal, 39*(1), 112–118.

Galadanci, N. A., Abdullahi, S. U., Abubakar, S. A., Jibir, B. W., Aminu, H., Tijjani, A., … Borodo, A. M. (2020). Moderate fixed-dose hydroxyurea for primary prevention of strokes in Nigerian children with sickle cell disease: Final results of the SPIN trial. *American Journal of Hematology, 95*(9), E247.

Gladwin, M. T. (2016). Cardiovascular complications and risk of death in sickle-cell disease. *The Lancet, 387*(10037), 2565–2574.

Gladwin, M. T., & Sachdev, V. (2012). Cardiovascular abnormalities in sickle cell disease. *Journal of the American College of Cardiology, 59*(13), 1123–1133.

Gladwin, M. T., Schechter, A. N., Ognibene, F. P., Coles, W. A., Reiter, C. D., Schenke, W. H., … Cannon III, R. O. (2003). Divergent nitric oxide bioavailability in men and women with sickle cell disease. *Circulation, 107*(2), 271–278.

Greenough, A., & Inusa, B. (2016). Pulmonary complications and lung function abnormalities in children with sickle cell disease. In *Sickle cell disease-pain and common chronic complications*. IntechOpen.

Halphen, I., Elie, C., Brousse, V., Le Bourgeois, M., Allali, S., Bonnet, D., & de Montalembert, M. (2014). Severe nocturnal and postexercise hypoxia in children and adolescents with sickle cell disease. *PloS One, 9*(5), e97462.

Hamideh, D., & Alvarez, O. (2013). Sickle cell disease related mortality in the United States (1999–2009). *Pediatric Blood & Cancer, 60*(9), 1482–1486.

Hammoudi, N., Arangalage, D., Djebbar, M., Stojanovic, K. S., Charbonnier, M., Isnard, R., … Lionnet, F. (2014). Subclinical left ventricular systolic impairment in steady state young adult patients with sickle-cell anemia. *The International Journal of Cardiovascular Imaging, 30*(7), 1297–1304.

Hammoudi, N., Lionnet, F., Redheuil, A., & Montalescot, G. (2020). Cardiovascular manifestations of sickle cell disease. *European Heart Journal, 41*(13), 1365–1373.

Hargrave, D. R., Wade, A., Evans, J. P., Hewes, D. K., & Kirkham, F. J. (2003). Nocturnal oxygen saturation and painful sickle cell crises in children. *Blood, The Journal of the American Society of Hematology, 101*(3), 846–848.

Harrington, J. K., Krishnan, U., Jin, Z., Mardy, C., Kobsa, S., & Lee, M. T. (2017). Longitudinal analysis of echocardiographic abnormalities in children with sickle cell disease. *Journal of Pediatric Hematology/Oncology, 39*(7), 500–505.

Hayes, M. M., Vedamurthy, A., George, G., Dweik, R., Klings, E. S., Machado, R. F., ... Thomson, C. C. (2014). Pulmonary hypertension in sickle cell disease. *Annals of the American Thoracic Society, 11*(9), 1488–1489.

Haymann, J. P., Hammoudi, N., Stankovic Stojanovic, K., Galacteros, F., Habibi, A., Avellino, V., ... Djebbar, M. (2017). Renin-angiotensin system blockade promotes a cardiorenal protection in albuminuric homozygous sickle cell patients. *British Journal of Haematology, 179*(5), 820–828.

Hebbel, R. P., Belcher, J. D., & Vercellotti, G. M. (2020). The multifaceted role of ischemia/reperfusion in sickle cell anemia. *The Journal of Clinical Investigation, 130*(3), 1062–1072.

Hernigou, P., Hernigou, J., & Scarlat, M. (2020). Shoulder osteonecrosis: Pathogenesis, causes, clinical evaluation, imaging, and classification. *Orthopaedic Surgery, 12*(5), 1340–1349.

Hulbert, M. L., McKinstry, R. C., Lacey, J. L., Moran, C. J., Panepinto, J. A., Thompson, A. A., ... Inusa, B. (2011). Silent cerebral infarcts occur despite regular blood transfusion therapy after first strokes in children with sickle cell disease. *Blood, The Journal of the American Society of Hematology, 117*(3), 772–779.

Indik, J. H., Nair, V., Rafikov, R., Nyotowidjojo, I. S., Bisla, J., Kansal, M., ... Oberoi, M. (2016). Associations of prolonged QTc in sickle cell disease. *PLoS One, 11*(10), e0164526.

Johnson, M. C., Kirkham, F. J., Redline, S., Rosen, C. L., Yan, Y., Roberts, I., ... DeBaun, M. R. (2010). Left ventricular hypertrophy and diastolic dysfunction in children with sickle cell disease are related to asleep and waking oxygen desaturation. *Blood, The Journal of the American Society of Hematology, 116*(1), 16–21.

Kalogeris, T., Baines, C. P., Krenz, M., & Korthuis, R. J. (2016). Ischemia/reperfusion. *Comprehensive Physiology, 7*(1), 113.

Kassim, A. A., Payne, A. B., Rodeghier, M., Macklin, E. A., Strunk, R. C., & DeBaun, M. R. (2015). Low forced expiratory volume is associated with earlier death in sickle cell anemia. *Blood, The Journal of the American Society of Hematology, 126*(13), 1544–1550.

Kassim, A. A., Pruthi, S., Day, M., Rodeghier, M., Gindville, M. C., Brodsky, M. A., ... Jordan, L. C. (2016). Silent cerebral infarcts and cerebral aneurysms are prevalent in adults with sickle cell anemia. *Blood, The Journal of the American Society of Hematology, 127*(16), 2038–2040.

Kato, G. J., Gladwin, M. T., & Steinberg, M. H. (2007). Deconstructing sickle cell disease: Reappraisal of the role of hemolysis in the development of clinical subphenotypes. *Blood Reviews, 21*(1), 37–47.

Kaur, H., Aurif, F., Kittaneh, M., Chio, J. P. G., & Malik, B. H. (2020). Cardiomyopathy in sickle cell disease. *Cureus, 12*(8).

King, A. A., Rodeghier, M. J., Panepinto, J. A., Strouse, J. J., Casella, J. F., Quinn, C. T., ... Woods, G. M. (2014). Silent cerebral infarction, income, and grade retention among students with sickle cell anemia. *American Journal of Hematology, 89*(10), E188–E192.

Kinney, T. R., Sleeper, L. A., Wang, W. C., Zimmerman, R. A., Pegelow, C. H., Ohene-Frempong, K., ... Moser, F. G. (1999). Silent cerebral infarcts in sickle cell anemia: A risk factor analysis. *Pediatrics, 103*(3), 640–645.

Kirkham, F., Hewes, D., Prengler, M., Wade, A., Lane, R., & Evans, J. (2001). Nocturnal hypoxaemia and central-nervous-system events in sickle-cell disease. *The Lancet, 357*(9269), 1656–1659.

Klings, E. S., Machado, R. F., Barst, R. J., Morris, C. R., Mubarak, K. K., Gordeuk, V. R., … Castro, O. (2014). An official American thoracic society clinical practice guideline: Diagnosis, risk stratification, and management of pulmonary hypertension of sickle cell disease. *American Journal of Respiratory and Critical Care Medicine*, *189*(6), 727–740.

Kwiatkowski, J. L., Zimmerman, R. A., Pollock, A. N., Seto, W., Smith-Whitley, K., Shults, J., … Ohene-Frempong, K. (2009). Silent infarcts in young children with sickle cell disease. *British Journal of Haematology*, *146*(3), 300–305.

Lamina, M. O., Animasahun, B. A., Akinwumi, I. N., & Njokanma, O. F. (2019). Doppler echocardiographic assessment of pulmonary artery pressure in children with sickle cell anaemia. *Cardiovascular Diagnosis and Therapy*, *9*(3), 204.

Lansberg, M. G., Albers, G. W., Beaulieu, C., & Marks, M. P. (2000). Comparison of diffusion-weighted MRI and CT in acute stroke. *Neurology*, *54*(8), 1557–1561.

Laurin, L.-P., Nachman, P. H., Desai, P. C., Ataga, K. I., & Derebail, V. K. (2014). Hydroxyurea is associated with lower prevalence of albuminuria in adults with sickle cell disease. *Nephrology Dialysis Transplantation*, *29*(6), 1211–1218.

Lebensburger, J. D., Aban, I., Pernell, B., Kasztan, M., Feig, D. I., Hilliard, L. M., & Askenazi, D. J. (2019). Hyperfiltration during early childhood precedes albuminuria in pediatric sickle cell nephropathy. *American Journal of Hematology*, *94*(4), 417–423.

Lebensburger, J. D., Cutter, G. R., Howard, T. H., Muntner, P., & Feig, D. I. (2017). Evaluating risk factors for chronic kidney disease in pediatric patients with sickle cell anemia. *Pediatric Nephrology*, *32*(9), 1565–1573.

Lebensburger, J., Johnson, S. M., Askenazi, D. J., Rozario, N. L., Howard, T. H., & Hilliard, L. M. (2011). Protective role of hemoglobin and fetal hemoglobin in early kidney disease for children with sickle cell anemia. *American Journal of Hematology*, *86*(5), 430–432.

Liem, R. I., Lanzkron, S., D. Coates, T., DeCastro, L., Desai, A. A., Ataga, K. I., … Lebensburger, J. D. (2019). American Society of Hematology 2019 guidelines for sickle cell disease: Cardiopulmonary and kidney disease. *Blood Advances*, *3*(23), 3867–3897.

Lunt, A., McGhee, E., Sylvester, K., Rafferty, G., Dick, M., Rees, D., … Greenough, A. (2016). Longitudinal assessment of lung function in children with sickle cell disease. *Pediatric Pulmonology*, *51*(7), 717–723.

McLaren, A., Klingel, M., Behera, S., Odame, I., Kirby-Allen, M., & Grasemann, H. (2017). Effect of hydroxyurea therapy on pulmonary function in children with sickle cell anemia. *American Journal of Respiratory and Critical Care Medicine*, *195*(5), 689–691.

Mehari, A., Gladwin, M. T., Tian, X., Machado, R. F., & Kato, G. J. (2012). Mortality in adults with sickle cell disease and pulmonary hypertension. *Jama*, *307*(12), 1254–1256.

Mehari, A., & Klings, E. S. (2016). Chronic pulmonary complications of sickle cell disease. *Chest*, *149*(5), 1313–1324.

Mehrad, B., Burdick, M. D., Wandersee, N. J., Shahir, K. S., Zhang, L., Simpson, P. M., … Field, J. J. (2017). Circulating fibrocytes as biomarkers of impaired lung function in adults with sickle cell disease. *Blood Advances*, *1*(24), 2217–2224.

Merle, N. S., Grunenwald, A., Rajaratnam, H., Gnemmi, V., Frimat, M., Figueres, M.-L., … Roumenina L.T. (2018). Intravascular hemolysis activates complement via cell-free heme and heme-loaded microvesicles. *JCI Insight*, *3*(12). https://doi.org/10.1172/jci.insight.96910

Miller, A. C., & Gladwin, M. T. (2012). Pulmonary complications of sickle cell disease. *American Journal of Respiratory and Critical Care Medicine*, *185*(11), 1154–1165.

Miller, S. T., Macklin, E. A., Pegelow, C. H., Kinney, T. R., Sleeper, L. A., Bello, J. A., … Moser, F. G. (2001). Silent infarction as a risk factor for overt stroke in children with sickle cell anemia: A report from the cooperative study of sickle cell disease. *The Journal of Pediatrics*, *139*(3), 385–390.

Mukisi-Mukaza, M., Manicom, O., Alexis, C., Bashoun, K., Donkerwolcke, M., & Burny, F. (2009). Treatment of sickle cell disease's hip necrosis by core decompression: A prospective case-control study. *Orthopaedics & Traumatology: Surgery & Research, 95*(7), 498–504.

Mushemi-Blake, S., Melikian, N., Drasar, E., Bhan, A., Lunt, A., Desai, S. R., ... Shah, A. M. (2015). Pulmonary haemodynamics in sickle cell disease are driven predominantly by A high-output state rather than elevated pulmonary vascular resistance: A prospective 3-dimensional echocardiography/Doppler study. *PLoS One, 10*(8), e0135472.

Naik, R. P., & Derebail, V. K. (2017). The spectrum of sickle hemoglobin-related nephropathy: From sickle cell disease to sickle trait. *Expert Review of Hematology, 10*(12), 1087–1094.

Nath, K. A., & Hebbel, R. P. (2015). Sickle cell disease: Renal manifestations and mechanisms. *Nature Reviews Nephrology, 11*(3), 161–171.

Nielsen, L., Canouï-Poitrine, F., Jais, J. P., Dahmane, D., Bartolucci, P., Bentaarit, B., ... Matignon, M. (2016). Morbidity and mortality of sickle cell disease patients starting intermittent haemodialysis: A comparative cohort study with non-Sickle dialysis patients. *British Journal of Haematology, 174*(1), 148–152.

Niss, O., Quinn, C. T., Lane, A., Daily, J., Khoury, P. R., Bakeer, N., ... Taylor, M. D. (2016). Cardiomyopathy with restrictive physiology in sickle cell disease. *JACC: Cardiovascular Imaging, 9*(3), 243–252.

Noronha, S. A., Sadreameli, S. C., & Strouse, J. J. (2016). Management of sickle cell disease in children. *Southern Medical Journal, 109*(9), 495–502.

Nouraie, M., Lee, J. S., Zhang, Y., Kanias, T., Zhao, X., Xiong, Z., ... Gibbs, J. S. R. (2013). The relationship between the severity of hemolysis, clinical manifestations and risk of death in 415 patients with sickle cell anemia in the US and Europe. *Haematologica, 98*(3), 464.

Ohene-Frempong, K., Weiner, S. J., Sleeper, L. A., Miller, S. T., Embury, S., Moohr, J. W., ... Gill, F. M. (1998). Cerebrovascular accidents in sickle cell disease: Rates and risk factors. *Blood, The Journal of the American Society of Hematology, 91*(1), 288–294.

Pannu, R., Zhang, J., Andraws, R., Armani, A., Patel, P., & Mancusi-Ungaro, P. (2008). Acute myocardial infarction in sickle cell disease: A systematic review. *Critical Pathways in Cardiology, 7*(2), 133–138.

Parent, F., Bachir, D., Inamo, J., Lionnet, F., Driss, F., Loko, G., ... Adnot, S. (2011). A hemodynamic study of pulmonary hypertension in sickle cell disease. *New England Journal of Medicine, 365*(1), 44–53.

Patel, U., Desai, R., Hanna, B., Patel, D., Akbar, S., Zubair, M., ... Sachdeva, R. (2020). Sickle cell disease-associated arrhythmias and in-hospital outcomes: Insights from the national inpatient sample. *Journal of Arrhythmia, 36*(6), 1068–1073.

Pegelow, C. H., Colangelo, L., Steinberg, M., Wright, E. C., Smith, J., Phillips, G., & Vichinsky, E. (1997). Natural history of blood pressure in sickle cell disease: Risks for stroke and death associated with relative hypertension in sickle cell anemia. *The American Journal of Medicine, 102*(2), 171–177.

Powars, D. R., Chan, L. S., Hiti, A., Ramicone, E., & Johnson, C. (2005). Outcome of sickle cell anemia: A 4-decade observational study of 1056 patients. *Medicine, 84*(6), 363–376.

Powars, D., Wilson, B., Imbus, C., Pegelow, C., & Allen, J. (1978). The natural history of stroke in sickle cell disease. *The American Journal of Medicine, 65*(3), 461–471.

Puffer, E., Schatz, J., & Roberts, C. W. (2007). The association of oral hydroxyurea therapy with improved cognitive functioning in sickle cell disease. *Child Neuropsychology, 13*(2), 142–154.

Quinn, C. T., & Sargent, J. W. (2008). Daytime steady-state haemoglobin desaturation is a risk factor for overt stroke in children with sickle cell anaemia. *British Journal of Haematology, 140*(3), 336–339.

Rosen, C. L., Debaun, M. R., Strunk, R. C., Redline, S., Seicean, S., Craven, D. I., ... Roberts, I. (2014). Obstructive sleep apnea and sickle cell anemia. *Pediatrics, 134*(2), 273–281.

Rother, R. P., Bell, L., Hillmen, P., & Gladwin, M. T. (2005). The clinical sequelae of intravascular hemolysis and extracellular plasma hemoglobin: A novel mechanism of human disease. *JAMA, 293*(13), 1653–1662.

Sachdev, V., Sidenko, S., Wu, M. D., Minniti, C. P., Hannoush, H., Brenneman, C. L., ... Kato, G. J. (2017). Skeletal and myocardial microvascular blood flow in hydroxycarbamide-treated patients with sickle cell disease. *British Journal of Haematology, 179*(4), 648–656.

Sharpe, C. C., & Thein, S. L. (2014). How i treat renal complications in sickle cell disease. *Blood, The Journal of the American Society of Hematology, 123*(24), 3720–3726.

Shimoda, L. A., & Semenza, G. L. (2011). HIF and the lung: Role of hypoxia-inducible factors in pulmonary development and disease. *American Journal of Respiratory and Critical Care Medicine, 183*(2), 152–156.

Simonneau, G., Gatzoulis, M. A., Adatia, I., Celermajer, D., Denton, C., Ghofrani, A., ... Machado, R. F. (2013). Updated clinical classification of pulmonary hypertension. *Journal of the American College of Cardiology, 62*(25S), D34–D41.

Sokunbi, O. J., Ekure, E. N., Temiye, E. O., Anyanwu, R., & Okoromah, C. A. (2017). Pulmonary hypertension among 5 to 18 year old children with sickle cell anaemia in Nigeria. *PLoS One, 12*(9), e0184287.

Solovey, A., Somani, A., Belcher, J. D., Milbauer, L., Vincent, L., Pawlinski, R., ... O'Sullivan, M. G. (2017). A monocyte-TNF-endothelial activation axis in sickle transgenic mice: Therapeutic benefit from TNF blockade. *American Journal of Hematology, 92*(11), 1119–1130.

Steen, R. G., Miles, M. A., Helton, K. J., Strawn, S., Wang, W., Xiong, X., & Mulhern, R. K. (2003). Cognitive impairment in children with hemoglobin SS sickle cell disease: Relationship to MR imaging findings and hematocrit. *American Journal of Neuroradiology, 24*(3), 382–389.

Strouse, J. J., Lanzkron, S., & Urrutia, V. (2011). The epidemiology, evaluation and treatment of stroke in adults with sickle cell disease. *Expert Review of Hematology, 4*(6), 597–606.

Strunk, R. C., Cohen, R. T., Cooper, B. P., Rodeghier, M., Kirkham, F. J., Warner, J. O., ... Rosen, C. L. (2014). Wheezing symptoms and parental asthma are associated with a physician diagnosis of asthma in children with sickle cell anemia. *The Journal of Pediatrics, 164*(4), 821–826. e821.

Takano, M., Meneshian, A., Sheikh, E., Yamakawa, Y., Wilkins, K. B., Hopkins, E. A., & Bulkley, G. B. (2002). Rapid upregulation of endothelial p-selectin expression via reactive oxygen species generation. *American Journal of Physiology-Heart and Circulatory Physiology, 283*(5), H2054–H2061.

Thein, M. S., Igbineweka, N. E., & Thein, S. L. (2017). Sickle cell disease in the older adult. *Pathology, 49*(1), 1–9.

Thota, V., Paravathaneni, M., Konduru, S., Buragamadagu, B. C., Thota, M., & Lerman, G. (2021). Treatment of refractory lactic acidosis with thiamine administration in a non-alcoholic patient. *Cureus, 13*(7), e16267. https://doi.org/10.7759/cureus.16267

Van Avondt, K., Nur, E., & Zeerleder, S. (2019). Mechanisms of haemolysis-induced kidney injury. *Nature Reviews Nephrology, 15*(11), 671–692.

van Beers, E. J., van Tuijn, C. F., Mac Gillavry, M. R., van der Giessen, A., Schnog, J.-J. B., Biemond, B. J., & Group, C. S. (2008). Sickle cell disease-related organ damage occurs irrespective of pain rate: Implications for clinical practice. *Haematologica, 93*(5), 757–760.

van Geyzel, L., Arigliani, M., Inusa, B., Singh, B., Kozlowska, W., Chakravorty, S., … Gupta, A. (2020). Higher oxygen saturation with hydroxyurea in paediatric sickle cell disease. *Archives of Disease in Childhood, 105*(6), 575–579.

Vichinsky, E. (2017). Chronic organ failure in adult sickle cell disease. *Hematology 2014, the American Society of Hematology Education Program Book, 2017*(1), 435–439.

Vichinsky, E. P., Neumayr, L. D., Gold, J. I., Weiner, M. W., Rule, R. R., Truran, D., … McMahon, L. (2010). Neuropsychological dysfunction and neuroimaging abnormalities in neurologically intact adults with sickle cell anemia. *JAMA, 303*(18), 1823–1831.

Wang, W. C., Langston, J. W., Steen, R. G., Wynn, L. W., Mulhern, R. K., Wilimas, J. A., … Figueroa, R. E. (1998). Abnormalities of the central nervous system in very young children with sickle cell anemia. *The Journal of Pediatrics, 132*(6), 994–998.

Wang, W. C., Pavlakis, S. G., Helton, K. J., McKinstry, R. C., Casella, J. F., Adams, R. J., & Rees, R. C. (2008). MRI abnormalities of the brain in one-year-old children with sickle cell anemia. *Pediatric Blood & Cancer, 51*(5), 643–646.

Ware, R. E., Rees, R. C., Sarnaik, S. A., Iyer, R. V., Alvarez, O. A., Casella, J. F., … Miller, J. H. (2010). Renal function in infants with sickle cell anemia: Baseline data from the BABY HUG trial. *The Journal of Pediatrics, 156*(1), 66–70. e61.

Wedderburn, C. J., Rees, D., Height, S., Dick, M., Rafferty, G. F., Lunt, A., & Greenough, A. (2014). Airways obstruction and pulmonary capillary blood volume in children with sickle cell disease. *Pediatric Pulmonology, 49*(7), 716–722.

Whitesell, P., Owoyemi, O., Oneal, P., Nouraie, M., Klings, E., Rock, A., … Taylor, R. (2016). Sleep-disordered breathing and nocturnal hypoxemia in young adults with sickle cell disease. *Sleep Medicine, 22*, 47–49.

Wood, J. C. (2016). The heart in sickle cell disease, a model for heart failure with preserved ejection fraction. *Proceedings of the National Academy of Sciences, 113*(35), 9670–9672.

Zimmerman, R. A. (2005). MRI/MRA evaluation of sickle cell disease of the brain. *Pediatric Radiology, 35*(3), 249–257.

9 Management of Pain in Sickle Cell Disease

Ademola Samson Adewoyin

Introduction/Background

Sickle cell disease (SCD) is a chronic haemolytic syndrome often interspersed and characterized by episodic pain. According to the International Association for the Study of Pain (IASP), pain has been described as an unpleasant sensory and emotional experience associated with, or resembling that associated with, actual or potential tissue damage. Pain in SCD is largely episodic, presenting as acute complications often called vaso-occlusive (painful) crisis. However, chronic pain also occurs in SCD. Pain is said to account for over 70% of acute admissions in SCD. The commonest vaso-occlusive/painful crisis in SCD is bone pain. Vaso-occlusion can occur in virtually any organ system in SCD. As such, other presentations of pain in SCD include abdominal crisis/girdle syndrome, or chest pain which may be associated with acute chest syndrome.

Pain Burden in Sickle Cell Disease

In terms of epidemiology, sickle cell pain is largely acute or chronic in nature. Acute and chronic pain syndromes in SCD present with significant intra-individual and inter-individual variability. Pain remains the primary and consistent presentation of SCD. Sickle cell pain is directly related to disease severity. Pain is the commonest cause of hospital admissions and re-admissions in SCD globally. Factors that decrease SCD severity will also reduce pain severity. Such factors may include raised haemoglobin F levels, co-inheritance of the alpha thalassemia trait, haemoglobin SC phenotype, Haemoglobin Sbeta+ phenotypes and younger ages. In a cross-sectional survey of 60 adult subjects in Benin City, Nigeria, 98.6% of the participants reported painful crisis, which accounted for 71.4% of the hospital admissions. Rates of painful crisis were higher between ages 15 and 29 years, males, haemoglobin SS phenotypes and higher leucocyte counts (though not statistically significant perhaps due to the power of the study).

Mostly acute sickle pain in infancy is associated with dactylitis (hand and foot syndrome). In childhood, sickle pain is largely episodic. However, chronic pain syndromes are more common with adulthood. In a study of 100 young subjects in age ranges 8–18 years reported by Sil et al. (2016), 40% reported chronic pain,

DOI: 10.4324/9781003463931-10

while another 40% exhibited episodic pain, the remainder had no pain over the three-month period. In the PiSCES (Pain in Sickle cell Epidemiology Study), adult patients reported chronic pain on 54.5% of 31,017 days at home, suggesting significant pain burden.

As described above, pain in SCD is often assessed in terms of physicality. However, the concept of total pain goes beyond just physical (nociceptive or neuropathic pain) to include emotional, social, and spiritual pain. Emotional pain will include the gloom, anger, frustrations, fear and helplessness associated with the chronic disease. Social pain such as isolation and social withdrawal, stigmatization, relational issues, and financial difficulties are evident in SCD. Spiritual pain will include fear of living, insecurities, inferiority complex, loss of esteem, loss of identity, rejection of life, and lack of purpose. All pains (physical, emotional, social or spiritual) in SCD are real and should be assessed and managed as in other forms of chronic diseases. Emotional, social, and spiritual pain associated with SCD are somewhat collateral in nature, associated with the physical pain. It is therefore important to fully understand the mechanisms of somatic pain in SCD, in a bid to create and drive effective management protocols for them.

Pathophysiology of Physical Pain in Sickle Cell Disease

Pain refers to an unpleasant sensory and emotional experience associated with actual or potential tissue damage. Pain is a subjective reaction to an objective stimulus. It is important to understand the biologic and molecular mechanism of pain specific to genesis of sickle pain, as this promotes development of targeted treatments with potentials to improve disease outlook. There are currently three described mechanisms of pain in SCD. All somatic pains that patients with SCD experience are linked to vaso-occlusion, central sensitization, or opioid withdrawal pain.

In SCD, primary disease event remains haemoglobin polymerization leading to chronic heamolysis, vasculopathy, oxidant stress, infarction-reperfusion injury, increased adhesiveness, and procoagulant tendencies. In more specifics, vascular dysfunction, inflammations, ischaemic-reperfusion injury and oxidative stress evoke activation of nociceptive nerve fibres, leading to acute pain. Physical pain in SCD is largely infarctive and inflammatory in nature.

In central sensitization, there is heightened responsiveness of the nociceptive fibres to normal painful and non-painful stimuli. Hyperalgesia refers to increased pain perception incongruent to the degree of painful stimuli. Allodynia refers to pain associated with a non-painful stimulus such as light touch, pressure, crude touch, or temperature changes. In some patients, long-term opioid use has also been shown to trigger increased pain sensitivity, often described by patients as generalized, "pain all over." Moreover, some pain descriptions also suggest a significant contribution of neuropathic component, which may be related to the disease or damage to the somatosensory nervous system. Chronic inflammations, constant endothelial activations, and generation of reactive oxygen species (ROS) underlie the chronic inflammatory and neuropathic pains. Chronic pains are from extended hyperalgesia after acute episodes and central sensitization have been described.

Neuropathic pain may be related to central or peripheral nerve injury and protein kinase C may be associated with the pain. In central sensitization, neuroplasticity in the brain and activation of glial cells has been described by neurophysiological studies.

The concept of cyclic opioid withdrawal syndrome refers to a pattern of repeated cycles of pain exacerbations, coupled with opioid withdrawal symptoms. This occurs when high doses of opioids are suddenly discontinued or precipitously decreased. It also occurs when opioid use is suddenly terminated after long-term exposure. It may also be related to changes in route of opioid administration or even the opioid type with resultant change in efficacy/potency and plasma opioid levels. Sudden reductions in plasma opioid levels trigger the opioid withdrawal symptoms which include low grade fever, chills, nausea and vomiting, changes in bowel habits, abdominal cramps, and depressed mood. Failure to treat opioid withdrawal promptly with opioids triggers dehydration and autonomic distress, inciting another round of severe pain, warranting hospitalization and high dose opioids, and the cycle may continue.

Pain Presentations in Sickle Cell Disease

Pain in SCD can be categorized into acute and chronic. Acute pain presentations are often termed bone pain crisis, painful crisis or vaso-occlusive crisis. Chronic pain may be related to the chronic pain syndrome or other long-standing pain associated with complications such as leg ulcers, avascular necrosis, spine deformities, and so on. Some chronic pain experienced may be unassociated with SCD such as connective tissue diseases and other non-SCD-related pathologies. This requires a high index of suspicion, as the primary expectation of painful crisis or chronic pain in SCD may mask the consideration of other likely possibilities.

Vaso-occlusive Crisis

This refers to the acute syndrome/manifestation of pain in SCD, otherwise called painful crisis, and classically involves the bone and other tissues. It occurs for hours to days, less commonly weeks. VOC begins at about mid infancy when the haemoglobin switch (F to S) occurs and early childhood. VOC becomes more frequent in adolescent and younger adulthood and tends to reduce in older adulthood. Generally, VOC involves a variety of capillary vascular beds in the deep muscles, joints, and bones which are richly innervated by nociceptive receptors and activated by release of pain mediators in SCD. Commonly affected bones in sickle crisis include the extremity bones such as femur and humerus, vertebrae, pelvis, ribs, and sternum. Multiple sites may be involved. Dactylitis, an early manifestation of bone infarction, involves the small bones of the hand or foot, causing a diffuse swelling over the involved area. Dactylitis is rare after 2–3 years of life. Frequency of bone pain crisis is higher in patients with homozygous SCD, lower Hb F, and higher baseline haemoglobin. Painful crisis is more common in young adults and tends to wane at older ages. Known precipitants of painful crisis include extremes of temperature (heat or cold), extremes of emotions (gloom or happiness), dehydration, intercurrent infections such as malaria, physical exertion, tobacco smoke, alcohol use, hard drugs, high altitude, hypoxic conditions, other somatic pain, pregnancy, and onset of menses in some ladies. In some cases, as much as 57%, no known precipitant can be identified. Typical pain descriptors for vaso-occlusion includes sharp, throbbing, stabbing, debilitating, excruciating in nature. In neuropathic pain, patients often report feelings of burning, tingling, pins and needles and numbness in the affected parts of the body.

Chronic Pain

Generally, chronic pain is defined by the International Association for the Study of Pain (IASP, n.d.) as persistent or recurrent pain lasting more than three months or beyond the normal tissue healing period. In SCD, chronic pain has recently been defined as pain that is present on most days and has lasted at least six months. Prevalence of chronic pain in SCD increases with age. By adulthood, more than 55% experience pain on more than half of days lived, while 29% experience pain on 95% of their days, according to Smith et al. (2008).

In terms of clinical presentation, chronic pain is either SCD related or not. SCD-related chronic pain includes vaso-occlusion and pain associated with SCD complications such as leg ulcers, osteonecrosis, spine deformities, gall stones, etc. Also, non-SCD-related pathologies such as auto-immune diseases may also induce chronic pain. The pain descriptors depend on the origin of the pain: infarcive, inflammatory, or neuropathic. Chronic pain must be diagnosed and treated accordingly.

Management of Pain in Sickle Cell Disease

Management of pain in SCD requires short-term treatments for acute pain and long-term strategies for chronic pain issues. Often times, a multimodal pharmacologic approach is indicated, coupled with non-pharmacologic techniques for analgesia.

In any sort of painful manifestation in SCD, optimal analgesia is important. Pain control measures are largely pharmacologic. The choice of analgesics, their dosing and frequency depends on the individual patients, pain/analgesia history, severity of the pain, co-morbidities, and response to treatments. There is no straight-jacket protocol to achieving optimal analgesia, it is highly individualized. Pain thresholds differ among individuals, as such subjective assessments from affected persons, are a major guide in formulating pain control protocols. Non-pharmacologic measures that could be integrated to pharmacologic measures include massage, hot water bottle, acupuncture, oral analgesia, cognitive behavioural modifications, etc.

World Health Organisation (WHO) pain ladder of 1986 (revised in 1996) has been a very simple valuable protocol for management of pain, initially designed for management of cancer pain but has found a lot of relevance in management of acute pain including SCD. The pain ladder of 1986 (revised in 1996) is purely pharmacologic before the 2020 Modification (World Health Organization, 1986). There is a rising burden of opioid abuse and toxicity, the 2020 modification seeks to promote non-opioid modalities for pain control, but yet to be clearly validated in SCD though applicable in all types of pain. Beyond integrative medicine therapies in every step depending on pain severity, if the non-opioids and weak opioids fail (persistence of pain), minimally invasive interventions (such as nerve blocks, spinal/epidural administration of local anaesthetics, neuromodulation spinal cord stimulation) in step 3 can be recommended before upgrading to strong opioids.

Management of pain in SCD should begin with assessment, then treatment, re-assessment and then adjustment of treatment to optimal pain control. Assessment of pain will include asking the patient, a clinical assessment including physical examination, and laboratory investigations. From the foregoing, it is therefore important to be able to assess pain intensity when managing pain. Pain is a subjective feeling. In order to control/respond to the subjective feeling of pain, there needs to be an objective assessment. Commonly recommended is the numeric rating scale in adults and pain faces scale in children as depicted in Figure 9.1.

Objective pain scores are a good guide to optimal interventions. Treatment of vaso-occlusive crisis: Painful crisis may be uncomplicated or complicated. Uncomplicated painful crisis refers to straightforward vaso-occlusive event largely involving the bones, whereas, complicated painful crisis refers to painful infarctions coupled with other sickle co-morbidities such as hyper-haemolysis, acute chest syndrome, sequestration crisis, etc.

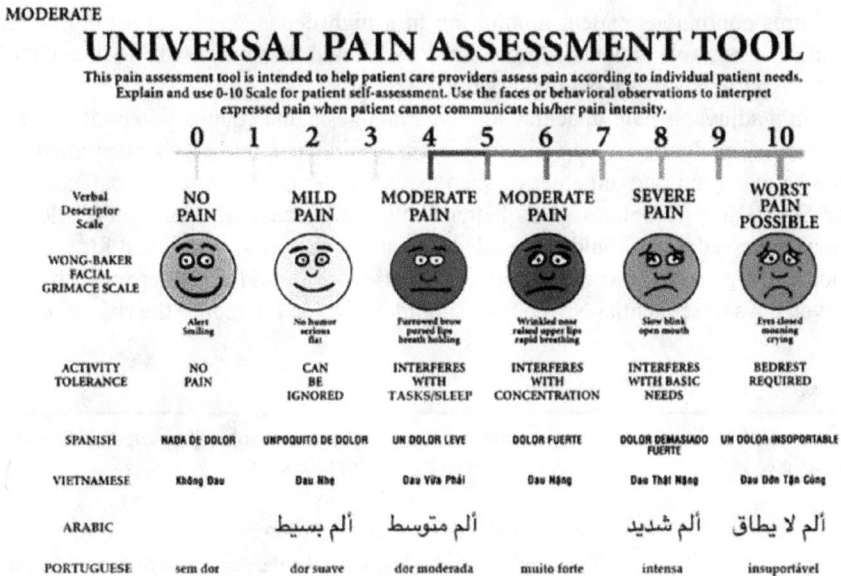

Figure 9.1 Universal pain assessment tool.

In principle, treatment of painful crisis includes adequate analgesia, hydration, warmth, prophylactic or therapeutic antibiotics if pyrexial after necessary culture samples are taken, as well as oxygenation if hypoxic (Sp O_2 < 90%). Oral hydration must be adequate with at least 1.5 L/m^2 of water-based fluid per day in children and 60–70 mL/kg in adults. If parenteral, not more than 1.5 times maintenance is given in order to prevent volume overload considering baseline anaemia in SCD. Home-based pain treatment should be initiated for mild-moderate pain levels with simple analgesics and weak opioids. Patients and parents should be encouraged to keep a stock of simple analgesics at home in event of a painful episode. If mild-to-moderate pain does not succumb to home-based oral analgesia and hydration within two days, in-hospital care may be warranted. Analgesia should be commenced within 15–30 minutes of presentation in the emergency room or day hospital. Effective analgesia should be achieved within one hour. There should be an ongoing assessment of analgesic efficacy every 30 minutes until pain is controlled, thereafter every two hours. Treatment should be individualized.

The choice of analgesia depends on the severity of the pain and the patient's prior analgesic needs/history. Generally, opioids are reserved for moderate to severe pains, while just simple analgesics and weak opioids may suffice for mild-moderate pains. Combination analgesia (two or more analgesics with different mechanisms of action) is often required in sickle cell for optimal analgesia. Categories of analgesics are listed in Table 9.1.

Opioids are a mainstay in control of sickle cell pain. Opioids are centrally acting drugs with potentials for central nervous system depression at toxic doses. Maximum doses of opioids should be used with caution. Strong opioid such as fentanyl requires continuous patient monitoring in a high dependency unit setting, especially for unstable patients. Opioid antidotes should be made available in event of any toxicities such as CNS depression.

Pain adjuvants help in achieving better analgesia and counter potential adverse effects of analgesic used. They may include mild sedatives such as promethazine or diazepam and antiemetics such as cyclizine. Combination of paracetamol or NSAIDS with opiates gives better analgesia because of their synergistic actions. Oversedation should be avoided. Laxatives should be prescribed for prevention and treatment of constipation, a side effect of opioid use. More than five to seven days of sequential NSAID use should be avoided to reduce the risk of peptic

Table 9.1 Categories of analgesics.

Non-opioids/peripherally acting	Non-steroidal anti-inflammatory	Diclofenac, Ketorolac, Ibuprofem, Naproxen, Ketoprofen, etc.
	COX2 inhibitors	Celecoxib
Non-opioids	Simple analgesics	Acetaminophen
Opioids	Weak opioids	Tramadol, Pentazocine, Dihydrocodeine, etc.
	Strong opioids	Morphine, Diamorphine, Pethidine, Fentanyl

ulceration and gut haemorrhage. Proton pump inhibitors such as Rabeprazole may be included to reduce the risk of peptic ulceration. NSAIDS are also potentially nephrotoxic and should be avoided in established renal disease.

The analgesic dose should be titrated with the pain severity until adequate control is achieved using a fixed dose schedule (FDS) of simple analgesics/NSAIDS/opioids, interspersed with short-acting agents for breakthrough pains. A prototype protocol is exemplified below for a severe painful crisis in a 37-year-old male haemoglobin SS phenotype presenting in the Emergency room:

- IM/IV Ketorolac 30 mg every 12 hours
- IV Omeprazole 40 mg daily
- Oral Pregabalin 50 mg every 12 hours
- Oral Bisacodyl 10 mg nocte
- Oral morphine 10 mg every 4 hours
- ±IV/Oral Paracetamol 1 g every 6 hours
- Anti-emetic, as required
- Anti-pruritic, as required

For patients who cannot be tolerated orally or in severe pains, parenteral analgesia is preferable. The type, dose, route of administration, duration and frequency of analgesics can be titrated as required after each pain assessments. For instance, continuous infusion of opioids may be more favoured compared to bolus injections in persistent pain. If available, patient-controlled analgesia (PCA) should be considered for severe pain. PCA reduces the risk of pain undertreatment. Where neuropathic pain component marked by tingling/burning sensation or numbness is suspected, drugs such as pregabalin or carbamazepine will be useful.

Prophylactic incentive spirometry is recommended for prevention of acute chest syndrome especially if painful crisis involves the chest wall. In the absence of a spirometer, ten deep breaths every two hours while awake between 8 a.m. and 10 p.m. are an alternative.

In difficult/intractable cases, where pain is unremitting after 48 hours of well-conducted analgesia, exchange blood transfusion (EBT) may be offered. EBT should be conducted with manual protocol or automated erythrocytapheresis using sickle negative, group specific (extended phenotype), packed red cells.

As largely depicted above, pain control in SCD is essentially pharmacologic. However, non-pharmacologic measures such as physical therapy with heat or ice packs, relaxation, distraction, music, menthol rub, meditation, and transcutaneous electrical nerve stimulation (TENS) are also helpful. Treatment of painful crisis in a dedicated day hospital is associated with better outcome due to prompt triage and familiarity with analgesic needs of individual patients, hence reduced risk of pain undertreatment. Invariably, there is reduction in overall patient admission rates and better outcomes compared to emergency room settings.

A multidisciplinary team (MDT) approach is required for optimal care of persons living with SCD, including pain manifestations. The team must include the physician haematologist, other sub-specialists depending on affected organ systems as well as dedicated nursing teams, mental health experts. Haematologists are not necessarily pain experts, inputs of a pain management physician must be sought in severe or intractable pain syndromes.

Associated Complications of Painful Crisis

In complicated painful crisis, bone pains may be associated with hyperhaemolysis (worsening anaemia). Hyperhaemolysis is often triggered by infections and may present with acute anaemia features of intravascular haemolysis with passage of dark coloured (coke coloured) urine. Infections such malaria and some bacterial sepsis are implicated in hyper-haemolytic crisis. Painful crisis may also be associated with sequestration crisis, especially in children. Acute chest syndrome is a potentially life-threatening complication of SCD. Pain in the chest wall may co-exist with acute chest syndrome, a lung pathology usually resulting from combined effects of vaso-occlusion/infarction within the pulmonary vasculature and infective origin. Acute chest syndrome is characterized by fever and/or new respiratory symptoms associated with new pulmonary infiltrates on chest imaging. Acute chest syndrome is clinically indistinguishable from pneumonia. The respiratory symptoms could include cough, expectoration, chest pain, fast breathing, wheezing, and difficult breathing. Acute chest syndrome should be identified in time and treated vigorously with exchange blood transfusion, hydration, analgesia, antibacterial therapy, supplemental oxygen support as required.

Painful crisis may also be associated with multi-organ failure syndrome (MOFS). MOFS is defined as sudden onset, severe organ dysfunction simultaneously involving at least two major organ systems (such as the liver, lung, and kidney) in the setting of an acute sickle cell crisis. MOFS is partly explained by significant vaso-occlusive events in vital organs with major functional compromise and organ failure. This life-threatening complication requires immediate intensive care and a multi-specialist attention including the intensivists, nephrologist, hepatologist, respiratory physicians, and others.

Prevention/Long-term Management of Painful Crisis

Painful crisis may or may not be associated with an identifiable inciting factor. However, avoidance of known precipitants of vaso-occlusive crisis is helpful in preventing crisis. These precipitants differ from person to person and may include cold, heat, physical exhaustion, fever, pregnancy, menstruation, and so on.

Hydroxyurea therapy has shown significant benefits in managing moderate-severe SCD. Hydroxyurea is an inhibitor of de novo purine and pyrimidine synthesis, acting on ribonucleotide reductase. Through stress erythropoiesis, hydroxyurea induces haemoglobin F production. Hydroxyurea also improves cell hydration, reduces leucocyte and platelet counts. In clinical effects, the resultant benefits of well-conducted hydroxyurea therapy will include reduced frequency and severity of bone pain crisis, reduced blood transfusion needs, and reduced hospitalization in SCD.

Where hydroxyurea is intolerable or contraindicated, hyper-transfusion or chronic transfusion therapy is also proven to be of immense benefit. Newer medications such as Crizanlizumab, Oxelotor and L-glutamine are also relevant for long-term control of sickle cell pain by ameliorating the disease. Clinical experiences with use of P selectin inhibitors such as Crizanlizumab are limited but hold great promise.

Future Therapies and Prognosis

As yet, no effective abortive therapies for sickle cell pain. Great impact on quality of life, impact of schooling, work and productivity and mental health issues are a major concern. More effective acute pain control and chronic pain management strategies currently suffice. Pain in sickle cell is not just physical, but bears psychologic consequences as well, as such need to offer total pain management to improve outcomes for affected persons and overall quality of life.

However, potentials for cure have been achieved through haemopoietic stem cell transplants for eligible cases. Stem cell therapy currently offers more hope for long-term management of pain (cure) in SCD.

References

Adewoyin, A. S. (2015). Management of sickle cell disease: A review for physician education in Nigeria (Sub-Saharan Africa). *Anemia*, e791498. https://doi.org/10.1155/2015/791498

Ballantyne, J. C., Kalso, E., & Stannard, C. (2016). WHO analgesic ladder: A good concept gone astray. *BMJ, 352*, i20. https://doi.org/10.1136/bmj.i20

Current Issues in Sickle Cell Pain and Its Management | Hematology, ASH Education Program | American Society of Hematology. (n.d.). Retrieved June 27, 2023, from https://ashpublications.org/hematology/article/2007/1/97/19153/Current-Issues-in-Sickle-Cell-Pain-and-Its

Delicou, S., & Maragkos, K. (2013). Pain management in patients with sickle cell disease – A review. *European Medical Journal: Hematology, 1*(1), 30–36. https://doi.org/10.33590/emjhematol/10310931

Evidence-Based Management of Sickle Cell Disease: Expert Panel Report, 2014 | NHLBI, NIH. (n.d.). Retrieved June 27, 2023, from https://www.nhlbi.nih.gov/health-topics/evidence-based-management-sickle-cell-disease

IASP announces revised definition of pain. (n.d.). Retrieved September 4, 2022, from https://www.iasp-pain.org/publications/iasp-news/iasp-announces-revised-definition-of-pain/

Management of chronic pain. (n.d.). SIGN. Retrieved June 27, 2023, from https://www.sign.ac.uk/our-guidelines/management-of-chronic-pain/

Marsh, A., & Vichinsky, E. P. (2015). Sickle cell disease. In *Postgraduate haematology* (pp. 98–113). Wiley & Sons. https://doi.org/10.1002/9781118853771.ch7

Okpala, I., & Tawil, A. (2002). Management of pain in sickle-cell disease. *Journal of the Royal Society of Medicine, 95*(9), 456–458. https://doi.org/10.1258/jrsm.95.9.456

Osunkwo, I., O'Connor, H. F., & Saah, E. (2020). Optimizing the management of chronic pain in sickle cell disease. *Hematology, 2020*(1), 562–569. https://doi.org/10.1182/hematology.2020000143

Overview | Sickle cell disease: Managing acute painful episodes in hospital | Guidance |
NICE. (2012, June 27). NICE. https://www.nice.org.uk/guidance/cg143

Sil, S., Cohen, L. L., & Dampier, C. (2016). Psychosocial and functional outcomes in youth
with chronic sickle cell pain. *The Clinical Journal of Pain, 32*(6), 527–533. https://doi.
org/10.1097/AJP.0000000000000289

Smith, W. R., Penberthy, L. T., Bovbjerg, V. E., McClish, D. K., Roberts, J. D., Dahman,
B., Aisiku, I. P., Levenson, J. L., & Roseff, S. D. (2008). Daily assessment of pain in
adults with sickle cell disease. *Annals of Internal Medicine, 148*(2), 94–101. https://doi.
org/10.7326/0003-4819-148-2-200801150-00004

World Health Organization (Ed.). (1986). *Cancer pain relief.* World Health Organization.
WHO Publications Center USA [distributor].

Yale, S. H., Nagib, N., & Guthrie, T. (2000). Approach to the vaso-occlusive crisis in adults
with sickle cell disease. *American Family Physician, 61*(5), 1349–1356.

Yang, J., Bauer, B. A., Wahner-Roedler, D. L., Chon, T. Y., & Xiao, L. (2020). The modified
WHO analgesic ladder: Is it appropriate for chronic non-cancer pain? *Journal of Pain
Research, 13*, 411–417. https://doi.org/10.2147/JPR.S244173

10 Management of Infections and Fever in Sickle Cell Disease (SCD)

Ahmed Mohammed Sarki, Lilian Nuwabaine and Sabrina Bakeera-Kitaka

Introduction: Infection and Fever in Sickle Cell Disease (SCD)

Sickle cell disease (SCD) remains a significant and often overlooked chronic illness, especially in regions like Western and Central Africa. People with SCD are notably susceptible to infections, particularly severe bacterial ones, which can lead to life-threatening fevers. Given the gravity of these fevers, their effective management in SCD patients is crucial. This chapter will provide an in-depth exploration of SCD and emphasize strategies and interventions specifically tailored for managing fevers in those affected by the disease.

Brief Overview about Sickle Cell Disease

SCD is a group of inherited haematological disorders caused by mutations in the sixth amino acid of the β-globin gene (Almahmoud et al., 2023). The mutation affects the structure and function of haemoglobin, a protein in red blood cells that carries oxygen throughout the body (Kato et al., 2018). SCD includes sickle cell anaemia (SCA) the most common genotype isinhomozygous haemoglobin SS (HbSS), and common heterozygous conditions are haemoglobin sickle beta zero thalassemia, haemoglobin sickle beta plus thalassemia, and haemoglobin SCD (HbSC) (Sedrak & Kondamudi, 2018; Ware et al., 2017). SCD is highly prevalent among the people of Sub-Saharan Africa, South Asia, the Middle East, and the Mediterranean (Sedrak & Kondamudi, 2018). There are approximately 300,000 new cases globally each year and the majority being in Sub-Saharan Africa (Almahmoud et al., 2023; Kato et al., 2018). SCA is the most prevalent form of SCD characterized by chronic haemolytic anaemia, unpredictable pain, and widespread organ damage. For example, the Global Burden of Disease 2021 Sickle Cell Disease Collaborators highlighted that between the year 2000 and 2021, the national incidence rates of SCD in most countries were relatively stable. However, total births of babies with SCD increased globally within the same period by 13.7% (95% uncertainty interval 11.1–16.5) to 515,000 primarily due to population growth in Western and Central Africa, and the Caribbean. In addition, the number of people living with SCD globally increased by 41.4% from approximately 5.5 million people in the year 2000 to over 7 million people in the year 2021 (Global Burden of Disease 2021 Sickle Cell Disease Collaborators, 2023).

DOI: 10.4324/9781003463931-11

Importance of Understanding Infection and Fever in SCD Patients

Most individuals with SCA (HbSS) are at an increased risk for infections due to weakened immune system and functional asplenia which usually develops at the age of five years (Almahmoud et al., 2023). People with SCD are more likely than others to get invasive infections (Koko et al., 2014). Therefore, it is imperative to understand infection and fever in SCD.

Pathophysiology of SCD and Susceptibility to Infections

The spleen is one of the first organs usually affected by SCD. In children with SCA, there is a reduction in the physiological function of the spleen, a condition called hypersplenism within the first year of life (Rogers et al., 2011). Vaso-occlusion of the spleen by sickled red blood cells, frequent ischaemia, and continuous atrophy of the organ could bring about splenic dysfunction (Tanabe et al., 2019). The spleen is a major filter of the blood and plays an important role in immune defence as well as in vascular and blood homeostasis by removing altered red blood cells, microorganisms, and blood-borne antigens. Splenic damage puts patients at risk for immune dysfunction, vascular narrowing and occlusion, and severe bacterial infection. People with SCD remain at high risk for infection and sepsis throughout life (Sobota et al., 2015).

Acute Splenic Sequestration Crisis

The splenic damage seen in patients with SCD is typically silent and progressive, but it becomes clinically apparent in acute splenic sequestration crisis (ASSC), a life-threatening complication involving rapid accumulation of sickled erythrocytes within the spleen (da Silva Filho et al., 2012). ASSC is defined as sudden splenomegaly, a reduction in Hb concentration of at least 2 g/dL, and a normal or elevated basal reticulocyte count. The spleen enlarges within a period of hours, trapping a large portion of circulating erythrocytes and acutely worsening the anaemia and circulatory failure. Symptoms include abdominal pain and distension, pallor, tachycardia, hypotension, and lethargy (Tanabe et al., 2019). Hypovolemic shock and death from cardiovascular collapse can occur within hours if untreated. In children with SCD, ASSC is one of the earliest life-threatening complications and may be the first clinical manifestation of the disease, occurring at a median age of 1.4 years, and as early as several weeks of age (Brousse et al., 2012). More than 12% of children with SCA experience ASSC, and 67% of those go on to have at least one more occurrence. In patients with HbSC, sequestration may occur in early and late adulthood (Koduri & Nathan, 2006).

Altered Spleen Function in SCD Patients

The spleen functions as a phagocytic filter that removes old and damaged cells plus blood microorganisms and also produces antibodies (Booth et al., 2010). Opsonized bacteria are removed efficiently by macrophages in the spleen or liver, but poorly opsonized bacteria are only cleared effectively by the spleen. Such pathogens include encapsulated bacteria, in particular *Streptococcus pneumoniae* (pneumococcus) and *Haemophilus influenzae* (Bohnsack & Brown, 1986).

Individuals with SCD typically suffer from functional hypo- or asplenism. The sluggish circulation through the spleen, high rates of O_2 extraction, and local acidosis cause deoxygenation of HbS, promoting sickling, which leads to congestion and engorgement of the sinusoids with sickled cells. This can cause change of course of blood via intrasplenic shunts, bypassing the normal filtering mechanisms. Macrophages that destroy the abnormally shaped cells may be blocked, affecting their phagocytic process. Hence, the hyposplenic state which can be reversed at first (William & Corozza, 2007). Over time, multiple episodes of sickling and ischemic damage may result to infarction of the spleen tissue (Booth, Inusa & Obaro, 2010). As a result, the spleen is unable to regenerate, becoming scared, atrophied, and non-functional culminating in autosplenectomy (Lucas, 2004).

Common Infections in SCD

Infection is a great contributor to morbidity and mortality in SCD, and it remains the leading cause of death worldwide especially in developing countries (Booth et al., 2010). In SCA, the spleen is the first organ injured by sickling in the microcirculation. At the age of 1, it is estimated that 30% of patients with SCA have functional asplenia and at six years 90% have functional asplenia. This leads to an increased risk for bacterial infection with encapsulated organisms (Driscoll, 2007). The most common bacterial infections are *Streptococcus pneumoniae*, salmonella, *Hemophilus Influenza* b, *Klebsiella pneumoniae*, and *Escherichia coli* (Shinde et al., 2015). In Sub-Saharan Africa, about one in two patients with SCD die from infection before the age of five years and children with SCD are 50 times more likely to suffer invasive pneumococcal disease (Ochocinski et al., 2020). Infections are less seen in adults compared to children with SCD (Sobota et al., 2015). Bacteraemia in adults is associated with severe clinical course and a poor prognosis. Bacteraemia is associated with immunosuppression, indwelling venous catheters, and a high frequency of associated bone and joint infections (Ochocinski et al., 2020; Sobota et al., 2015).

Streptococcus pneumoniae

The incidence of invasive streptococcus pneumoniae infection is 6.9 infections per 100 patients-year among children with SCA under five years (Wong et al., 1992). The risk of bacteraemia with *Streptococcus pneumoniae* is about 400-fold higher in patients who have SCD (Driscoll, 2007).

Haemophilus influenzae

People with SCD are at high risk of *Haemophilus influenzae* infection due to functional asplenia. In African countries, where vaccination rates are still low, Hib still remains the most significant cause of bacteraemias in people with SCD

(Allali et al.,2018). Children with SCD remain at risk for infection with bacterial stereotypes not covered by immunizations including non-b and non-typeable *H. influenzae* (Battersby et al.,2010). *H. influenza* is a devastating and fatal invasive bacterial infection especially among children under five years (Soeters et al., 2018).

Salmonella

Most Salmonella infections in SCD involve long bones and joints, can be symmetrical, and occur most frequently in early childhood (Chambers et al., 2000; Epps et al., 1991). SCD has classically been associated with Salmonella abscesses of the spleen (Neonato et al., 2000).

Osteomyelitis

Osteomyelitis is a frequent infection complication in patients with SCD and it is greatly due to altered function of the spleen, sickle cell induced damage to bone marrow and maybe bowel ischaemia (Sabota et al., 2015). In SCD, Salmonella species, other Gram-negative pathogens, and *S. aureus* are the most common isolates in adults. Salmonella is isolated most commonly, followed by *Staphylococcus aureus* and other Gram-negative pathogens in osteomyelitis (Driscoll, 2007). The clinical presentation of osteomyelitis is somewhat similar to that of vaso-occlusive (VOC) pain crisis. No definitive imaging modalities (bone scan, magnetic resonance imaging) can differentiate with certainty between osteomyelitis and VOC. The diagnosis still relies on clinical assessment fever, leukocytosis, erythrocyte sedimentation rate or positive blood cultures from blood or bone obtained by aspiration (Driscoll, 2007). Magnetic resonance imaging and bone scintigram can sometimes help identify foci of infection. Bone biopsy or aspiration of a suspected infection site is the gold standard for diagnosis, despite substantial false negative rates (Sabota et al., 2015).

Urinary Tract Infections

Patients with SCA have increased susceptibility to develop urinary tract infections (UTIs) because of altered blood flow in the renal vasculature which causes papillary necrosis and loss of urinary concentrating and acidifying ability of the nephrons with the consequent formation of abnormally dilute and alkaline urine which favours bacterial proliferation (Smith, 1972). This predisposes them to recurrent UTI and subsequent renal damage (Shinde et al., 2015).

Respiratory Infections: Pneumoniae, Bronchitis

Respiratory infections are a risk factor for triggering acute chest syndrome (ACS) in SCA patients and often lead to several complications (Alkindi et al., 2020).

Other Bacterial, Viral, and Fungal Infections

Parvovirus B19

In SCD, Parvovirus B19 usually causes a transient aplastic crisis which occurs in 65– 80% of infections, the virus infects erythroid progenitor cells resulting in temporary cessation of erythropoiesis resulting in severe anaemia (Servey et al., 2007). However, the Parvovirus infection does not recur due to long-lasting humoral immunity and most children recover within two weeks of infection (Cannas et al., 2019). Due to weak immune system among SCD patients, there is a high prevalence of protozoan and helminthic parasites; hence, the SCD patients should have regular stool examination (Ahmed & Uraka, 2011).

Malaria

Malaria infection is the most prevalent cause of crises in SCD in countries where malaria is endemic (Shinde et al., 2015). This confounds the standard response to fever in SCD through administering antibiotics with antimalarials to a well-appearing child with a positive malaria test (Cannas et al., 2019).

Fever in Sickle Cell Disease (SCD)

A fever represents an elevation in body temperature and often signifies the body's immune response to pathogens or other stimuli. In patients with SCD, fever is a critical symptom. According to Ellison et al. (2015), it's one of the most significant indicators of infection among this population. Fever in SCD is not merely a symptom; it is often a medical emergency. This urgency arises from the fact that fever can be a sign of other associated SCD complications, such as ACS (Guilcher et al., 2012). Given the potential consequences, any fever in an SCD patient, regardless of age, warrants immediate evaluation and intervention. An additional concern is that fever might precipitate a sickle cell crisis. As such, monitoring body temperature and adhering to antipyretic recommendations from healthcare professionals are paramount for these individuals.

Clinical Approach and Management

History and Physical Examination

Several protocols for guiding the management of fever in SCD patients exist. The consensus is that patients less than two months old with HbSS, HbSC, or HbSβ⁰, or HbSβ⁺ phenotypes who have a temperature ≥38.5°C or a history of temperature ≥38.5°C within two days of presentation should promptly visit a health facility (Guilcher et al., 2012). Furthermore, all SCD patients presenting with fever should be evaluated by a physician and have a complete blood count (CBC), blood culture, reticulocyte count, and given antibiotics within one hour of presentation (Guilcher et al., 2012). Typically, SCD patients presenting with fever can be managed on an outpatient basis if they meet low-risk clinical criteria, the term "low-risk" in this context generally refers to patients who, based on their clinical presentation and initial investigations, are deemed to have a lower likelihood of developing serious complications from their current illness. Otherwise, they should be admitted for inpatient antibiotics and observation. Some of the effective interventions include parenteral antibiotics therapy and transfusion.

Initial Investigations for SCD Patients Presenting with Fever

1 Peripheral IV access/port access

- Establish a peripheral intravenous (IV) line or access an existing port.

2 Blood tests

- CBC with differential to assess the different types of blood cells
- Reticulocyte count to evaluate the body's production of immature red blood cells
- Blood culture to check for the presence of bacteria or other pathogens in the blood
- Liver functional tests to assess the liver's health and functionality
- C-reactive protein (CRP) to measure the level of inflammation in the body
- Blood gas, particularly in cases with significant respiratory concerns

3 Urinalysis

- A test of the urine to check for signs of kidney disease and to evaluate the body's overall health

Other Investigations

1 Chest Radiograph (X-ray)

- Indicated if there are clinical respiratory symptoms.
- Should be considered if there's new onset hypoxia, which is defined as room air saturation dropping >3% below the patient's baseline or if the oxygen saturation drops below the 93% threshold in a patient whose baseline is unknown.

2 Clinical Observations and Assessments

- Check for altered mental status or new neurological findings.
- Evaluate for potential complications specific to SCD such as splenic sequestration, ACS, or Vaso-Occlusive Episode (VOE) that might require IV analgesia.
- Monitor the oxygen saturation continuously, especially in patients who exhibit new hypoxia or those with unknown baseline readings. Oxygen saturation levels should ideally remain ≥93%. If there's a decrease of more than 1% from the baseline saturation, further assessment and intervention may be warranted, unless the haemoglobin (Hgb) level is >10 g/dL.
- Monitor the White Blood Cell (WBC) count, as it can be indicative of an infection or another inflammatory process.

Empiric Antibiotic Therapy

Parenteral antibiotics therapy entail administering IV ceftriaxone 100 milligrams per kg or a maximum of 2 grams per dose should be administered as soon as possible within one hour after the blood draw to prevent overwhelming sepsis. The parenteral antibiotics should be administered before other investigations such as chest X-ray and they should not wait for blood test results. In case the child is allergic to ceftriaxone, it is advised to administer clindamycin 40 milligrams per kg per day intravenously every six hours and if meningitis is suspected or child is in sepsis administer Vancomycin 60 milligrams per kg per day every six hours (Guilcher et al., 2012).

Vaccinations

Use of conjugated vaccines against *Streptococcus pneumoniae*, meningococcal vaccine, and *Haemophilus influenzae* type B vaccine (Hib vaccine) based on recent guidelines is recommended (Sobota et al., 2015). All patients with SCD should receive at least one dose of pneumococcal conjugate vaccines (PCV). Children with SCD should receive PCV 23 at two years for supplementary protection against *Streptococcus pneumoniae* and a booster given at five years. Meningococcal vaccination is not recommended in SCD patients who are infected as it increases the risk for mortality, and both adults and children with SCD should receive an annual dose of *Haemophilus influenzae* vaccine each year starting at six months of age (Sobota et al., 2015).

Prophylactic Antibiotics

Prophylactic antibiotics such as penicillin or erythromycin may be prescribed to prevent bacterial infections in children with SCD (Sobota et al., 2015). Penicillin is a medicine that helps kill bacteria, administer 125 mg twice daily for children younger than three years; 250 mg twice daily for those three years and older once the diagnosis is established; this regimen should be continued until at least five years of age and continue in case they have had a splenectomy or invasive pneumococcal disease (Yawn & John-Sowah, 2015).

Patient and Caregiver Education

In addition to medical management, individuals with SCD should practice good hygiene, including frequent hand washing and avoiding close contact with people who are sick. They should also seek medical care promptly if they develop symptoms of infection, such as fever, cough, or shortness of breath. Individuals with SCD are recommended to drink plenty of fluids to prevent dehydration, which can increase the risk of infection. Staying hydrated can prevent a patient with SCD from getting vaso-occlusive crises, stroke, and infections (Brugnara, 2018). Individuals with SCD should avoid contact with people who are sick to reduce susceptibility to infection (Cannas et al., 2019).

Complications of Infections in SCD

Acute Chest Syndrome

Roughly 50% of patients who have SCD experience at least one episode of ACS. Although ACS is more common in children, it is more severe in adults. Patients with SCD present with fevers and pulmonary infiltrates when experiencing an episode of ACS. Approximately 29% of ACS episodes are due to infection, with agents including bacteria, viruses, Mycoplasma, and Chlamydia (Sobota et al., 2015). The treatment for ACS includes broad-spectrum antibiotics, including a cephalosporin and macrolide, as well as oxygen, hydration, incentive spirometry, and early intervention with simple transfusion therapy for associated hypoxia or a haematocrit less than 18% (0.18) (Yawn & John-Sowah, 2015).

Multiple Organ Failure

Multisystem organ failure is thought to result in part from diffuse microvascular occlusion and tissue ischaemia (Tanabe et al., 2019). The most serious emerging complication is pulmonary artery hypertension (PAH). PAH may occur in up to 30% of young adults who have HbSS and is associated with chronic hypoxia, dyspnea, and syncope. In the early stages, however, it is asymptomatic. PAH is a disease of the large pulmonary artery, which histology is similar to the cerebral arteriopathy of stroke in SCD. Other chronic organ damage commonly seen in SCD includes osteonecrosis of the femoral and humeral heads, which occurs in 50% of those who have HbSS by age 35 years, with an increased risk for those who have Hb-SS and alpha thalassemia. Approximately 60% of patients who have HbSC develop osteonecrosis by age 60 years. Proliferative retinopathy is more common in HbSC; approximately 50% of patients develop retinopathy. Renal abnormalities of glomerular and tubular functions leading to hyposthenuria are common in all sickle syndromes, and nephrotic syndrome and end stage renal disease can occur in 5–10% of HbSS patients. Chronic leg ulcers occur in 10–25% of HbSS patients, priapism in 10–40% of adult males.

Overwhelming Sepsis

All SCD genotypes put patients at increased risk for severe infection – particularly invasive bacterial infection – throughout life. This increased susceptibility is largely due to splenic and immune dysfunction. Young children with SCA in particular are at elevated risk for pneumoniae, septicaemia, and meningitis and other infections are also common in SCD. Risk of catheter-related infections is also higher in SCD. Infection is a common precipitant of VOE and the most common cause of ACS.

Vaso-occlusive Crisis

Vaso-occlusive crisis (VOC) is a common complication of SCD with episodes that present with sudden onset of excruciating pain, often localized in the extremities, chest or back. VOC is a clinical diagnosis with no objective diagnostic tests and almost all SCD patients will encounter VOC in their lifetime. VOC can present as early as six months of age and recurrences have variable presentations and frequency (Driscoll, 2007).

Prolonged Hospitalizations

SCA is a chronic haematologic condition that requires frequent hospitalization representing a significant economic burden on the health services (Abd El-Ghany et al., 2021). The hospital admission pattern of children with SCA varies in different parts of the world. The most common causes of hospitalization in these cases include painful crisis and infection. Also, acute sequestration crisis and ACS were reported in many cases. In addition, the hospitalization might be for blood transfusion (Abd El-Ghany et al., 2021).

Conclusion

In summary, SCD patients are highly prone to bacterial infections and these infections can be severe often leading to death, especially among children. Thus, it is a medical emergency. Therefore, there is a need for both preventive and curative interventions for preventing SCD patients from getting infections including vaccination, prophylactic antibiotics, hydration, parenteral antibiotics therapy, and transfusion. Frontline health workers require training and capacity-building about requisite guidelines for managing infections and fever among SCD patients. Policymakers and public health planners need to establish a mechanism for raising awareness regarding the prevention of infection among SCD patients and their support networks.

References

Ahmed, S. G., & Uraka, J. (2011). Impact of intestinal parasites on haematological parameters of sickle cell anaemia patients in Nigeria. *Eastern Mediterranean Health Journal, 17*, 710–713. https://doi.org/10.26719/2011.17.9.710.

Alkindi S., Al-Yahyai T., Raniga S., Boulassel M. R., & Pathare A. (2020). Respiratory viral infections in sickle cell anemia: Special emphasis on H1N1 co-infection. *Oman Medical Journal, 35*(6), e197.

Allali, S., Chalumeau, M., Launay, O., Ballas, S. K., & de Montalembert, M. (2018). Conjugate Haemophilus influenzae type b vaccines for sickle cell disease. *The Cochrane database of systematic reviews, 8*(8), CD011199. https://doi.org/10.1002/14651858.CD011199.pub3

Almahmoud, T., Alnashwan, T., Al Kuhaimi, L., Essa, M. F., Al Balawi, N., Al Jamaan, K., & Al-Harthy, N. (2023). Management of fever and acute painful crises in children with sickle cell disease in emergency departments: A tertiary hospital experience. *Frontiers in Pediatrics, 11*, 1195040.

Battersby, A. J., Knox-Macaulay, H. H., & Carrol, E. D. (2010). Susceptibility to invasive bacterial infections in children with sickle cell disease. *Pediatric Blood Cancer, 55*(3), 401–406.

Bohnsack, J. F., & Brown, E. J. (1986). The role of the spleen in resistance to infection. *Annual Review of Medicine, 37*, 49–59.

Booth, C., Inusa, B., & Obaro, S. K. (2010). Infection in sickle cell disease: A review. *International Journal of Infectious Diseases, 14*(1), 2–12.

Brousse, V., Elie, C., Benkerrou, M., Odièvre, M. H., Lesprit, E., Bernaudin, F., Grimaud, M., Guitton, C., Quinet, B., Dangiolo, S., & de Montalembert, M. (2012). Acute splenic sequestration crisis in sickle cell disease: Cohort study of 190 paediatric patients. *British Journal of Haematology, 156*(5), 643–648. https://doi.org/10.1111/j.1365-2141.2011.08999.x

Brugnara C. (2018). Sickle cell dehydration: Pathophysiology and therapeutic applications. *Clinical Hemorheology and Microcirculation, 68*(2–3), 187–204. https://doi.org/10.3233/CH-189007

Cannas, G., Merazga, S., & Virot, E. (2019). Sickle cell disease and infections in high- and low-income countries. *Mediterranian Journal of Hematology and Infectious Diseases, 11*(1), e2019042. https://doi.org/10.4084/MJHID.2019.042

Chambers, J. B., Forsythe, D. A., Bertrand, S. L., Iwinski, H. J., & Steflik, D. E. (2000). Retrospective review of osteoarticular infections in a pediatric sickle cell age group. *Journal of Pediatric Orthopedics, 20*(5), 682–685. https://doi.org/10.1097/00004694-200009000-00025

da Silva Filho, I. L., Ribeiro, G. S., Moura, P. G., Vechi, M. L., Cavalcante, A. C., & de Andrada-Serpa, M. J. (2012). Sickle cell disease: Acute clinical manifestations in early childhood and molecular characteristics in a group of children in Rio de Janeiro. *Revista Brasileira de Hematologia e Hemoterapia, 34*(3), 196–201. https://doi.org/10.5581/1516-8484.20120049

Driscoll, C. (2007). Sickle cell disease. *Pediatrics in Review, 28*, 259–268. https://doi.org/10.1542/pir.28-7-259.

Abd El-Ghany, S. M., Tabbakh, A. T., Nur, L. I., & Abdelrahman, R. Y. (2021). Analysis of causes of hospitalization among children with sickle disease in a group of private hospitals in Jeddah, Saudi Arabia. *Journal of Blood Medicine, 12*, 733–740. https://doi.org/10.2147/JBM.S318824

Ellison, A. M., Thurm, C., Alessandrini, E., Jain, S., Cheng, J., Black, K., Schroeder, L., Stone, K., & Alpern, E. R. (2015). Variation in paediatric emergency department care of sickle cell disease and fever. *Academic Emergency Medicine, 22*(4), 423–430.

Epps, C. H. Jr., Bryant, D. D. 3rd, Coles, M. J., & Castro, O. (1991). Osteomyelitis in patients who have sickle-cell disease. Diagnosis and management. *The Journal of Bone & Joint Surgery, 73*(9), 1281–1294.

GBD 2021 Sickle Cell Disease Collaborators. (2023). Global, regional, and national prevalence and mortality burden of sickle cell disease, 2000–2021: A systematic analysis from the global burden of disease study 2021. *The Lancet Haematology, 10*(8), e585–e599. https://doi.org/10.1016/S2352-3026(23)00118-7

Guilcher, G., Purves, E., McCartney, H., & Wu, J. (2012). Guidelines for the Management of Fever in Sickle Cell Patients. Division of Hematology/Oncology, BC's Children's Hospital. https://www.childhealthindicatorsbc.ca/sites/default/files/BCCH_ED_Sickle%20Cell%20Fever%20Guidelines%20(Jan%202012).pdf. Accessed July 12, 2023.

Jenerette, C. M., & Brewer, C. (2010). Health-related stigma in young adults with sickle cell disease. *Journal of the National Medical Association, 102*(11), 1050–1055. https://doi.org/10.4236/ojped.2014.44036

Kato, J. G., Piel, F. B., Reid, C. D., Gaston, M. H., & Frempong, K. O. (2018). Sickle cell disease. *Nature Reviews Disease Primers, 4*(1), 1–22.

Kaur, M., Dangi, C. B. S., & Singh, M. (2013). An overview on sickle cell disease profile. *Asian Journal of Pharmaceutical and Clinical Research*, *6*(Suppl 1), 25–37.

Koduri, P. R., & Nathan, S. (2006). Acute splenic sequestration crisis in adults with hemoglobin S-C disease: A report of nine cases. *Annals of Hematology*, *85*, 239–243.

Koko, J., Gahouma, D., Ategbo, S., Seilhan, C., Pambou, A., & Moussavou, A. (2014). Fever among children with sickle-cell disease: Findings from the general pediatric ward of the Owendo pediatric hospital in Libreville, Gabon. *Open Journal of Pediatrics*, *4*, 262–268. https://doi.org/10.4236/ojped.2014.44036/

Lucas, S. (2004). The morbid anatomy of sickle cell disease and sickle cell trait. In I. Okpala (Ed.), *Practical management of haemoglobinopathies*. Oxford: Blackwell.

Mantadakis, E., Cavender, J. D., Rogers, Z. R., Ewalt, D. H., & Buchanan, G. R. (1999). Prevalence of priapism in children and adolescents with sickle cell anemia. *Journal of Pediatric Hematology/Oncology*, *21*(6), 518–522.

Nath, K. A., & Hebbel, R. P. (2015). Sickle cell disease: Renal manifestations and mechanisms. *Nature Reviews Nephrology*, *11*(3), 161–171. https://doi.org/10.1038/nrneph.2015.8

Neonato, M.G., Guilloud-Bataille, M., Beauvais, P., Begue, P., Belloy, M., Benkerrou, M., Ducrocq, R., Maier-Redelsperger, M., De Montalembert, M., Quinet, B., Elion, J., Feingold, J. & Girot, R. (2000). Acute clinical events in 299 homozygous sickle cell patients living in France. French Study Group on Sickle Cell Disease. European. *Journal of Haematology*, *65*, 155–164.

Ochocinski, D., Dalal, M., Black, L. V., Carr, S., Lew J., Sullivan, K., & Kissoon, N. (2020). Life-threatening infectious complications in sickle cell disease: A concise narrative review. *Frontiers in Pediatrics*, *8*(38). https://doi.org/10.3389/fped.2020.00038

Rogers, Z. R., Wang, W. C., Luo, Z., Iyer, R. V., Shalaby-Rana, E., Dertinger, S. D., Shulkin, B. L., Miller, J. H., Files, B., Lane, P. A., Thompson, B. W., Miller, S. T., & Ware, R. E. (2011) Biomarkers of splenic function in infants with sickle cell anemia: Baseline data from the BABY HUG trial. *Blood*, *117*, 2614–2617.

Sobota, A., Sabharwal, V., Fonebi, G., & Steinberg, M. (2015). How we prevent and manage infection in sickle cell disease. *British journal of haematology*, *170*(6), 757–767. https://doi.org/10.1111/bjh.13526

Sedrak, A., & Kondamudi, N. P. (2018). Sickle cell disease. In *StatPearls*. Treasure Island (FL): Stat Pearls Publishing. Available from https://www.ncbi.nlm.nih.gov/books/NBK482384/. Accessed July 18, 2023.

Servey, J. T., Reamy, B. V., & Hodge, J. (2007). Clinical presentation of parvovirus B19 infection. *American Family Physician*, *75*, 373–376.

Shinde, S., Bakshi, A. P., & Shrikhande, A. V. (2015). Infections in sickle cell disease. *IAIM*, *2*(11), 26–34.

Smith, C. H. (1972). *Blood diseases of infancy and childhood* (pp. 376–377). St. Louis: C. V. Mosby Company.

Sobota, A., Sabharwal, V., Fonebi, G., & Steinberg, M. (2015). How we prevent and manage infection in sickle cell disease. *British Journal of Haematology*, *170*(6), 757–767.

Soeters, H. M., Blain, A., Pondo, T., Doman, B., Farley, M. M., Harrison, L. H. et al. (2018). Epidemiology and trends in invasive *Haemophilus infleuenza* disease United States 2009–2015. *Clinical Infectious Diseases*, *67*(6), 881–889.

Tanabe, P., Spratling, R., Smith, D., Grissom, P., & Hulihan, M. (2019). Understanding the complications of sickle cell disease. *American Journal of Nursing*, *119*(6), 26–35.

Ware, E.R., Montalembert, M., Tshilolo, L., & Abboud, M. R. (2017). Sickle cell disease. *The Lancet*, *390* (10091), 311–323.

William, B. M., & Corazza, G. R. (2007). Hyposplenism: A comprehensive review. Part I: Basic concepts and causes. *Haematology*, *12*, 1–13.

Wong, W. Y., Overturf, G. D., & Powars, D. R. (1992). Infection caused by Streptococcus pneumoniae in children with sickle cell disease: epidemiology, immunologic mechanisms, prophylaxis, and vaccination. *Clinical Infectious Diseases*, *14*(5), 1124–1136. https://doi.org/10.1093/clinids/14.5.1124

Yawn, B. P., & John-Sowah J. (2015). Management of sickle cell disease: Recommendations from the 2014 expert panel report. *American Family Physician*, *92*(12), 1069–1076.

Yeruva, S. L., Paul, Y., Oneal, P., & Nouraie, M. (2016). Renal failure in sickle cell disease: Prevalence, predictors of disease, mortality and effect on length of hospital stay. *Hemoglobin*, *40*(5), 295–299. https://doi.org/10.1080/03630269.2016.1224766

11 Transfusion in Sickle Cell Disease (SCD)

Complications Including Iron Overload

Kanayo Nwankwo and Sophie Uyoga

Introduction

Blood transfusion therapy is an integral component of the management of sickle cell anemia (SCA). While recent improvements in the diagnosis and management of sickle cell disease (SCD) have resulted in survival improvements in Africa, this has led to increasing levels of hospital admission for the management of crises, which often involve transfusions. However, blood transfusion is not a completely benign process. Risk benefit assessment must be weighed, as frequent transfusions can lead to iron overload as well as erythrocyte alloimmunization, transfusion reactions and infections. Alloimmunization is caused by the induction of antibodies to minor or variant antigens, typically within the Rh or Kell systems, on donor red blood cells, and is an important cause of intravascular hemolysis following subsequent transfusions. Iron overload can be managed by various strategies but if left unmonitored can result in organ damage.

Notwithstanding the recent advances, blood transfusion in SCD in Africa is not without its myriad of challenges including low availability of safe blood, lack of voluntary, non-remunerated donors, difficulties in accessing health care as patients often have to pay out of pocket for this, and the inadequacies of the transfusion system all plays a key role in the standard of care of patients with SCD. Improved efforts and strategies to overcome these challenges and optimize blood transfusion practices will reduce the morbidity and mortality hence reducing the disease burden in Africa.

Recruitment blood donor programs like "Haima health initiative", a youth-led non-governmental organization established in 2016, have not only improved access to matched units but helped curb the menace of chronic blood shortage in Nigeria. We encourage efforts to educate African communities about the importance of blood donation to diversify the blood transfusion therapy pool.

This chapter focuses on description of transfusion in SCD, guidelines available on when and how to transfuse, types of blood products in use, collation and quantification of data on transfusion for the management of SCD, description and mechanism of complications and their prevalence, monitoring and impact of transfusion in SCD.

DOI: 10.4324/9781003463931-12

Description of Transfusion in SCD

Red cell transfusions play an important role in management. In hypoxic conditions, sickled erythrocytes increase blood viscosity through polymerization, intracellular precipitation, and increased adhesiveness with the vascular endothelium. Transfusion of sickle-negative red blood cells (RBCs) is indicated to improve oxygen-carrying capacity during acute severe exacerbations of anemia, as occurs during episodes of splenic sequestration or aplastic crisis. It is imperative to state here that the clinical benefit of transfusing sickle-negative RBCs in SCD (as compared to sickle trait RBCs) has not been specifically studied. However, sickle hemoglobin (HgbS) in blood from individuals with sickle cell trait will make it difficult for the clinician to predict the anticipated HgbS level after the transfusion.

For example, in SSA as high as 25–40 percent of the donor population in some countries carry the sickle cell gene (Piel, F. B. et al., 2013. Global burden of sickle cell anaemia in children under five). This has resulted in a reduced number of the potential sickle-free donor pool. This requirement for sickle-free blood puts more strain on the transfusion service in the areas of high prevalence of SCD. Obtaining sickle cell trait-negative blood should not delay transfusion in the setting of acute anemia.

Donor erythrocytes may be administered as a simple transfusion or as an exchange transfusion Simple transfusion is the infusion of donor erythrocytes without removal of recipient blood. It is simple, more convenient, and less expensive and requires one point of peripheral venous access and associated with reduced risk of alloimmunization as less unit of donor's blood required.

Exchange transfusion involves removal of recipient blood before and/or during donor erythrocyte infusion. This can be manual or automated, and also called erythrocytapheresis. The Manual Method is performed using a series of repeated phlebotomies and transfusions. It is time-consuming and provides less consistent control of fluid balance during the procedure. Erythrocytapheresis requires apheresis machines and operators with technical expertise and are very limited in many centers in SSA. Benefits over simple transfusion include increased HB-A containing erythrocytes and reduced risk of iron overload. The decision regarding the type of transfusion technique to employ should be guided by patient acuity, institutional expertise, and compatible blood supply.

In most countries in SSA, maintaining a safe and adequate blood supply is challenging. Therefore, a conservative transfusion policy appears to be most appropriate (Osaro & Charles, 2011).

Guidelines Available on When and How to Transfuse

Blood transfusion is primarily for therapeutic (for acute and life-threatening SCD-related complications) or prophylactic purposes. This helps in hemodilution of the sickled erythrocytes and increasing HB-A containing erythrocytes, suppression of new production of HgbS cells via negative feedbacks, and increased in oxygen delivery to the tissues. Red cell transfusions are not indicated for treatment of chronic steady-state anemia or for uncomplicated episodes of vaso-occlusive pain. The

Table 11.1 Expert panel's recommendations for transfusion therapy.

Indication	How To transfuse	Quality of evidence	Strength of recommendation
Symptomatic ACS combined with a decreased Hb of 1 g/dL below baseline	Simple transfusion	Low	Weak
Symptomatic severe ACS (as defined by an oxygen saturation less than 90% despite supplemental oxygen)	Exchange transfusion	Low	Strong
Acute splenic sequestration plus severe anemia	Simple transfusion	Low	Strong
Stroke	Simple or exchange transfusion	Low	Moderate
Hepatic sequestration	Exchange or simple transfusion		
Intrahepatic cholestasis	Exchange or simple transfusion		
Multisystem organ failure (MSOF)	Exchange or simple transfusion		
Aplastic crisis	Simple transfusion		
Symptomatic Anemia	Simple transfusion		

Table 11.2 Acute complications – graded recommendations when transfusion is not indicated.

Indication	Quality of evidence	Strength of recommendation
Uncomplicated painful crisis	Low	Moderate
Priapism	Low	Moderate

most common indications for therapeutic transfusions are acute stroke, acute chest syndrome (ACS), acute drop in hemoglobin from base line without reticulocytosis, acute hepatic sequestration, splenic sequestration crisis, and acute multi-organ failure. Transfusion can also be used prophylactically for perioperative transfusion (Tables 11.1–11.5).

Recommendations (*Evidence-Based Management of Sickle Cell Disease: Expert Panel Report, 2014 | NHLBI, NIH, pp. 81–85*)

1 In adults and children with SCA, transfuse RBCs to bring the hemoglobin level to 10 g/dL prior to undergoing a surgical procedure involving general anesthesia.
   (Strong Recommendation, Moderate-Quality Evidence)
2 In patients with HbSS disease who require surgery and who already have a hemoglobin level higher than 8.5 g/dL without transfusion, are on chronic hydroxyurea therapy, or who require high-risk surgery (e.g., neurosurgery, prolonged anesthesia, cardiac bypass), consult a sickle cell expert for guidance as to the appropriate transfusion method.
   (Strong Recommendation, Low-Quality Evidence)

3   In adults and children with HbSC or HbSB+-thalassemia, consult a sickle cell expert to determine if full or partial exchange transfusion is indicated before a surgical procedure involving general anesthesia.

*(**Moderate Recommendation, Low-Quality Evidence**)*

Transfusion Goals

1   RBC units that are to be transfused to individuals with SCD should include matching for C, E, and K antigens.

*(**Moderate Recommendation, Low-Quality Evidence**)*

2   In patients with SCA, who are not chronically transfused and who are therefore at risk for hyperviscosity due to high percentages of circulating HbS-containing erythrocytes, avoid transfusing to a target hemoglobin above 10 g/dL.

*(**Moderate Recommendation, Low-Quality Evidence**)*

3   In chronically transfused children with SCA, the goal of transfusion should be to maintain a HbS level of below 30 percent immediately prior to the next transfusion.

*(**Moderate Recommendation, Moderate-Quality Evidence**)*

4   The expert panel recommends that clinicians prescribing chronic transfusion therapy follow an established monitoring protocol.

*(**Moderate Recommendation, Low-Quality Evidence**)*

Table 11.3 Acute complications – consensus recommendations when transfusion is not indicated.

Indication
Asymptomatic anemia
Acute kidney injury, unless MSOF

Table 11.4 Chronic complications – graded recommendations for when to initiate a chronic transfusion program.

Indication	How to transfuse	Quality of evidence	Strength of recommendation
Child with transcranial Doppler (TCD) reading[a] >200 cm/sec	Exchange or simple transfusion	High	Strong
Adults and children with previous clinically overt Stroke	Exchange or simple transfusion	Low	Moderate

[a]   TCD reading is the time averaged mean maximal cerebral blood flow velocity.

Table 11.5 Chronic complications – graded recommendations for when transfusion is not indicated.

Indication	Quality of evidence	Strength of recommendation
♣ Recurrent splenic sequestration	Low	Weak

Before Transfusion

1 Obtain patient treatment history to include locations where prior transfusions were received and any adverse effects.
2 Notify the blood bank that the patient being initiated on chronic transfusion therapy has SCD.
3 Type and screen: This is done to assess whether the patient has developed any new RBC antibodies from the prior transfusion. Leukocyte depleted, red cells negative for C, E, and Kell antigens reduce the incidence of alloimmunization.
4 Complete blood count (CBC) and reticulocyte count should be done to help guide the frequency and volume of transfusions.

Volume to be Transfused

The volume of blood required can be estimated based on patient weight and hematocrit; these are particularly important for children.

In children, transfusion of 10 mL/kg will increase the Hgb 2.5 to 3.0 g/dL and the hematocrit by 7–9 percentage points.

For adults, each unit of RBC transfused will increase the Hgb concentration by approximately 1 g/dL and the hematocrit by three percentage points.

$$\text{Packed RBC volume for simple transfusion (mL)}$$
$$= \left([\text{dHCT} - \text{iHCT}] \times \text{TBV}\right) \div \text{rpHCT}$$

$$\text{Manual partial exchange volume} (\text{mL}) = \left([\text{dHCT} - \text{iHCT}] \times \text{TBV}\right)$$
$$\div \left(\text{rpHCT} - \left[(\text{iHCT} + \text{dHCT}) \div 2\right]\right)$$

d-HCT and iHCT as desired hematocrit and initial hematocrit in percentage, respectively; TBV is the estimated total blood volume in mL (i.e., 60 mL/kg in adult women, 70 mL/kg in adult men, 80 mL/kg in children, 100 mL/kg in infants); and rpHCT is the hematocrit of the replacement packed RBC (typical range, 55–60 percent).

Complications Associated with Transfusion Including Iron Overload

The use of blood transfusion in SCD is for the management of crisis or to prevent the development of complications. The aim of transfusion is to correct anemia and in turn improve oxygen-carrying capacity. Use of non-sickle blood also helps reversal of vaso-occlusion and hemolysis. Indications for acute transfusion in SCD include symptomatic anemia, stroke, hepatic sequestration, ACS, acute multiorgan failure, surgery, and pregnancy. Indications for chronic transfusions include recurrent vaso-occlusive crisis, primary and secondary stroke prevention (Davis et al., 2017b; Han, Hensch, & Tubman, 2021).

Blood transfusion is associated with a number of complications in recipients, this is not limited to; immune modulation, transfusion-associated acute lung injury (TRALI), transfusion-related circulatory overload, acute hypotensive transfusion reactions, febrile non-hemolytic transfusion reaction, massive transfusion-associated reactions (Delaney et al., 2016) that may present as mild or severe reactions and transfusion-transmitted infections. In addition to the usual transfusion risks SCD patients are at higher risk for serious transfusion complications including delayed hemolytic transfusion reactions (DHTRs) and iron overload. (a review by Fasano et al., inconsistent, and poor reporting of transfusion reactions, Fasano et al., 2019).

Delayed Hemolytic Transfusion Reaction

DHTRs occur in transfusion recipients' days to weeks post-transfusion. This is as a result of the development of alloantibodies to red cell antigens of the Rh, Kell, Duffy, Kidd, MNS, and Diego blood group systems, on donor red blood cells from previous transfusions. Re-exposure to the antigen in a subsequent transfusion results in increased antibody production. The IgG antibodies will bind to red blood cells expressing the foreign antigen and the cells are subsequently removed by the spleen causing extravascular hemolysis. Symptoms of DHTRs include a decline in hemoglobin and hematocrit levels post-transfusion, jaundice, fever, hemoglobinuria, and renal failure. Markers of hemolysis may also be elevated post-transfusion. In some cases, alloantibodies may be detected while clinical features are absent, and the patient will be at high risk of developing a transfusion reaction.

The incidence of DHTRs is 1:12,500 transfusions; however, individuals with SCD have a higher risk (4–11%) for developing DHTR as they higher rates of alloimmunization post-transfusion compared to those without SCD. A systematic review of studies conducted in SSA highlighted that the proportion of alloimmunization was 7.4 (95% confidence interval: 5.1–10.0) per 100 transfused SCD patients (Boateng, Ngoma, Bates, & Schonewille, 2019). Studies conducted in developed countries have shown that alloimmunization is due to the differences in the red cell genetic diversity of the donors that are of Caucasian descent with that of SCD patients that are mainly of African descent. Extended serological matching for red cell antigens has been shown to reduce rates of alloimmunization (Chou et al., 2013; Delaney et al., 2016; Fasano et al., 2019; Vichinsky et al., 1990).

Iron Overload

The amount of iron in a unit of packed RBCs is about 200–250 micrograms. In the absence of transfusion iron in blood binds to transferrin and gets transported to the liver where it is stored as ferritin or to the bone marrow for erythropoiesis (Figure 11.1). Depending on the number, frequency, and type of transfusion, chronic blood transfusion can result in iron overload in individuals with SCD. Iron turnover post-transfusion is due to destruction of RBCs that subsequently result in transferrin bound iron being directed to the bone marrow and hepatocytes. Continued

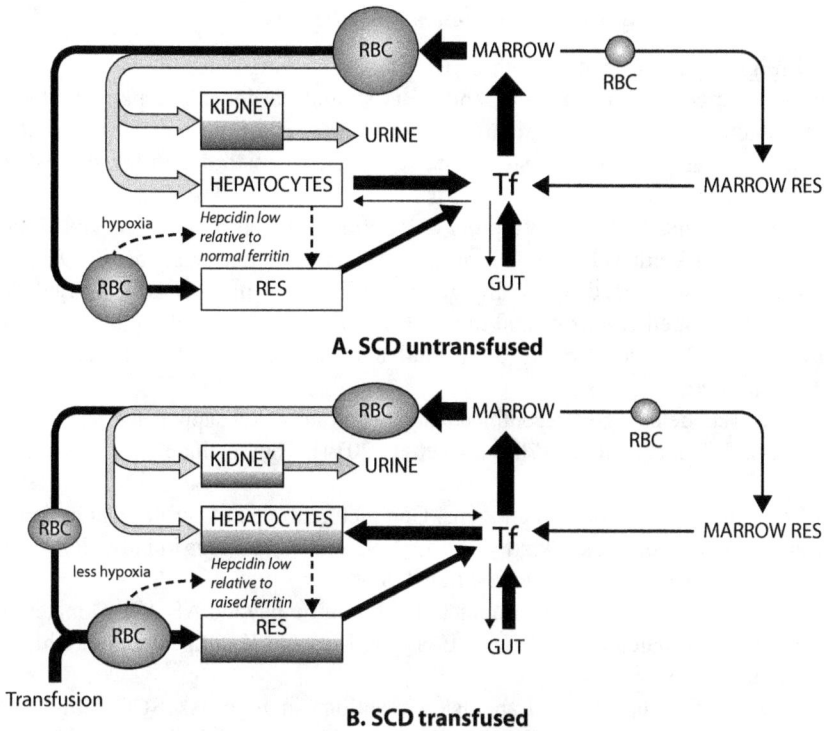

Figure 11.1 Summary of differences in iron turnover in SCD triggered by transfusion (Porter & Garbowski, 2013).

destruction of RBCs results in saturation of serum transferrin and subsequent presence of non-transferrin bound iron (NTBI) in circulation that has high redox ability and gets into cells through ion transporters regardless of the cytosolic iron levels. The NTBI then deposits in the liver, heart, and endocrine organs. Heart failure, endocrine disorders, hepatic fibrosis, and cirrhosis are some of the clinical complications associated with iron overload in SCD. These complications result in organ damage which subsequently increase hospital admissions for management of the complications and a place these individuals at a higher risk of mortality.

Hyperviscosity

Hyperviscosity arises due to an increment in hematocrit as a result of receiving red blood cells via transfusion. Increased viscosity of blood reduces its flow and may result in vascular occlusion, it also impairs oxygen delivery to the deep tissue. The risk of developing hyperviscosity depends on hematocrit and %HbS. Worth noting is the fact that exchange transfusion reduces %HbS and viscosity while simple transfusions on the other hand result in higher hematocrit and increased viscosity (Davis et al., 2017a).

Prevention and Management of Transfusion Complications

Before giving an individual with SCD baseline investigations blood group, allo-antibody screening, reticulocyte, and CBC should be done. The patient's blood transfusion history of alloimmunization and previous DHTR episodes as well as number of past transfusions should be reviewed so as to determine the risk of developing DHTR.

Extended matching of recipient RBC antigens with those of the donor reduces the likelihood of developing alloantibodies and subsequent DHTRs. However, this is faced by challenges including low number of potential donors in developed countries and the cost implications to transfusion services in developing countries for the additional antigen matching beyond ABO and RhD matching.

Several guidelines give recommendations for transfusion support for SCD (Chou et al., 2020; Davis et al., 2017b; Yawn et al., 2014). They include

- Profiling of red blood cell antigens. Conduct genotype of serological typing of at least C/c, E/e, K, Jka/Jkb, Fya/Fyb, M/N, and S/s antigens in individuals with SCD if possible before their first transfusion.
- Prophylactic red cell antigen matching should be beyond ABO/RhD matching and include matching for Rh (C, E or C/c, E/e) and K antigens that are highly immunogenic.
- Prevention of hemolytic transfusion reactions in high-risk SCD individuals using immunosuppressive therapy (intravenous immunoglobulin [IVIg], steroids, and/or rituximab) in emergency transfusions without compatible blood or in patients with history of severe hemolytic transfusion reactions.
- Identification of Rh system variants in SCD individuals by genotyping as antibodies may not always be present.
- On identification of RBC antibodies that are clinically significant, blood selected for transfusion should be devoid of the corresponding antigens.

Once transfused, patients should be monitored for fever, jaundice, anemia, and painful crisis. CBC and determination of hemolysis markers and alloantibodies should be done when there is suspicion of a DHTR (Davis et al., 2017a)

Monitoring of iron overload pre- and post-transfusion in SCD patients can be done through determination of hepatic iron content in blood by quantifying serum ferritin and iron levels, through magnetic resonance imaging (MRI) or a liver biopsy. Serum ferritin is measured every three weeks post-transfusion and is associated with limitations of not increasing in a linear manner between values of 10 and 30 milligrams/gram dry weight liver (Adamkiewicz et al., 2009). Serum ferritin levels are also influenced by inflammation and increase with increasing levels of IL-6. Hence serial measurements are advised for the assessment of iron overload. Determination of liver and cardiac iron concentrations by MRI imaging is done annually, however this test is not accessible in most of SSA. Liver function tests will help to determine organ function in patients with iron overload.

The management of iron overload in SCD patients receiving regular transfusions is part of the treatment process, but this is not the case for those receiving episodic transfusions. Iron chelation therapy aims to reduce levels of plasma and cytosolic NTBI. The treatment is recommended when patients have received more than 20 units of blood, have a liver iron content >7 milligrams/gram dry weight liver or serum ferritin levels more than 1,000 micrograms/liter. Excess iron forms complexes with iron chelators and enables excretion in urine and stool. Deferoxamine (Desferal; DFO), deferasirox (Exjade or Jadenu™; DFX), and deferiprone (Ferriprox; DFP) are the three approved iron chelators. DFX and DFO have been licensed for the management of iron overload in SCD (Coates & Wood, 2017; Porter & Garbowski, 2013).

Chelation therapy comes with its own set of challenges. Toxicity associated with the use of chelators includes local reaction at injection site, anaphylaxis, infection and visual impairment for DFO while DFX may cause nausea, gastrointestinal bleeding, impaired renal and liver function. The use of chelation therapy should be accompanied with monitoring of several parameters including platelet and neutrophil counts, creatinine, and liver function. The use of MRI imaging during iron chelation therapy with has been shown to improve the management of IC therapy (Alkindi, Panjwani, Al-Rahbi, Al-Saidi, & Pathare, 2021). Another challenge is adherence to the treatment, and this is heavily reliant on the support given to the patient by the clinical team providing treatment (Coates & Wood, 2017).

Red cell exchange transfusion as opposed to top-up transfusions reduces the risk of iron overload and subsequent need for iron chelation therapy.

References

Diop, S., Pirenne, F., Transfusion and sickle cell anemia in Africa. Transfus Clin Biol. 2021. **28**(2): p. 143–145. doi:10.1016/j.tracli.2021.01.013

Piel, F. B., Hay, S.I., Gupta, S., Weatherall, D.J., Williams, T.N., Global burden of sickle cell anaemia in children under five, 2010-2050: modelling based on demographics, excess mortality, and interventions. PLoS Med. 2013. **10**(7): p. e1001484. doi:10.1371/journal.pmed.1001484

Adamkiewicz, T.V., et al., Serum ferritin level changes in children with sickle cell disease on chronic blood transfusion are nonlinear and are associated with iron load and liver injury. Blood. 2009. **114**(21): p. 4632–4638.

Alkindi, S., et al., Iron overload in patients with heavily transfused sickle cell disease-correlation of serum ferritin with cardiac T2(*) MRI (CMRTools), liver T2(*) MRI, and R2-MRI (Ferriscan(R)). Front Med (Lausanne). 2021. **8**: p. 731102.

Boateng, L.A., et al., Red blood cell alloimmunization in transfused patients with sickle cell disease in Sub-Saharan Africa; A systematic review and meta-analysis. Transfus Med Rev, 2019. **33**(3): p. 162–169.

Chou, S.T., et al., High prevalence of red blood cell alloimmunization in sickle cell disease despite transfusion from Rh-matched minority donors. Blood, 2013. **122**(6): p. 1062–1071.

Chou, S.T., et al., American Society of Hematology 2020 guidelines for sickle cell disease: Transfusion support. Blood Adv, 2020. **4**(2): p. 327–355.

Coates, T.D., Wood, J.C., How we manage iron overload in sickle cell patients. Br J Haematol, 2017. **177**(5): p. 703–716.

Davis, B.A., Allard, S., Qureshi, A., Porter, J.B, Pancham, S., Win, N., Cho, G., Ryan, K., British Committee for Standards in Hematology, Guidelines on red cell transfusion in sickle cell disease. Part I: Principles and laboratory aspects. Br J Haematol, 2017a. **176**(2): p. 179–191.

Davis, B.A., Allard, S., Qureshi, A., Porter, J.B, Pancham, S., Win, N., Cho, G., Ryan, K., British Committee for Standards in Hematology, Guidelines on red cell transfusion in sickle cell disease. Part II: Indications for transfusion. Br J Haematol, 2017b. **176**(2): p. 192–209.

Delaney, M., et al., Transfusion reactions: Prevention, diagnosis, and treatment. Lancet, 2016. **388**(10061): p. 2825–2836.

Fasano, R.M., et al., Impact of red blood cell antigen matching on alloimmunization and transfusion complications in patients with sickle cell disease: A systematic review. Transfus Med Rev, 2019. **33**(1): p. 12–23.

Han, H., Hensch, L., Tubman, V.N. Indications for transfusion in the management of sickle cell disease. Hematology Am Soc Hematol Educ Program, 2021. **2021**(1): p. 696–703.

Howard, J., Malfroy, M., Llewelyn, C., Choo, L., Hodge, R., Johnson, T., et al., The transfusion alternatives preoperatively in sickle cell disease (TAPS) study: A randomised, controlled, multicentre clinical trial. Lancet. 2013. **381**(9870): p. 930–938.

National Heart, Lung and Blood Institute. Evidence-Based Management of Sickle Cell Disease: Expert Panel Report. 2014. http://www.nhlbi.nih.gov/health-pro/guidelines/sickle-cell-disease-guidelines.

Osaro, E.,Charles, A.T., The challenges of meeting the blood transfusion requirements in Sub-Saharan Africa: The need for the development of alternatives to allogenic blood. J Blood Med, 2011. **2**: p. 7–21. https://doi.org/10.2147/JBM.S17194

Porter, J., Garbowski, M., Consequences and management of iron overload in sickle cell disease. Hematology Am Soc Hematol Educ Program, 2013. **2013**: p. 447–456.

Vichinsky, E.P., et al., Alloimmunization in sickle cell anemia and transfusion of racially unmatched blood. N Engl J Med, 1990. **322**(23): p. 1617–1621.

Yawn, B.P., et al., Management of sickle cell disease: Summary of the 2014 evidence-based report by expert panel members. JAMA, 2014. **312**(10): p. 1033–1048.

12 Pregnancy in Women with Sickle Cell Disorder

Bosede Bukola Afolabi

Introduction

The natural history of sickle cell disorder (SCD) has always included high mortality with very few people with the disorder living past the age of five. A review of the latest National Demographic Health Survey (NDHS, 2018) in Nigeria estimated the average under-five mortality to be 490 per 1,000 live births (Nnodu et al., 2021). This has changed somewhat in high-income countries, where there are optimal medical facilities and appropriate access to them. However, the majority of individuals with the condition actually live in low- and middle-income countries (LMICs), with Nigeria having the largest number worldwide. Despite the fact that the under-five mortality rates are still quite high, more women with the condition are now surviving till adulthood and achieving pregnancy.

Pregnancy in women with this disorder is fraught with complications, for both the mother and her baby, with an increased risk of maternal and perinatal mortality (Boafor et al., 2021; Olamijulo, Olorunfemi, & Okunola, 2022). The common complications that occur in pregnancy can be divided into those specific to SCD and those that are non-specific. The non-specific ones can be further broken into obstetric and non-obstetric complications (Table 12.1) (Babah, Aderolu, Oluwole, & Afolabi, 2019; Figueira, Surita, Fertrin, Nobrega, & Costa, 2022). Those that are sickle cell specific include vaso-occlusive and other crises, and acute chest syndrome. A prospective comparative study of 50 women with SCD found them to have significantly more frequent admissions than age, gestational age and parity matched haemooglobin AA women (Babah et al., 2019); yet as in the non-pregnant, there is a lot of variability with 32% of haemoglobin (Hb) SS women having a normal course in a large cohort study from Jamaica (Lewis, Thame, Howitt, Hambleton, & Serjeant, 2021). In some of the few studies done, specifically in women of reproductive age, women with SCD have been reported to have a lower ovarian reserve than women with Hb AA, when matched for age and parity (Garba et al., 2021) and are also more prone to miscarriage, as seen in the Jamaican cohort study (Lewis et al., 2021). Cardiac size in pregnant Hb SS women was found to be larger than that of Hb AA women in the third trimester, with no difference in cardiac function as measured by ejection fraction. The women were also found to have a significant reduction in their left ventricular diameter in systole at six weeks postpartum,

DOI: 10.4324/9781003463931-13

Table 12.1 Common complications of sickle cell disorder in pregnancy in LMIC.

Sickle specific	Non-sickle specific	
	Obstetric	*Non-obstetric*
Vaso-occlusive crises	Pregnancy-induced hypertension	Urinary tract infection
Haemolytic crises	Preeclampsia/eclampsia	Respiratory tract infection
Sequestration crises	Intrauterine growth restriction	Surgical site infection
Acute chest syndrome	Preterm delivery	Malaria
	Still birth	
	Perinatal death	

when compared to the size in the third trimester, in a longitudinal study carried out in Nigeria, suggesting a positive adaptation of cardiac function during pregnancy (Aliyu et al., 2022).

Despite the challenges, pregnancy can be managed successfully most of the time. Pre-conceptual care with appropriate counselling and tests, frequent, multi-disciplinary antenatal care when they do get pregnant, and prompt diagnosis and treatment of their various complications is key to their management.

Pre-conception Care in LMIC

The ideal situation would be for women with SCD to attend a pre-conception clinic before attempting pregnancy. However, health-seeking behaviour is poor in LMIC due to poverty and lack of awareness. In the few situations where women seek counselling before conception, the following management plan may be instituted.

Although there were no randomised controlled trials showing the effect of genetic risk assessment on reproductive outcomes as reported in a recent systematic review (Hussein, Henneman, Kai, & Qureshi, 2021), there have been reports of a reduction of births affected by haemoglobinopathies including SCD, in countries where screening programmes have been instituted (Chakravorty & Dick, 2019). It is therefore recommended to carry out partner screening when a woman with SCD presents at the pre-conception clinic. This is to enable the couple to make informed decisions including whether to have children together as a couple, and whether to have prenatal diagnosis when they do get pregnant, if the partner is found to be a sickle trait carrier. Such counsel should be given in the context of the prevailing abortion laws in the state or country as many LMIC countries have restrictive abortion laws, allowing abortion only to save the mother's life.

Renal function tests to include creatinine concentration and urinary protein: creatinine ratio should be done to assess renal function and microscopic or gross proteinuria. This is because majority of individuals with SCD develop renal disease during their lifetime (Ataga, Saraf, & Derebail, 2022; Olaniran et al., 2020) and any woman with pre-existing renal disease entering pregnancy has a higher risk of hypertensive disease including preeclampsia/eclampsia, and possible deterioration of the renal disease. A study examining pregnant women with SCD, with and without preeclampsia, found a significant risk of deteriorating renal function in those with preeclampsia one year after delivery (Boudhabhay et al., 2021). They should be referred to nephrologists if they have abnormal renal function test results, before trying to conceive. Regarding cardiovascular complications, pulmonary hypertension is also common in SCD (Isa et al., 2020) and pregnancy in women with pulmonary hypertension is associated with a high maternal mortality rate. Despite the findings of a lower maternal mortality rate of approximately 12% in two recent systematic reviews of pulmonary hypertension in pregnancy (Jha, Jha, Mishra, & Sagili, 2020; Low et al., 2021), it is important to note that these studies were mostly carried out in high-income countries and women with SCD with pulmonary hypertension in LMIC should be counseled about the substantial risk of maternal death.

The steady-state haemoglobin concentration, or packed cell volume (PCV), and whether there is a history of transfusions or frequent crises should be noted. If the steady-state Hb is not known, it should be established before pregnancy to have a baseline rate to monitor changes in the haemoglobin concentration during pregnancy. Plasma volume expansion is seen in normal pregnancy and correlates well with an optimal pregnancy outcome in terms of maternal well-being and optimal birth weight. However, plasma volume expansion is blunted in sickle cell pregnancy (Abudu & Sofola, 1988; Afolabi et al., 2016) and the haemoglobin concentration does not change significantly during pregnancy in steady-state pregnant Hb SS women (Afolabi, Akanmu, Oluwole, Kehinde, & Abudu, 2014). Thus any significant drop in haemoglobin concentration should warrant investigation and treatment, especially since their steady-state haemoglobin concentration is usually below 8g/dl (Afolabi et al., 2014; Agbaje, Adeyomoye, Omidiji, Oboke, & Afolabi, 2018).

The women's current medication use should also be reviewed. They should be encouraged to take 5 mg of folic acid a day as this is sufficient to replenish their folate stores as required in haemolytic conditions. It also helps prevent neural tube defects in the fetus of pregnant women, when taken before conception and in the first 12 weeks. They should be instructed to start or continue on their malaria prophylaxis as malaria is a common cause of morbidity in pregnant women with SCD. Daily proguanil is commonly prescribed to individuals with SCD in Nigeria although monthly sulphadoxine-pyrimethamine has been found to be more effective in a randomised controlled trial conducted in non-pregnant individuals, albeit with small numbers (Dawam et al., 2016). As there are no randomised trials in pregnant women with SCD, they should be prescribed 200-mg proguanil daily, or monthly sulphadoxine-pyrimethamine from the second trimester of pregnancy.

Hydroxyurea is an antineoplastic drug that has been found useful in reducing the frequency of complications such as vaso-occlusive crises and acute chest syndrome by raising the concentration of fetal haemoglobin (Rankine-Mullings & Nevitt, 2022). However, it is not recommended in pregnancy as the risk to the fetus is unclear. A large cohort study examining the effects of hydroxyurea use in SCD reported on the effects of inadvertent use in early pregnancy. Of 125 pregnancies, there was no evidence of an increased risk of miscarriage or congenital malformations (de Montalembert et al., 2021). A more recent report found hydroxyurea to be safe up till the time of conception but found higher odds of miscarriage or stillbirth in the women who took hydroxyurea during pregnancy and conception (Kroner et al., 2022). The use of hydroxyurea during pregnancy should therefore still be restricted but in the event of severe and frequent crises, experienced maternal medicine specialists may decide to prescribe it with individual consideration, after counselling the woman on the risks and benefits. In the postpartum period, however, it is relatively safe during breastfeeding and should be prescribed for women with severe recurrent crises or acute chest syndrome in pregnancy (Ware et al., 2020).

Antenatal Care

During pregnancy, encouraging frequent antenatal visits and obstetric scans where feasible, and individualised care with careful attention to their vital signs, increases the chances of detecting complications before they become difficult to reverse. Multidisciplinary care is important if available as the affected women benefit from haematology, microbiology, respiratory and intensive care input as required.

Table 12.2 depicts an antenatal clinic routine in an LMIC. It is particularly important to ensure that the woman's vital signs are checked each visit. This should include the pulse and respiratory rates, and blood pressure, as well as their oxygen saturation. The latter can be achieved with relatively inexpensive handheld finger pulse oximeters (Figure 12.1) and is important because knowledge of the value often helps to diagnose respiratory insufficiency earlier than the subjective assessment of the women. A value of less than 95% should be viewed as abnormal and she should be carefully questioned and examined appropriately, to decide whether to investigate further or to admit her. The woman with SCD should be questioned specifically for symptoms of vaso-occlusive crises and respiratory symptoms and given prompt treatment as required. She should be informed about the relative high risk of complications during pregnancy and requested to drink water liberally and avoid extremes of temperature, especially low temperatures. Urine microscopy, culture, and sensitivity may be done at the first visit if affordable as urinary tract infection is common in pregnant women with SCD (Lewis et al., 2021; Proske et al., 2021). However, as bacteriology is relatively expensive, urinalysis may be done instead and repeated every visit, to screen for bacteriuria, as well as proteinuria and glycosuria.

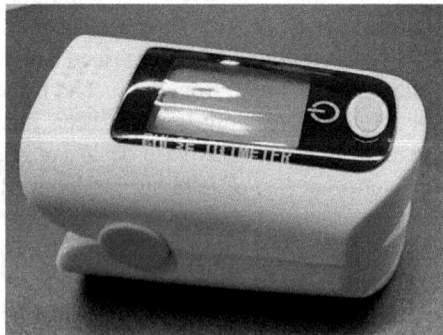

Figure 12.1 Finger pulse oximeter.

Table 12.2 Pragmatic cost-effective approach to providing antenatal care to pregnant sickle cell disease women in Nigeria.

Visit	History	Examination	Investigations	Drugs	Counselling
First	Detailed history	Blood pressure Weight measurement Height measurement Oxygen saturation Detailed physical examination including general examination, cardiovascular system check, and abdominal examination to examine the uterus and its content and check for hepatosplenomegaly Breast examination	Blood group Complete blood count Urinalysis HIV screening Hepatitis B and C VDRL Obstetric ultrasound scan for dating and to confirm fetal viability if date of last menstrual period is unknown	Malaria prophylaxis (usually proguanil 200 mg till delivery) Folic acid 5–10 mg daily till delivery Tetanus toxoid injection[a] Low dose aspirin[b]	Counselling for prenatal diagnosis for fetal genotype if indicated and if the facility exists Plan on mode of delivery and for pain relief during labour are discussed. Specific instructions are documented on the front of the case-folder if applicable
Subsequent – Two weekly till 28 weeks, thereafter weekly till delivery	Enquiries about new symptoms and resolution of previous symptom if any	Weight measurement Oxygen saturation Blood pressure General physical examination Abdominal examination with focus on uterus and its content, liver, and splenic enlargement	Packed cell volume or Hb concentration Urinalysis Complete blood count if indicated Fetal anomaly scan at 18–20 weeks	Malaria prophylaxis and folic acid as above Repeat tetanus toxoid if due[a]	Reminder on previous counselling; also, on birth preparedness, complication readiness, and family planning Conclusion on mode of delivery at 37 weeks

Notes: Additional care instituted is dependent on symptoms and signs elicited at presentation in the hospital.

[a] Tetanus toxoid is administered as per WHO protocol. First dose is given at first contact, second dose four weeks after, third dose six months after second dose, and fourth and fifth dose at yearly intervals after the third dose.

[b] Low dose aspirin is not routinely prescribed for pregnant women with SCD in Nigeria. Decision to prescribe low dose aspirin is based on physician's expert opinion and often individualised. When used, it is commenced at 12 weeks and continued till 36 weeks in women with an additional risk factor such as age >40 or multiple pregnancy. Ongoing clinical trial on its use with details below.

Source: Reproduced from a manuscript accepted for publication in Hematology, the American Society of Hematology Education Program.

Routine drugs including folic acid 5 mg daily and proguanil 200 mg daily (or monthly sulphadoxine-pyrimethamine – see preconception care above) are to be continued or commenced during pregnancy and taken throughout. Empirical iron use is not indicated as individuals with SCD often have enough iron, due to recurrent haemolysis as well as transfusions (Sukla et al., 2021). As there is an increased iron requirement in pregnancy, however, it is important to investigate appropriately and treat women with proven iron deficiency (ferritin < 30 ng/ml or low transferrin saturation), especially in those whose haemoglobin concentrations drop without any other obvious sign of illness.

Specific Complications

Pregnancy is unique in the fact that its management has to take two "patients" into account – the mother and her unborn fetus. This affects diagnostic tests as well as treatment options as the safety of the fetus has to be considered. However, in situations where the mother's life is at risk, it is important to ensure the most effective tests and medication are prescribed regardless of the safety concerns, while ensuring that the mother is aware of the risks involved, and verbally consents to the management decisions before they are carried out.

Maternal Complications

Vaso-occlusive Crisis

The extremely distressing vaso-occlusive "pain" crises should be promptly treated as it may be a precursor to acute chest syndrome, which is a life-threatening complication, and is one of the commonest causes of death in SCD (Klings & Steinberg, 2022; Lewis et al., 2021). Carefully administered hydration and adequate analgesia from acetaminophen to non-steroidal anti-inflammatory drugs (NSAIDs) and opiates should be administered as appropriate for gestational age and degree of pain. NSAIDs should be avoided in the first trimester as there are concerns about a possible increased risk of miscarriage (Li, Ferber, Odouli, & Quesenberry, 2018), and after 30 weeks' gestation, because of the risk of premature closure of the ductus arteriosus (Dathe et al., 2022). Pregnant women with SCD can often be maintained and weaned off oral morphine, and this should not be withheld for fear of addiction as the benefits outweigh the risks. It is however important to enquire about previous history of opiate addiction and, if present, care should be taken to administer such drugs restrictively and in collaboration with a psychiatrist. A practical approach to managing vaso-occlusive crises in pregnancy is as follows:

1 **Assess:** Take a history to ascertain if this is typical sickle pain or not, and if there are precipitating factors. Examine with focus on the site of pain, any atypical features of the pain, and any precipitating factors, in particular for any signs of infection.

Assess for precipitating factors such as infection, including malaria, or dehydration.

2 **Analgesia:** Start with paracetamol for mild pain; NSAIDs for mild to moderate pain between 12 and 30 weeks; weak opioids such as co-dydramol, co-codamol, or dihydrocodeine for moderate pain; and stronger opiates such as morphine for severe pain.

Pethidine is contraindicated due to the risk of toxicity and seizures.

3 **Investigations:** Full blood count, tests for malaria, reticulocyte count and renal function, blood cultures, chest X-ray, urine culture, and liver function tests.

Transfuse with packed red cells, HbAA blood if PCV is less than 18%, aiming to raise the haematocrit to steady state if known, or 26–28%.

4 **Fluid and oxygen:** Fluid balance – ensure fluid intake of an appropriate amount of fluid. Administer IV fluids, preferably hypotonic fluids such as 4.3% dextrose in 0.18 normal saline, based on the woman's clinical status and urine output. Avoid overhydration and be especially careful in women with cardiac or renal disease.

5 **Transfusion:** Transfuse with packed red cells ensuring blood is haemoglobin AA genotype, in cases of severe anaemia below 18% PCV, aiming to raise the haematocrit to between 26% and 28%. Also transfuse if there is a sudden drop in haemoglobin concentration below the steady state.

6 **Treatment:** Therapeutic antibiotics if there is evidence of infection as seen by a high white cell count and neutrophilia, or a positive culture. However, leucocytosis should be interpreted with caution as white cell count is commonly raised in both SCD and pregnancy. Pneumonia is often due to atypical organisms and initial treatment should be with azithromycin and co-amoxiclav. If malaria is diagnosed, it should be treated with artemisinin combination therapy.

7 **Monitoring:** Invite a multidisciplinary team – maternal medicine, haematology, anaesthetist, and pulmonologist, as required. Monitor vital signs, including pain score and oxygen saturation and provide facial oxygen if oxygen saturation falls below the woman's baseline or <95%. Daily or twice daily haematocrit or haemoglobin concentration checks are required in order to detect a rapid fall early. There should be early recourse to intensive care if satisfactory saturation cannot be maintained with facial oxygen.

Blood Transfusion

Prophylactic blood transfusion to keep the haemoglobin concentration at a specific level is not advocated during pregnancy in women with SCD as there is no evidence available regarding its effectiveness or otherwise. A Cochrane review concluded that the available single randomised controlled trial evidence was not of sufficient quality to determine a change in existing policy (Okusanya & Oladapo, 2016). The trial found that prophylactic transfusions reduced the incidence of painful crises but did not have any impact on maternal or perinatal mortality (Koshy, Burd, Wallace, Moawad, & Baron, 1988). As there are many complications associated with blood transfusion, including transfusion reactions, allo-immunisation, iron overload, and infections, it is important to determine if the expected benefits outweigh the risks. Blood products and detailed cross matching such as extended Kell are not commonly available in LMICs. In the author's institution, top-up transfusions are given when required, e.g. a sudden drop in haemoglobin concentration between visits or below 5g/dl, a drop of ≥3g/dl from the woman's known steady state, or in situations when the woman has associated symptoms of anaemia or a drop in oxygen saturation, even without a significant drop in haemoglobin concentration. When transfusion is indicated, haemoglobin AA blood is recommended. In situations of frequent recurrent vaso-occlusive crises or severe acute chest syndrome, exchange blood transfusion is recommended as in the non-pregnant (Davis et al., 2017).

Pneumonia and Acute Chest Syndrome

Pregnant women with SCD often present with pneumonia and treatment should involve the input of a pulmonologist. A chest X-ray is mandatory for any woman presenting with respiratory symptoms such as cough and chest pain, together with a fever, or other evidence of clinical compromise such as reduced oxygen saturation or increase in respiratory rate. The X-ray can be done with abdominal shielding in the second trimester and beyond but should not be omitted when required in the first trimester, as the benefits or accurate diagnosis and treatment usually outweigh the minimal risks of radiation (Mattsson, Leide-Svegborn, & Andersson, 2021).

Acute chest syndrome is difficult to differentiate from pneumonia and often coincides with it. New pulmonary infiltrates on chest X-ray in combination with cough, chest pain, and fever are highly suggestive, especially with the background of a severe vaso-occlusive crisis and treatment and supportive therapy should be started promptly and aggressively. Anaesthetists or intensivists should be consulted early in the management and exchange blood transfusion is often required. This can be manual or automated depending on availability of equipment and infrastructure as it has been found that manual exchange blood transfusion EBT is also effective for the treatment of acute chest syndrome (Mukherjee, Sahu, Ray, Maiti, & Prakash, 2022).

Non-sickle-Related Complications

Pregnancy-Induced Hypertension (PIH) and Preeclampsia/eclampsia

PIH is frequently seen in pregnant women with SCD and is documented in several studies. Preeclampsia is also more common in these women as reported in meta-analyses and some recent reports although some individual prospective studies in Nigeria and Germany did not find a significant difference in the incidence of preeclampsia or eclampsia in pregnant women with SCD (Babah et al.,

2019; Proske et al., 2021). Sickle cell pregnancy can thus be seen as a mild or moderate risk factor for preeclampsia. Low dose aspirin has been found to be effective in preventing preeclampsia in women at high risk for the condition and is relatively safe for this purpose. However, it has not been tested in pregnant women with SCD and a meta-analysis found a slightly increased risk of placental abruption and vaginal bleeding with the use of low dose aspirin. Although it has been recommended in some guidelines, low dose aspirin is not yet in universal use for preventing preeclampsia in sickle cell pregnancy and thus women should be considered on an individual basis. A randomised controlled trial on its use for this purpose is currently underway (Afolabi et al., 2021), the results of which should be useful in this regard. In the meantime, it would be expedient to administer between 75 and 150 mg of low dose aspirin to pregnant women with SCD if there is an additional moderate risk factor such as multiple pregnancy or pregnancy conceived by in vitro fertilisation, as recommended by UK NICE guidelines (NICE, 2019).

If facilities exist, a risk factor assessment for preeclampsia should also be carried out using uterine artery doppler assessment, mean arterial pressure, PAPP-A, SFlt-1, PLGF and maternal characteristics and medical history (Poon et al., 2019, 2021), depending on which of the biomarkers are available. If high risk for preeclampsia, $\geq$100 mg of low dose aspirin should be administered from before 16 weeks' gestation and stopped at 36 weeks' gestation (NICE, 2019).

If a pregnant woman with SCD develops PE, she should be managed like any other woman with PE, with treatment of the hypertension with antihypertensives such as alpha methyldopa, nifedipine, or labetalol, and the use of magnesium sulphate to prevent eclampsia as well as for neuroprotection of the prematurely delivered infant (NICE, 2019). Delivery is the only truly effective treatment but the timing is often weighed against the maturity of the fetus, with a tendency to delay delivery in favour of the latter. As women with SCD complicated by preeclampsia are likely to have an even higher likelihood of adverse maternal outcome, caution should be taken with expectant management and delivery may need to be effected earlier rather than later (Magee, Nicolaides, & von Dadelszen, 2022).

Fetal Complications

Intrauterine growth restriction (IUGR) is common in SCD and can lead to still birth and perinatal morbidity and mortality. Several meta-analyses report a 3–4-fold increase in IUGR, small for gestational age and perinatal mortality in SCD. IUGR is often considered to be due to uteroplacental insufficiency but is also associated with a lack of plasma volume expansion in pregnancy, a situation that has been found in reports of plasma volume measurement in pregnant women with SCD, as mentioned above. It is therefore important to monitor the growth of the fetus in these women, although the frequent and specialised ultrasound scan examinations required including umbilical artery, ductus venosus and cerebral artery dopplers, are not easily accessible in LMIC due to cost as well as availability of requisite skill. In areas with poor access, the following should be done:

Baseline ultrasound scan at booking
Anomaly scan at 20 weeks
Growth scan at 28–30 weeks
Four weekly growth scans

If evidence of growth restriction is detected, umbilical artery doppler scans should be performed as well as non-stress tests, from 28 weeks onwards with a view to delivery at the appropriate time in order to reduce the incidence of still-birth. A reasonable delivery cut-off in the absence of an experienced feto-maternal medicine team is the presence of absent or reversed end-diastolic flow in an umbilical artery doppler examination, or an abnormal non-stress test. If there are no resource constraints in the particular context, the usual expectant management of IUGR should be carried out in order to delay the timing of delivery and reduce the complications of prematurity.

Delivery

Timing of delivery is important. Although there is no clear evidence to support early delivery, it is expedient to deliver women with SCD after 38 weeks as there is a higher risk of complications such as vaso-occlusive crises, which may be further complicated by acute chest syndrome, at later gestational ages (Oteng-Ntim et al., 2021). Delivery should be by the vaginal route unless there are obstetric reasons not to do so, as there is a higher risk of infections, anaesthetic complications, and thromboembolic disease with caesarean section. Examples of indications for caesarean section include previous caesarean section, severe IUGR with a need for early delivery, or in the event that a woman has a severe vaso-occlusive crisis and is adjudged not to be able to withstand the stress of labour. Some women with SCD may also have had avascular necrosis of the head of the femur, a relatively common complication in individuals with SCD and may be unable to abduct their hips sufficiently to deliver vaginally. As these indications are frequently seen, women with SCD often end up being delivered by caesarean section.

Induction of labour should be offered between 38- and 39-weeks' gestation, for women that are not scheduled for elective caesarean section, using mechanical methods with transcervical extra-amniotic foley catheter insertion overnight for cervical ripening, or 25-µg oral misoprostol administered after dissolving a 200-µg tablet in water and dividing the solution into eight parts. Artificial rupture of membranes is done once the cervix is favourable and oxytocin used to stimulate contractions if the woman does not start to contract within an hour of ARM. As oral misoprostol avoids vaginal examinations and consequent infection, and as it does not appear to increase the risk of uterine tachysystole at low doses of 25 µg compared to foley catheter (Kerr et al., 2021), it may be preferable to foley catheter in pregnant SCD women. There are concerns about induction of labour after previous caesarean birth, in women with

SCD. Caution should be exercised in such cases because of the risk of uterine rupture and haemorrhage in a group of women known to have chronic anaemia, particularly in resource-limited environments with paucity of blood products.

Labour should be monitored carefully with special attention to the reduction of stress as well as adequate pain relief. Companionship and respectful maternity care should be emphasised and good pain relief in the form of epidural analgesia if available, or strong opiates such as parenteral pentazocine or morphine should be used during labour. Pethidine is however contraindicated as it is known to cause seizures in SCD. Labour should not be prolonged and the woman should be well hydrated throughout labour either with oral or intravenous fluids. Antibiotics are not required unless there is empirical evidence to administer them such as a sudden rise or unexplained white cell count, and positive cultures.

If there is maternal exhaustion, evidence of maternal compromise or delay during the second stage of labour, delivery can be assisted with vacuum or forceps delivery. If caesarean section is required, anaesthesia should be by a regional block technique preferably, in order to avoid the effects of general anaesthesia, which could increase their risk of respiratory compromise.

Prevention of thromboembolic disease is essential regardless of mode of delivery and women with SCD who are admitted for vaso-occlusive crises or any other reason should be given unfractionated heparin or low molecular weight heparin for thromboprophylaxis, throughout the period of admission. This is because both pregnancy and SCD are independent risk factors for venous thromboembolism (RCOG, 2015). Risk assessment guidelines for prevention and treatment of thromboembolic disease should also be used to determine whether to start preventive therapy from earlier on in pregnancy.

Postpartum Period

As the risk of complications is still high within the first few days of the puerperium, it is advised that women with SCD are observed in hospital for at least four days postpartum, regardless of mode of delivery. Although there is no clear evidence supporting this, postpartum crises are common and blood pressure is known to rise on the third day postpartum in all women (Nelson-Piercy, 2015). Their oxygen saturation and hydration status should be continuously monitored, as well as the rest of their vital signs, in order to spot complications early and treat appropriately. Women should be reminded to ensure they keep well hydrated even after they have been discharged from hospital.

The neonate should be screened for SCD early, in places where universal newborn screening is not done. Breastfeeding is encouraged unless the woman is too unwell to do so and the regular types of pain relief including paracetamol, opiates and non-steroidal anti-inflammatory drugs can be safely used during breastfeeding. As individuals with SCD have a higher risk of infections, it appears wise to give antibiotics for the therapeutic period of five days after caesarean section, to aid wound healing, especially in environments in which the infection prevention and control chain can't be guaranteed.

Prevention of thromboembolic disease should be continued throughout admission and for as long as necessary after discharge, based on local available guidelines for the prevention of thromboembolism in pregnancy and the postpartum period. If there are no available guidelines, the RCOG Green top guidelines on the topic can be followed (RCOG, 2015).

Contraception

Women with SCD should be encouraged and counselled to space their families and limit the total number of pregnancies, because of the high risk of complications in pregnancy. Progesterone-based contraceptives have been found to be effective and safe in SCD and may decrease frequency of crises (Legardy & Curtis, 2006). Intramuscular depot progesterone contraceptives such as Depo Provera, progesterone implants such as Implanon, levonorgestrel intrauterine systems, and progesterone only pills are therefore recommended, depending on how long the contraception is required for. Combined oral contraceptives are not usually advised because of the oestrogen content and the additional risk of thromboembolism. They may however be considered on an individual basis if there is no other option especially as there are no studies showing direct evidence of complications with the use of combined contraceptives (Carvalho et al., 2017; Haddad, Curtis, Legardy-Williams, Cwiak, & Jamieson, 2012). As copper-based intrauterine contraceptive devices often cause heavier periods and have a small risk of pelvic infection, they are not first line for women with SCD (De Sanctis et al., 2020). If the couple have completed their family, they should also be counselled about male or female sterilisation. Bilateral tubal ligation can be carried out during delivery if a caesarean section is planned. If there is no plan for a surgical procedure at delivery or any other time, it is safer to use non-surgical, long-acting means of contraception, as described above.

References

Abudu, O. O., & Sofola, O. A. (1988). Intravascular volume expansion and fetal outcome in pregnant Nigerians with hemoglobin SS and SC. *J Natl Med Assoc, 80*(8), 906–912. Retrieved from https://www.ncbi.nlm.nih.gov/pubmed/3246704

Afolabi, B. B., Akanmu, A. S., Oluwole, A. A., Kehinde, M. O., & Abudu, O. O. (2014). Evaluation of haematological parameters in pregnant Nigerian women with sickle cell anaemia. *Niger Quart J Hospital Med, 24*(2), 91–95.

Afolabi, B. B., Babah, O. A., Adeyemo, T. A. (2022). Evidence-based obstetric management of women with sickle cell disease in low-income countries. *Hematology Am Soc Hematol Educ Program, 2022*(1), 414–420.

Afolabi, B. B., Babah, O. A., Adeyemo, T. A., Odukoya, O. O., Ezeaka, C. V., Nwaiwu, O., … Ogunnaike, B. A. (2021). Low-dose aspirin for preventing intrauterine growth restriction and pre-eclampsia in sickle cell pregnancy (PIPSICKLE): A randomised controlled trial (study protocol). *BMJ Open, 11*(8), e047949. https://doi.org/10.1136/bmjopen-2020-047949

Afolabi, B. B., Oladipo, O. O., Akanmu, A. S., Abudu, O. O., Sofola, O. A., & Broughton Pipkin, F. (2016). Volume regulatory hormones and plasma volume in pregnant women with sickle cell disorder. *J Renin Angiotensin Aldosterone Syst, 17*(3). https://doi.org/10.1177/1470320316670444

Agbaje, O. A., Adeyomoye, A. A. O., Omidiji, O. A. T., Oboke, O. S., & Afolabi, B. B. (2018). Evaluation of umbilical artery Doppler indices in pregnant women with sickle cell anemia disease at a Nigerian Tertiary Hospital. *J Diagnost Med Sonography, 34*(6), 466–478. https://doi.org/10.1177/8756479318791157

Aliyu, Z., Kushimo, O. A., Oluwole, A. A., Amadi, C., Oyeyemi, N., Mbakwem, A., & Afolabi, B. B. (2022). Effects of pregnancy on cardiac structure and function in women with sickle cell anemia: A longitudinal comparative study. *J Matern Fetal Neonatal Med*, 1–6. https://doi.org/10.1080/14767058.2022.2089549

Ataga, K. I., Saraf, S. L., & Derebail, V. K. (2022). The nephropathy of sickle cell trait and sickle cell disease. *Nat Rev Nephrol, 18*(6), 361–377. https://doi.org/10.1038/s41581-022-00540-9

Babah, O. A., Aderolu, M. B., Oluwole, A. A., & Afolabi, B. B. (2019). Towards zero mortality in sickle cell pregnancy: A prospective study comparing haemoglobin SS and AA women in Lagos, Nigeria. *Niger Postgrad Med J, 26*(1), 1–7. https://doi.org/10.4103/npmj.npmj_177_18

Boafor, T. K., Ntumy, M. Y., Asah-Opoku, K., Sepenu, P., Ofosu, B., & Oppong, S. A. (2021). Maternal mortality at the Korle Bu Teaching Hospital, Accra, Ghana: A five-year review. *Afr J Reprod Health, 25*(1), 56–66. https://doi.org/10.29063/ajrh2021/v25i1.7

Boudhabhay, I., Boutin, E., Bartolucci, P., Bornes, M. I., Habibi, A., Lionnet, F., ... Audard, V. (2021). Impact of pre-eclampsia on renal outcome in sickle cell disease patients. *Br J Haematol, 194*(6), 1053–1062. https://doi.org/10.1111/bjh.17606

Carvalho, N. S., Braga, J. P., Barbieri, M., Torloni, M. R., Figueiredo, M. S., & Guazzelli, C. A. (2017). Contraceptive practices in women with sickle-cell disease. *J Obstet Gynaecol, 37*(1), 74–77. https://doi.org/10.1080/01443615.2016.1225023

Chakravorty, S., & Dick, M. C. (2019). Antenatal screening for haemoglobinopathies: Current status, barriers and ethics. *Br J Haematol, 187*(4), 431–440. https://doi.org/10.1111/bjh.16188

Dathe, K., Frank, J., Padberg, S., Hultzsch, S., Beck, E., & Schaefer, C. (2022). Fetal adverse effects following NSAID or metamizole exposure in the 2nd and 3rd trimester: An evaluation of the German Embryotox cohort. *BMC Pregnancy Childbirth, 22*(1), 666. https://doi.org/10.1186/s12884-022-04986-4

Davis, B. A., Allard, S., Qureshi, A., Porter, J. B., Pancham, S., Win, N., ... British Society for, H. (2017). Guidelines on red cell transfusion in sickle cell disease. Part II: Indications for transfusion. *Br J Haematol, 176*(2), 192–209. https://doi.org/10.1111/bjh.14383

Dawam, J. A., Madaki, J. K. A., Gambazai, A. A., Okpe, E. S., Lar-ndam, N., Onu, A., & Gyang, M. (2016). Monthly sulphadoxine-pyrimethamine combination versus daily proguanil for malaria chemoprophylaxis in sickle cell disease: A randomized controlled study at the Jos University Teaching Hospital. *Niger J Med, 25*(2), 119–127. Retrieved from https://www.ncbi.nlm.nih.gov/pubmed/29944308

de Montalembert, M., Voskaridou, E., Oevermann, L., Cannas, G., Habibi, A., Loko, G., ... All, E. H. U. I. (2021). Real-life experience with hydroxyurea in patients with sickle cell disease: Results from the prospective ESCORT-HU cohort study. *Am J Hematol, 96*(10), 1223–1231. https://doi.org/10.1002/ajh.26286

De Sanctis, V., Soliman, A. T., Daar, S., Canatan, D., Di Maio, S., & Kattamis, C. (2020). Current issues and options for hormonal contraception in adolescents and young adult women with sickle cell disease: An update for health care professionals. *Mediterr J Hematol Infect Dis, 12*(1), e2020032. https://doi.org/10.4084/MJHID.2020.032

Figueira, C. O., Surita, F. G., Fertrin, K., Nobrega, G. M., & Costa, M. L. (2022). Main complications during pregnancy and recommendations for adequate antenatal care in sickle cell disease: A literature review. *Rev Bras Ginecol Obstet, 44*(6), 593–601. https://doi.org/10.1055/s-0042-1742314

Garba, S. R., Makwe, C. C., Osunkalu, V. O., Kalejaiye, O. O., Soibi-Harry, A. P., Aliyu, A. U., & Afolabi, B. B. (2021). Ovarian reserve in nigerian women with sickle cell anaemia: A cross-sectional study. *J Ovarian Res, 14*(1), 174. https://doi.org/10.1186/s13048-021-00927-5

Haddad, L. B., Curtis, K. M., Legardy-Williams, J. K., Cwiak, C., & Jamieson, D. J. (2012). Contraception for individuals with sickle cell disease: A systematic review of the literature. *Contraception, 85*(6), 527–537. https://doi.org/10.1016/j.contraception.2011.10.008

Hussein, N., Henneman, L., Kai, J., & Qureshi, N. (2021). Preconception risk assessment for thalassaemia, sickle cell disease, cystic fibrosis and Tay-Sachs disease. *Cochrane Database Syst Rev, 10*, CD010849. https://doi.org/10.1002/14651858.CD010849.pub4

Isa, H., Adegoke, S., Madu, A., Hassan, A. A., Ohiaeri, C., Chianumba, R., … Nnodu, O. (2020). Sickle cell disease clinical phenotypes in Nigeria: A preliminary analysis of the Sickle Pan Africa Research Consortium Nigeria database. *Blood Cells Mol Dis, 84*, 102438. https://doi.org/10.1016/j.bcmd.2020.102438

Jha, N., Jha, A. K., Mishra, S. K., & Sagili, H. (2020). Pulmonary hypertension and pregnancy outcomes: Systematic review and meta-analysis. *Eur J Obstet Gynecol Reprod Biol, 253*, 108–116. https://doi.org/10.1016/j.ejogrb.2020.08.028

Kerr, R. S., Kumar, N., Williams, M. J., Cuthbert, A., Aflaifel, N., Haas, D. M., & Weeks, A. D. (2021). Low-dose oral misoprostol for induction of labour. *Cochrane Database Syst Rev, 6*, CD014484. https://doi.org/10.1002/14651858.CD014484

Klings, E. S., & Steinberg, M. H. (2022). Acute chest syndrome of sickle cell disease: Genetics, risk factors, prognosis, and management. *Expert Rev Hematol, 15*(2), 117–125. https://doi.org/10.1080/17474086.2022.2041410

Koshy, M., Burd, L., Wallace, D., Moawad, A., & Baron, J. (1988). Prophylactic red-cell transfusions in pregnant patients with sickle cell disease. A randomized cooperative study. *N Engl J Med, 319*(22), 1447–1452. https://doi.org/10.1056/NEJM198812013192204

Kroner, B. L., Hankins, J. S., Pugh, N., Kutlar, A., King, A. A., Shah, N. R., … Sickle Cell Disease Implementation, C. (2022). Pregnancy outcomes with hydroxyurea use in women with sickle cell disease. *Am J Hematol, 97*(5), 603–612. https://doi.org/10.1002/ajh.26495

Legardy, J. K., & Curtis, K. M. (2006). Progestogen-only contraceptive use among women with sickle cell anemia: A systematic review. *Contraception, 73*(2), 195–204. https://doi.org/10.1016/j.contraception.2005.08.010

Lewis, G., Thame, M., Howitt, C., Hambleton, I., & Serjeant, G. R. (2021). Pregnancy outcome in homozygous sickle cell disease: Observations from the Jamaican birth cohort. *BJOG, 128*(10), 1703–1710. https://doi.org/10.1111/1471-0528.16696

Li, D. K., Ferber, J. R., Odouli, R., & Quesenberry, C. (2018). Use of nonsteroidal antiinflammatory drugs during pregnancy and the risk of miscarriage. *Am J Obstet Gynecol, 219*(3), 275.e1–275.e8. https://doi.org/10.1016/j.ajog.2018.06.002

Low, T. T., Guron, N., Ducas, R., Yamamura, K., Charla, P., Granton, J., & Silversides, C. K. (2021). Pulmonary arterial hypertension in pregnancy – a systematic review of outcomes in the modern era. *Pulm Circ, 11*(2), 20458940211013671. https://doi.org/10.1177/20458940211013671

Magee, L. A., Nicolaides, K. H., & von Dadelszen, P. (2022). Preeclampsia. *N Engl J Med, 386*(19), 1817–1832. https://doi.org/10.1056/NEJMra2109523

Mattsson, S., Leide-Svegborn, S., & Andersson, M. (2021). X-ray and molecular imaging during pregnancy and breastfeeding-when should we be worried? *Radiat Prot Dosimetry*, *195*(3–4), 339–348. https://doi.org/10.1093/rpd/ncab041

Mukherjee, S., Sahu, A., Ray, G. K., Maiti, R., & Prakash, S. (2022). Comparative evaluation of efficacy and safety of automated versus manual red cell exchange in sickle cell disease: A systematic review and meta-analysis. *Vox Sang*. https://doi.org/10.1111/vox.13288

National Population Commission Nigeria. National Demographic and Health Survey Nigeria 2018 [Available from: https://dhsprogram.com/pubs/pdf/FR359/FR359.pdf.

Nelson-Piercy, C. (2015). *Handbook of obstetric medicine* (fifth ed.). Boca Raton, FL: CRC Press.

NICE. (2019). Hypertension in pregnancy: Diagnosis and management. *National Institute for Health and Clinical Excellence Clinical Guideline*, *133*, 1–57.

Nnodu, O. E., Oron, A. P., Sopekan, A., Akaba, G. O., Piel, F. B., & Chao, D. L. (2021). Child mortality from sickle cell disease in Nigeria: A model-estimated, population-level analysis of data from the 2018 demographic and health survey. *Lancet Haematol*, *8*(10), e723–e731. https://doi.org/10.1016/S2352-3026(21)00216-7

Okusanya, B. O., & Oladapo, O. T. (2016). Prophylactic versus selective blood transfusion for sickle cell disease in pregnancy. *Cochrane Database Syst Rev*, *12*, CD010378. https://doi.org/10.1002/14651858.CD010378.pub3

Olamijulo, J. A., Olorunfemi, G., & Okunola, H. (2022). Trends and causes of maternal death at the Lagos University teaching hospital, Lagos, Nigeria (2007–2019). *BMC Pregnancy Childbirth*, *22*(1), 360. https://doi.org/10.1186/s12884-022-04649-4

Olaniran, K. O., Allegretti, A. S., Zhao, S. H., Achebe, M. M., Eneanya, N. D., Thadhani, R. I., … Kalim, S. (2020). Kidney function decline among black patients with sickle cell trait and sickle cell disease: An observational cohort study. *J Am Soc Nephrol*, *31*(2), 393–404. https://doi.org/10.1681/ASN.2019050502

Oteng-Ntim, E., Pavord, S., Howard, R., Robinson, S., Oakley, L., Mackillop, L., … British Society for Haematology, G. (2021). Management of sickle cell disease in pregnancy. A british society for haematology guideline. *Br J Haematol*, *194*(6), 980–995. https://doi.org/10.1111/bjh.17671

Poon, L. C., Magee, L. A., Verlohren, S., Shennan, A., von Dadelszen, P., Sheiner, E., … Hod, M. (2021). A literature review and best practice advice for second and third trimester risk stratification, monitoring, and management of pre-eclampsia: Compiled by the pregnancy and non-communicable diseases committee of FIGO (the International Federation of Gynecology and Obstetrics). *Int J Gynaecol Obstet*, *154*(Suppl 1), 3–31. https://doi.org/10.1002/ijgo.13763

Poon, L. C., Shennan, A., Hyett, J. A., Kapur, A., Hadar, E., Divakar, H., … Hod, M. (2019). The International Federation of Gynecology and Obstetrics (FIGO) initiative on pre-eclampsia: A pragmatic guide for first-trimester screening and prevention. *Int J Gynaecol Obstet*, *145*(Suppl 1), 1–33. https://doi.org/10.1002/ijgo.12802

Proske, P., Distelmaier, L., Aramayo-Singelmann, C., Koliastas, N., Iannaccone, A., Papathanasiou, M., … Alashkar, F. (2021). Pregnancies and neonatal outcomes in patients with sickle cell disease (SCD): Still a (high-)risk constellation? *J Pers Med*, *11*(9). https://doi.org/10.3390/jpm11090870

Rankine-Mullings, A. E., & Nevitt, S. J. (2022). Hydroxyurea (hydroxycarbamide) for sickle cell disease. *Cochrane Database Syst Rev*, *9*, CD002202. https://doi.org/10.1002/14651858.CD002202.pub3

RCOG. (2015). Reducing the risk of venous thromboembolism during pregnancy and the puerperium. *Royal Coll Obstet Gynaecol Green-Top Guideline*, 1–40. Retrieved from https://www.rcog.org.uk/media/qejfhcaj/gtg-37a.pdf

Sukla, S. K., Mohanty, P. K., Patel, S., Das, K., Hiregoudar, M., Soren, U. K., & Meher, S. (2021). Iron profile of pregnant sickle cell anemia patients in Odisha, India. *Hematol Transfus Cell Ther*. https://doi.org/10.1016/j.htct.2021.06.012

Ware, R. E., Marahatta, A., Ware, J. L., McElhinney, K., Dong, M., & Vinks, A. A. (2020). Hydroxyurea exposure in lactation: A pharmacokinetics study (HELPS). *J Pediatr, 222*, 236–239. https://doi.org/10.1016/j.jpeds.2020.02.002

13 Sickle Cell Disease and Nutrition

Vivian Omuemu

Introduction

Sickle cell disease (SCD) results from a genetic substitution that leads to the body making abnormal haemoglobin (Hb) which is the oxygen-carrying substance in the blood. This increases its tendency to polymerise and cause sickling of the red blood cells (RBCs) (Hyacinth et al., 2013). These sickled RBCs adhere to the endothelium of blood vessels causing vasospasms, vasoconstriction and triggering inflammation (Khan et al., 2016) which produces oxygen deficiency at the target tissue or organ. This causes tissue damage which leads to ischaemia, infarction and a compromised reduced lifespan (Chakravorty & Williams, 2015; Khan et al., 2016).

In most of the cases, it requires immediate hospitalisation and medical intervention with anti-inflammatory drugs, non-steroidal analgesics, hydroxyurea (HU), opioid analgesics, rehydration and in severe cases blood transfusion (Stevens et al., 1986) which may cause other long-term side effects. Repeated sickling of these RBCs increases their fragility and tendency for breakdown causing haemolytic anaemia (Hyacinth et al., 2013). The increased premature destruction of these red cells leads to a shortening of their lifespan (8–25 days as opposed to the normal (100–120 days)) in patients with SCD. This creates a need for increased erythropoiesis (RBC production) which leads to increased protein turnover and metabolic rate in SCD patients compared to individuals without the disease, thus leading to increased energy demand (Borel et al., 1998; Hibbert et al., 2006; Hyacinth et al., 2013; Umeakunne & Hibbert, 2019). Furthermore, increased haemolysis results in decreased red cell count and anaemia. As a compensatory mechanism to maintain tissue oxygenation, the heart rate increases, leading to greater myocardial energy demand (Hibbert et al., 2006; Hyacinth et al., 2013) with the net effect of a higher myocardial energy requirement and total energy requirement (Umeakunne & Hibbert, 2019).

Mechanism for Developing Nutritional Deficiencies in Sickle Cell Disease

Several macro- and micronutrients are deficient in patients with SCD and may occur either due to lowered intake of specific nutrients or abnormalities in the

DOI: 10.4324/9781003463931-14

metabolic pathway or alterations at the genetic level (Kawchak et al., 2007; Khan et al., 2016). These nutritional deficiencies affect the concentration of foetal hae-moglobin (HbF) in SCD patients and are associated with the clinical manifestations and severity of the disease (Khan et al., 2016; Martyres et al., 2016).

The occurrence of nutritional deficiencies in SCD patients has been attributed to protein hypermetabolism (increased catabolism), decreased dietary intake, in-testinal malabsorption, increased cardiac energy expenditure and increased red cell turnover (Hyacinth et al., 2010). All the above mechanisms manifest as increased resting energy expenditure (REE) (Hyacinth et al., 2013).

The reduction in food intake is thought to be due to raised interleukins (IL-6 pro-inflammatory cytokine) levels in individuals with SCD (Hibbert et al., 2005). This protein acts on the brain to cause a decrease in appetite leading to decreased food intake (Hyacinth et al., 2010; Khan et al., 2016; Taylor et al., 1995). In addi-tion, repeated ill health and frequent hospitalisations are also thought to be associ-ated with varying degrees of anorexia and reduced feeding time in SCD patients (Hyacinth et al., 2010).

Psychological and social stresses, extreme pain as well as restricted activity may drive the SCD child to dysfunctional eating. This may manifest as difficulty in eating or consuming non-food items which are characteristic symptoms of pica, leading to nutritional deficiencies. Although one quarter of children with SCD are affected by pica, the biological explanation remains unclear (Khan et al., 2016; Lemanek et al., 2002).

The most widely reported mechanism for explaining nutritional deficiencies in SCD patients is increased metabolic requirement and relative nutrient deficiency. SCD is associated with hypermetabolism (Barden et al., 2000; Hyacinth et al., 2010; Hibbert et al., 2005, 2006; Singhal et al., 2002) which is due to increased inflammation, myocardial energy demand from an increased heart rate and eryth-ropoiesis linked to increased haemolysis (Ganong, 2003; Hyacinth et al., 2010, Hyacinth, 2018; Hibbert et al., 2006).

Hypermetabolism is a state of increased caloric demand with a high rate of catabolism (nutrient breakdown) and anabolism (nutrient build-up). How-ever, in SCD, there is a shift towards increased nutrient breakdown, leading to increased nutrient demand (Hibbert et al., 2006; Hyacinth et al., 2013; Khan et al., 2016).

The patient with SCD is in a state where catabolism exceeds anabolism, re-sulting in an energy requirement that exceeds the apparently adequate nutrient intake in the absence of SCD. This hypermetabolism is associated with an in-crease in REE, which is a measure of the energy consumption of an individual at rest (Umeakunne & Hibbert, 2019). The shortened lifespan of sickled blood cells and haemolysis accompanied by erythropoiesis causes increased energy demand of the body and the resting energy required (Barden et al. 2000; Borel et al., 1998; Hibbert et al., 2005, 2006; Khan et al., 2016). Hence, their requirement for energy to sustain the normal functions of growth, physiological functioning and physical activity is not met.

Increased energy requirements that are not followed by an increase in caloric intake lead to impaired growth status in SCD patients (Khan et al., 2016; Singhal et al., 2002). Also in order to maintain and supply oxygen to the different tissues of the body, workload on the cardiac system is increased, thereby triggering a state of chronic inflammation. The high REE among SCD patients is determined primarily by energy needs for increased protein metabolism in addition to compromised protein utilisation due to deficiencies of some amino acids (Khan et al., 2016; Singhal et al., 2002). The increase in protein turnover leads to a state of relative nutritional insufficiency because the flow of nutrients for other essential metabolic needs is limited (Enwonwu & Lu, 1991; Hyacinth et al., 2013; Nelson et al., 2002; Prasad and Cossack, 1984; Umeakunne & Hibbert, 2019; Williams et al., 2004).

In SCD patients, nutrients from the diet and amino acids from body protein catabolism are diverted to support the rapid red cell production, increased myocardial energy demand due to increased heart rate (a compensatory mechanism for anaemia) and propagation of the state of chronic subclinical inflammation reported among SCD patients rather than being available for normal growth and development in children and for maintaining adequate muscle mass in adults. This increases the energy requirement which manifests as a relative nutrient deficiency (Akohoue et al., 2007; Hyacinth et al., 2013; Hibbert et al., 2005, 2006; Umeakunne & Hibbert, 2019).

This means that even when food intake might be adequate, it is still not sufficient to maintain normal body function and metabolism for the individual with SCD due to the increased nutritional and energy demand imposed by the disease. This results in poor nutritional status which manifests as poor or delayed growth, low weight-for-age, height-for-age (Al-Saqladi et al., 2008; Hyacinth et al., 2010; Heyman et al., 1985; Prasad, 1997; Zemel et al., 2007), delayed sexual maturity and poor immunologic function (Bao et al., 2008; Hyacinth et al., 2013) in individuals with this disease.

The individuals with SCD are in a state where their body breaks down nutrients quicker than they build them up, resulting in higher than normal energy requirements for both macronutrients and micronutrients and therefore need to eat more to avoid being deficient in nutrients. This nutritional insufficiency has a significant impact on the severity of the clinical manifestations of the disease which further increases the energy expenditure and decreases the calorie intake, thus resulting in a vicious cycle of poor dietary intake, severity of the disease and poor nutritional status.

Role of Macronutrient Deficiencies

Evidence has shown that macro- and micronutrients deficiencies are a critical feature of SCD (Al-Saqladi et al., 2008; de Franceschi et al., 2000; Hyacinth et al., 2010; Prasad, 1997; Reed et al., 1987; Tomer et al., 2001). Protein energy malnutrition and micronutrient deficiencies underlie some of the metabolic and physiological irregularities observed in SCD, including arginine dysregulation and reduced endothelial function, among others (Cox et al., 2018).

Arginine

Arginine is an amino acid which plays a vital role in the synthesis of nitric oxide in the endothelial cells. Nitric oxide causes dilatation of the blood vessels thereby allowing blood to flow easily. It reduces the adhesiveness of sickled erythrocytes to the vascular wall, platelet aggregation and protects the blood vessels from oxidative stress (Khan et al., 2016). In patients with SCD, low plasma arginine is common (Cox et al., 2011) and is further decreased during vaso-occlusive episodes and acute chest syndrome. This is because the enzyme arginase is released from ruptured erythrocytes, platelets, and the liver, and high concentrations of this enzyme reduce plasma arginine, thereby decreasing nitric oxide production (Cox et al., 2018).

Arginase degradation produces ornithine which is a competitive inhibitor of arginine uptake by endothelial cells. Thus, the arginine to ornithine ratio is crucial for endothelial nitric oxide synthase activity (Cox et al., 2018). Low arginine to ornithine ratios are associated with increased pulmonary artery pressure and death (Cox et al., 2018; Enwonwu et al., 1990; Kato et al., 2009; Khan et al., 2016; Morris, 2014; Umeakunne & Hibbert, 2019). This impairment in arginine metabolism in SCD contributes to endothelial dysfunction, vaso-occlusive crises (VOCs) and pulmonary hypertension. Therefore, arginine becomes an essential amino acid in SCD (Cox et al., 2018; Khan et al., 2016; Morris, 2014; Umeakunne & Hibbert, 2019).

Glutamine

Glutamine is a non-essential amino acid whose synthesis is ATP-dependent. Glutamine becomes conditionally essential in SCD due to its increased requirement. Deficiency for glutamine availability may result in metabolic stress, increased REE, muscle wasting and decreased immune function (Umeakunne & Hibbert., 2019).

Interleukins

Higher levels of interleukins (IL-1 and IL-6) affect taste, smell, and suppress the appetite thereby affecting their dietary intakes (Khan et al., 2016).

Lipids

In SCD, there is abnormality in the phospholipids composition of the membrane in sickled erythrocytes due to deficiencies of certain polyunsaturated fatty acids such as omega-3 and omega-6 fatty acids. This is associated with dehydration as well as abnormal sodium and potassium transport in sickled erythrocytes and has an effect on cellular function (Connor et al., 1997; Khan et al., 2016).

The increased permeability of sodium and potassium in the deoxygenated sickle cell leads to an overload on the renal system causing its damage (Agoreyo & Nwanze, 2010; Khan et al., 2016).

In combination with the protein abnormality of Hb, these molecular changes in membrane phospholipids composition may accentuate sickling of the cells in these patients.

Water

One of the important factors affecting cell sickling is the loss of water in the cell. The abnormally high red cell permeability and migration of potassium and chloride ions carrying water across the cells causes dehydration, which consequently increases the tendency of the Hb to polymerise and sickle (Hyacinth et al., 2010; Khan et al., 2016). Poor hydration status of the erythrocytes leads to increased viscosity and may contribute to the VOC associated with SCD (Umeakunne & Hibbert et al., 2019).

Role of Micronutrients – Minerals

Iron

Iron deficiency is a relatively common occurrence in SCD, especially in children and pregnant women who live in developing countries (Hyacinth et al., 2010; Mohanty et al, 2008; Okeahialam & Obi, 1982; Rao & Sur, 1981; Vichinsky et al., 1981). Some controversies, however, exist with the role of iron in SCD. It has been suggested that iron deficiency, through the reduction of the mean corpuscular Hb concentration (MCHC), may actually be beneficial in SCD. This is based on the observation that Hb polymerisation and cell sickling is closely correlated to MCHC (Reed et al., 1987). A second iron-related problem in SCD is that of iron overload which may be primarily caused by the administration of large numbers of transfusions, although some aspects of iron metabolism may also contribute to this condition (Reed et al., 1987). Although it is an important component of red cells, excess iron has also been shown to contribute to the generation of free radicals, which lead to lipid peroxidation, severe membrane damage and worsening of haemolysis in patients with SCD (Belcher et al., 1999; Hyacinth et al., 2010).

Zinc

Zinc deficiency is common and significant in SCD. Reduced zinc levels in plasma erythrocytes are a consequence of hyperzincuria (increased urinary excretion of zinc), caused by increased haemolysis (Hyacinth et al., 2010; Khan et al., 2016).

Zinc deficiency is associated with abnormalities in growth and sexual development, defects in the immune system, impaired healing of chronic leg ulcers (Hibbert et al., 2005; Hyacinth et al., 2010) and increased painful crisis in patients with SCD (Khan et al., 2016).

Copper

Copper is a key ingredient for functioning of ceruloplasmin, a metalloenzyme which helps to mobilise stored iron in the liver and make it more available for Hb synthesis. Therefore, in copper deficiency, the synthesis of Hb is reduced, despite increased iron levels in the liver (Khan et al., 2016; Okochi & Okpurzor, 2005).

Copper level is also determined by zinc levels occurring in an inverse inter-active role (King & Cousins, 2006). In patients with SCD, low circulating zinc and concomitant high copper levels is a consistent feature (Hyacinth et al., 2010). Excess copper is associated with free radical production and oxidative damage in SCD, therefore, the need for an adequate balance between zinc and copper sup-plementation in general and for patients with severe SCD in particular (Hyacinth et al., 2010).

Magnesium

Magnesium deficiency is associated with increased sickling due to dehydration of sickled erythrocytes erythrocytes (Khan et al., 2016 and hence increased HbS polymerisation (de Franceschi et al., 2000; Hyacinth et al., 2010).

Role of Micronutrients – Vitamins

Antioxidant Vitamins

Red cells are rich in unsaturated fatty acids that are sensitive to oxidative injury (Reed et al., 1987) and abnormal red cells generate excessive oxidation products which play a role in the formation of irreversibly sickled cells (ISC). Antioxidant vitamins such as vitamin E play a role in protecting the erythrocytes against oxi-dant stress. There are several reports indicating deficiency of antioxidant vitamins A, C and E in patients with SCD (Ohnishi et al., 2000; Reed et al., 1987; Vichinsky et al., 1981).

This has been linked to the formation of ISC which is associated with shortened red cell survival and increased haemolysis (Reed et al., 1987).

This contributes to the poor growth and weight seen in children with SCD and susceptibility to bacterial infections (Khan et al., 2016) as well as VOC-related acute chest syndrome (Klings & Farber, 2001).

Vitamin B6 (Pyridoxine)

Low vitamin B6 status has also been reported in patients with SCD, and this is as-sociated with high reticulocyte counts (Hyacinth et al., 2010; Nelson et al., 2002).

Vitamin B9 (Folate)

Patients with SCD are at an increased risk for folate deficiency due to increased erythropoiesis (Dixit et al., 2017).

Vitamin C

Reduced levels of vitamin C and riboflavin have also been documented in SCD. This latter finding is further supported by a low activity of the riboflavin-dependent enzyme glutathione reductase in sickle erythrocytes (Reed et al., 1987).

Vitamin D

Vitamin D is vital for calcium homeostasis and essential for bone mineralisation. Vitamin D also functions to regulate immune responses and inflammation (Umeakunne & Hibbert, 2019).

Patients with SCD are prone to bone fractures and often their vitamin D status is found to be very low, putting them at great risk. Routine supplementation with vitamin D helps maintain the vitamin levels in such patients (Khan et al., 2018).

Deficiencies in vitamin D contribute to osteopenia and osteoporosis which affect up to 80% of patients with SCD. Patients with low serum vitamin D are also reported to have more crisis-related hospital visits per year than those with normal levels (Umeakunne & Hibbert, 2019).

Manifestations of Nutritional Deficiencies in Sickle Cell Disease

In SCD, the increased energy requirements due to macro- and micronutrient deficiencies have a negative effect on growth and maturation (in children and adolescents) as well as on immune functions (Hyacinth et al., 2013; Reed et al., 1987).

This often manifests as growth retardation (underweight, stunting, wasting and decreased skinfold thickness) (Heyman et al., 1985) and delay in maturational milestones such as menarche or adrenarche (Hyacinth et al., 2013; Zemel et al., 2007). Nutritional insufficiency is also associated with low serum immunoglobulin level which can account in part for the increased susceptibility to infection seen in patients with the disease (Hyacinth et al., 2013; Lesourd & Mazari, 1997).

Nutritional Interventions for Patients with Sickle Cell Disease

Potential Benefits of Nutrition-Related Interventions in SCD

There is no definitive effective treatment or cure for SCD, and there are several interventions to prevent the disease or reverse the sickling phenomenon (Khan et al., 2016; Umeakunne & Hibbert, 2019). However, these do not possess the ideal combination of efficacy, safety and ease of use. For example, hydroxyurea raises the levels of HbF and is associated with decreased morbidity in children and adults, but can have devastating side effects (Khan et al., 2016; Pace et al., 2015).

Also the newer therapies using blood and bone marrow stem cell transplant can be curative but are expensive and unaffordable to the majority of affected patients (Khan et al., 2016; Talano & Cairo, 2015). Thus, more sustainable, affordable and evidence-based interventions would be beneficial.

There is a relative shortage of macro- and micronutrients for normal growth and development in patients with SCD, even with adequate dietary intake because of their much higher energy requirements (Hyacinth et al., 2010; Khan et al., 2016; Umeakunne & Hibbert, 2019). Therefore, nutritional interventions addressing this increased energy expenditure should be an important aspect of supportive management for patients with SCD. With some evidence indicating improvement in growth parameters and clinical course following single or multiple nutrients supplementation (Hyacinth et al, 2013; Heyman et al., 1985; Khan et al., 2016; Prasad & Cossack, 1984; Zemel et al., 2002), nutritional interventions could be of immense benefits in the management of patients with SCD since it would be relatively easy to apply and affordable to most of those affected by the disease.

Therefore, this knowledge should motivate promoting nutritional interventions for managing individuals with this disease. Thus, in African and other low-to-middle income countries (LMICs), a holistic, sustainable and affordable strategy incorporated into the healthcare structure that combines these nutrients will be beneficial. This is because more complex approaches (such as bone marrow transplant and gene therapy) for managing SCD are either too expensive or not readily accessible or have side effects (Hyacinth, 2018; Hyacinth et al., 2013; Khan et al., 2016).

Specific Nutritional Interventions

Nutrition Education

The aim of nutrition education is to develop sustainable positive behavioural changes. It is an important strategy as it has the potential to ensure the success of other nutritional interventions. This is because poor nutrition knowledge, attitudes and practices apart from economic limitations or low availability of foods are major barriers that affect healthy nutritional practices.

In order to participate in a sustained and effective way, patients and their families should receive information and education on specific nutrient and calorie needs. Information should be provided about the role of nutritional insufficiency in the complications of SCD, adequate dietary intake and ways of preparing nutritious meals (particularly among the low income groups) (Khan et al., 2016).

Food Supplementation

Identifying and recommending foods needed to supplement the increased energy demand of individuals with SCD will improve growth and development, promote weight maintenance, conserve muscle mass and reduce inflammation in these patients (Hyacinth et al., 2013). Supplementation with a high protein diet, dietary lipids and micronutrients (minerals and vitamins) will ensure that the extra caloric requirement due to the pathological processes of the disease is adequately compensated for (Hyacinth et al., 2013).

Dietary sources of foods rich in these macro- and micronutrients are shown in Table 13.1.

Table 13.1 Dietary sources of nutrients suggested for nutritional management of SCD.

Nutrients	Food sources
Protein	Eggs, fish, chicken, meat, beans or tofu, nuts, peas, kidney beans, chickpeas, soya beans, peanuts, lentils, whole grains
Carbohydrate	Whole grains (e.g., wheat, sorghum, millet oatmeal, brown rice), beans, lentils, peas, potatoes, fruits, vegetables
Omega-3 fatty acids	Fish, sea foods, fatty fish (salmon, tuna, mackerel), avocado, walnuts, flaxseeds
Dietary fibre	Tubers and roots, sweet potatoes, wheat, millet, sorghum, bean, nuts, apples, kidney beans, chickpeas, soya beans, peanuts, green leafy vegetables, almonds, banana, apples, pears, avocado, yams
Vitamin B6	Potatoes, yam, plantain, chickpeas, bananas, fortified cereals, tuna fish, salmon fish
Vitamin B12	Liver, fortified cereals, tuna fish, salmon fish
Folate	Beetroot, chickpeas, avocado, spinach, broccoli, wheat, kidney beans
Vitamin A	Avocado, green vegetables, sweet potato, carrots, broccoli, spinach, pumpkin, mango, red peppers, sweet potatoes, papaya
Vitamin C	Potatoes, broccoli, oranges, kiwi, guava, strawberries, green vegetables, cauliflower, bell peppers, tomatoes, apples
Vitamin D	Salmon fish, tuna fish, mackerel, cod liver oil, sardines, fortified cereals, fortified milk and yoghurt, fortified soy milk, eggs, fortified orange juice, mushrooms
Vitamin E	Wheat, sunflower seeds, almonds, spinach, broccoli, peanut butter
Dietary antioxidants	Cinnamon, thyme, rosemary, turmeric, black raspberries, blueberries, black currants, blackberries, strawberries, pomegranates, apples
Iron	Avocado Spinach, liver, kidney, tofu, turkey, plantain
Calcium	Milk, yoghurt, cheese, leafy green vegetables, yoghurt, cheese, sardines, milk, fortified soymilk, fortified cereals, fortified orange juice, salmon
Magnesium	Plantain, almonds, cashews, peanuts, spinach, whole wheat cereal, soymilk, oatmeal, avocado, dark chocolate, baked potato with skin, brown rice, kidney beans
Zinc	Oysters, crab, beef, fortified cereals, chickpeas, oatmeal, beans, lentils, almonds, cashews
Dietary Nitrates	Spinach, lettuce, beetroot, celery, cabbage, turnips, parsley
Vitamins and minerals	Kidney beans, chickpeas, soya beans, peanuts, tomatoes, bananas, pawpaw, pineapple, cucumber, carrots, water melon, pumpkin, avocado

Source: Modified from Bolarinwa (2020); Umeakunne and Hibbert (2019).

Macronutrients

Amino Acids

Supplementation of a high protein diet decreases infection (Umeakunne & Hibbert, 2019), improves clinical status and growth by significantly reducing inflammation, oxidative stress, pain episodes and enhancing microvascular function (Cox et al., 2018; Hyacinth et al., 2010; Morris et al., 2003; Tomer et al., 2001; Umeakunne & Hibbert, 2019).

Amino-acids (L-phenylalanine benzyl) have been shown to display their anti-sickling action by increasing the cell volume of the RBCs (Acquaye et al., 1982; Khan et al., 2016).

Arginine supplementation improves liver function, increases plasma arginine concentration and nitric oxide metabolite levels in individuals with and without SCD, thereby reducing oxidative stress (Hyacinth et al., 2010; Kehinde et al., 2015; Umeakunne & Hibbert, 2019).

Arginine supplementation has also been shown to be successful in treating leg ulcers, pulmonary hypertension and pain associated with VOC in SCD patients (Bakshi & Morris, 2016; Khan et al., 2016; Morris et al., 2003). Glutamine supplementation decreases REE suggesting a reduced protein turnover and improved glutamine nutritional status (Umeakunne & Hibbert, 2019; Williams et al., 2004).

Other amino acids such as L-histidine, leucine, valine, and cysteine are also insufficient in SCD (Minniti, 2018; Umeakunne & Hibbert, 2019) and higher dietary intake is recommended. Foods high in essential amino acids include red meat, eggs, fish, poultry, milk, yoghurt, fish, nuts, legumes and beans.

Dietary Lipids and Omega-3 Fatty Acids

Supplementation with omega-3 fatty acids has also been shown to decrease the painful haemolytic and VOCs and improve the membrane fatty acid composition (Daak et al., 2013; Khan et al., 2016; Okpala et al., 2011; Tomer et al., 2001). The diverse anti-aggregatory, anti-adhesive, and anti-inflammatory roles of omega-3 fatty acids makes it beneficial for the prevention of cell sickling and reduction of the painful crisis in SCD (Khan et al., 2016; Okpala et al., 2011; Umeakunne & Hibbert, 2019). Therefore, dietary intake of foods rich in this compound is essential. Examples include fish and other seafoods (salmon, mackerel), walnuts and soybean oil.

Water

Hydration plays an essential role in reducing cell sickling in the disease (Umeakunne & Hibbert, 2019). Therefore, it is crucial to promote proper hydration by frequent intake of water and other fluids, as well as avoiding physical activity and extreme weather that result in excessive sweating. Patients with SCD should avoid or reduce intake of dietary sodium (salt) to maintain good hydration status by limiting high sodium, processed foods and snacks while consuming water and fluids throughout the day (Umeakunne & Hibbert, 2019; Williams-Hooker et al., 2013).

Micronutrients

Supplementation with other micronutrients like vitamin A, vitamin B, and magnesium results in clinical benefits such as improved growth, decreased hospital emergency room visits, decreased frequency of pain crisis and reduced frequency of infections; in addition to improvement in muscle function, cognition and coordination; decreased inflammation; and improvement in antioxidant and anaemia status.

Minerals

Zinc therapy has been reported to increase the oxygen affinity of sickle erythrocytes, decrease the ISC count (Reed et al., 1987) and reduce oxidative stress (Bao et al., 2008; Hyacinth et al., 2010). Zinc supplementation is effective in reducing red cell dehydration, sickle cell crises, pain and other life-threatening complications associated with the disease (Khan et al., 2016). It is also beneficial in wound healing of chronic leg ulcers among SCD patients (Hyacinth et al., 2010; Serjeant et al., 1970). Zinc supplementation improves growth (weight and height) and boosts immunity of pre-pubertal aged children with the SCD (Hyacinth et al., 2010; Khan et al., 2016). It is also reported to increase serum testosterone and reduce infections and hospital admissions in adult SCD patients (Hyacinth et al., 2010; Khan et al., 2016).

Chromium helps in the management of SCD as it plays a role in carbohydrate metabolism which is the body's much required energy source (Khan et al., 2016). Manganese which helps in glycoprotein synthesis and bone formation is also important for management of SCD due to its role in the respiratory chain reaction required for the much needed energy production in these patients (Khan et al., 2016).

Magnesium supplementation improves several haematological indices in adult SCD patients, including improvement of red cell hydration (indicated by reduction in number of dense sickle erythrocytes, absolute reticulocyte count and immature reticulocytes) (Hyacinth et al, 2010). It also improves the erythrocyte membrane transport abnormalities in patients with SCD (Khan et al., 2016; Oladipo et al., 2005) as well as decreasing the length of hospital stay in children admitted for painful crises (Brousseau et al., 2004; Hyacinth et al., 2010).

Vitamins

SCD is one of the many diseases in which oxidative stress plays a significant role affecting the RBCs and leading to inflammation and the resulting pain. Therefore, the use of antioxidants to improve clinical status is essential. Supplementation with natural antioxidants vitamins such as A, C and E either alone or in combination have been shown to decrease the number of ISC, protecting the erythrocytes against oxidative stress (Reed et al., 1987) thereby reducing the sickling pain crisis (Khan et al., 2016).

Vitamin B6 (Pyridoxine) is known for its crucial roles in the metabolism of lipids and proteins (Khan et al., 2016).

Routine folic acid supplementation is common in the long-term management of SCD. This treatment is based mainly on preventing deficiency from increased folate turnover, as in any chronic haemolytic anaemia responsive to folate supplementation (Dixit et al., 2017; Hyacinth et al., 2010; Lindenbaum, 1977). This will replace depleted folate stores and reduce the symptoms of anaemia (Dixit et al.,

2017). Folate supplementation is also beneficial in reducing the risk of endothelial damage in SCD patients (Khan et al., 2016; Ohnishi et al., 2000).

The low vitamin D status in patients with SCD makes them prone to bone fractures. Therefore, routine supplementation with vitamin D and calcium in patients helps to maintain the vitamin levels (Adewoye et al., 2008; Hyacinth et al., 2010), in addition to causing a decrease in the number of pain days and an increase in the quality-of-life scores (Hyacinth et al., 2013; Osunkwo et al., 2012).

Dietary intake of fish has also been linked with these improved clinical status (Umeakunne & Hibbert, 2019). Vitamin D supplementation also has a protective effect against respiratory infections commonly found in children with SCD (Lee et al., 2018; Umeakunne & Hibbert, 2019). Sources of dietary vitamin D include fortified milk, plant milk and yoghurt, fortified orange juice, fortified breakfast cereals, mushrooms, fatty fish, cheese, egg yolks and liver (Umeakunne & Hibbert, 2019).

Food Fortification

Consuming foods fortified with various nutrients including amino acids, vitamins and minerals is also valuable in increasing nutrients stores. Examples include milk or breakfast cereals fortified with vitamin D, calcium and other essential amino acids; calcium-fortified foods like cereals, powdered milk, soymilk and orange juice.

Dietary Diversification

Since persons with SCD have increased requirement for both micronutrients and micronutrients, a balanced diet that includes a variety of healthful foods from all the food groups can provide the body with energy, fibre, vitamins, minerals and other essential nutrients. Example of food timetable suitable for persons with SCD is shown in Table 13.2.

These will, in addition to meeting their health needs, also support growth and other essential functions as well as being beneficial in making more healthy RBCs. It has been shown that nutritional interventions which combine micronutrients and macronutrients (proteins carbohydrates and fats) help to achieve optimal nutritional and immunological status. This improves the clinical condition and reduces hospital admissions in individuals with SCD, in addition to reducing the associated inflammation which drives disease severity and ultimate organ damage (Hyacinth et al., 2010, 2013; Umeakunne & Hibbert, 2019).

This is because nutrient utilisation in the body is a multistep process, with different nutrients feeding into the process at various points. Insufficient quantities of one component of this multistep process could have a deleterious effect on the entire body (Hyacinth et al., 2013). Therefore, increased intake of food sources of all these nutrients is essential to provide the needed energy requirements for patients with SCD.

Table 13.2 Example of food timetable suitable for persons with SCD.

Meals	Examples
Breakfast	*Acha* (millet) porridge Coconut rice pudding Spiced oatmeal with fruits and nuts Parfait: Greek yoghurt and fruit bowl Sweet potato frittata Egg and cress sandwiches *Moin Moin* (steamed bean pudding)
Lunch	Pumpkin vegetable (*Ugu*) sauce Apple fish stew – served with any of these: kidney beans, bulgur wheat, whole wheat pasta, couscous, rice, beans, plantain, sweet potatoes, quinoa, yam, etc. Jollof bulgur wheat Carrot jollof rice – serve with fried plantain (*dodo*) Peanut butter chicken – serve with roasted peanuts and fried rice or noodles Garden egg (eggplant) sauce – serve with boiled plantain, yam, sweet potatoes or rice Sautéed greens with melon (*egusi*) – serve with rice, yam or plantain Scent leaf flatbread – serve with soups or use as flatbreads for stuffing Beef fried quinoa Gizdodo (gizzard and fried plantain) with *Ugu* (pumpkin leaf)
Dinner	Oxtail carrot soup Couscous and kidney beans bowl Meatballs in tomato sauce – serve with pasta, rice or any other side Chicken skewers – serve with rice or fries, vegetables and sauces Vegetable soup – serve with warm bread or flat bread Frejon [brown/black beans (*Ewa Oloyin*/Honey beans)] – serve with fish sauce or fried plantain and beef Fish soup – serve with rice or boiled yam, plantain Coconut shrimp curry – serve with brown rice, white rice, steamed *acha* or couscous
Smoothies and drinks	Peanut butter smoothie Green smoothie Zobo (hibiscus) and pineapple drink Pineapple iced tea Spiked water with cucumbers and apples or citrus Avocado banana smoothie

Source: Modified from Bolarinwa (2020).

Conclusion

Nutritional interventions as supportive management in SCD can be beneficial for improving the clinical outcome, quality of life, and future prospects of those with the disease. Therefore, it would be valuable to determine specific recommended dietary allowances (RDAs) that will meet the increased energy and nutrients requirements for individuals (children, adults, and pregnant women) with SCD.

References

Acquaye, C. T., Young, J. D., Ellory, J. C., Gorecki, M., Wilchek, M. (1982). Mode of transport and possible mechanism of action of L-phenylalanine benzyl ester as an anti-sickling agent. Biochim Biophys Acta. 693: 407–16.

Adewoye, A. H., Chen, T. C., Ma, Q., McMahon. L., Mathieu, J., Malabanan, A. (2008). Sickle cell bone disease: Response to vitamin D and calcium. Am J Hematol. 83(4): 271–4. https://doi.org/10.1002/ajh.21085

Agoreyo, F., Nwanze, N. (2010). Plasma sodium and potassium changes in sickle cell patients. Int J Genet Mol Biol. 2: 14–9.

Akohoue, S. A., Shankar, S., Milne, G. L., Morrow, J., Chen, K. Y., Ajayi, W. U. (2007). Energy expenditure, inflammation, and oxidative stress in steady-state adolescents with sickle cell anaemia. Paediatr Res. 61: 233–8.

Al-Saqladi, A. W. M., Cipolotti, R., Fijnvandraat, K., Brabin, B. J. (2008). Growth and nutritional status of children with homozygous sickle cell disease. Ann Trop Paediatr Internat Child Health. 28: 165–89. https://doi.org/10.1179/146532808X335624

Bakshi, N., Morris, C. R. (2016). The role of the arginine metabolome in pain: Implications for sickle cell disease. J Pain Res. 9: 167–75.

Bao, B., Prasad, A. S., Beck, F. W. J., Snell, D., Suneja, A., Sarkar, F. H. (2008). Zinc supplementation decreases oxidative stress, incidence of infection, and generation of inflammatory cytokines in sickle cell disease patients. Transl. Res. 152(2): 67–80. https://doi.org/10.1016/j.trsl.2008.06.001

Barden, E. M., Zemel, B. S., Kawchak, D. A., Goran, M. I., Ohene-Frempong, K., Stallings, V. A. (2000). Total and resting energy expenditure in children with sickle cell disease. J Pediatr. 136: 73–9.

Belcher, J. D., Marker, P. H., Geiger, P., Girotti, A. W., Steinberg, M. N., Hebbel, R. P. (1999). Low-density lipoprotein susceptibility to oxidation and cytotoxicity to endothelium in sickle cell anemia. J Lab Clin Med. 133(6): 605–12. https://doi.org/10.1016/s0022-2143(99)90191-9.

Bolarinwa, B. editors. (2020). The healthy warrior's cookbook. Sickle Cell Aid Foundation. Bookcraft.

Borel, M. J., Buchowski, M. S., Turner, E. A., Goldstein, R. E., Flakoll, P. J. (1998). Protein turnover and energy expenditure increase during exogenous nutrient availability in sickle cell disease. Am J Clin Nutrit. 68: 607–14.

Brousseau, D. C., Scott, J. P., Hillery, C. A., Panepinto, J. A. (2004). The effect of magnesium on length of stay for paediatric sickle cell pain crisis. Acad Emerg Med. 11(9): 968–72. https://doi.org/10.1197/j.aem.2004.04.009.

Chakravorty, S., Williams, T. N. (2015). Sickle cell disease: A neglected chronic disease of increasing global health importance. Arch Dis Child. 100: 48–53.

Connor, W. E., Lin, D. S., Thomas, G., Ey, F., DeLoughery, T., Zhu, N. (1997). Abnormal phospholipid molecular species of erythrocytes in sickle cell anemia. J Lipid Res. 38: 2516–28.

Cox, S. E., Ellins, E. A., Marealle, A. I., Newton, C.R., Soka, D., Sasi, P. (2018). Lancet Haematol. 5: e147–60. https://doi.org/10.1016/S2352-3026(18)30020-6

Cox, S. E., Makani, J., Komba, A. N., Soka, D., Newton, C. R., Kirkham, F. J. (2011). Global arginine bioavailability in Tanzanian sickle cell anaemia patients at steady-state: A nested case control study of deaths versus survivors. Br J Haematol. 155: 522–4. https://doi.org/10.1111/j.1365-2141.2011.08715.x.

Daak, A. A., Ghebremeskel, K., Hassan, Z., Attallah, B., Azan, H. H., Elbashir, M. I. (2013). Effect of omega-3 (n − 3) fatty acid supplementation in patients with sickle cell anaemia: Randomised, double-blind, placebo-controlled trial. Am J Clin Nutr. 97: 37–44.

De Franceschi, L., Bachir, D., Galacteros, F., Tchernia, G., Cynober, T., Neuberg, D. (2000). Oral magnesium pidolate: Effects of long-term administration in patients with sickle cell disease. Br J Haematol. 108: 284–9. https://doi.org/10.1046/j.1365-2141.2000.01861.x

Dixit, R., Nettem, S., Madan, S. S., Soe, H. H. K., Abas, A. B. L., Vance, L. D. (2017). Folate supplementation in people with sickle cell disease. Cochrane Database Syst Rev. 2: 1–35. CD011130. https://doi.org/10.1002/14651858.CD011130.pub2.

Enwonwu, C. O., Lu, M. (1991). Elevated plasma histamine in sickle cell anaemia. Clinica Chimica Acta. 203: 363–8. https://doi.org/10.1016/0009-8981(91)90309-z

Enwonwu, C. O., Xu, X. X., Turner, E. (1990). Nitrogen metabolism in sickle cell anaemia: Free amino acids in plasma and urine. Am J Med Sci. 300: 366–71.

Ganong, W. F. (2003). Abnormalities of haemoglobin production. (Chapt. 27) In: Review of medical physiology (21 ed). New York, NY: Lange Medical Books/McGraw Hill. p. 912

Heyman, M., Katz, R., Hurst, D., Chiu, D., Ammann, A., Vichinsky, E. (1985). Growth retardation in sickle cell disease treated by nutritional support. The Lancet. 325: 903–6. https://doi.org/10.1016/s0140-6736(85)91677-0

Hibbert, J. M., Creary, M. S., Gee, B. E., Buchanan, I., Quarshie, A., Hsu, L. L. (2006). Erythropoiesis and myocardial energy requirements contribute to the hypermetabolism of childhood sickle cell anaemia. J Paediatr Gastroenterol Nutrit. 43: 680–7.

Hibbert, J. M., Hsu, L. L., Bhathena, S. J., Irune, I., Sarfo, B., Creary, M. S. (2005). Pro-inflammatory cytokines and the hypermetabolism of children with sickle cell disease. Exp Biol Med. 230: 68–74.

Hyacinth, H. I. (2018). Sickle-cell anaemia needs more food? Haematology 5(4): e130–e131. doi: 10.1016/S2352-3026(18)30032-2.

Hyacinth, H. I., Adekeye, O. A., Yilgwan, C. S. (2013). Malnutrition in sickle cell anaemia: Implications for infection, growth, and maturation. J Soc Behav Health Sci. 7(1): 1–11. https://doi.org/10.5590/JSBHS.2013.07.1.02.

Jaja, S. I., Kehinde, M. O., Ogungbemi, S. I. (2008). Cardiac and autonomic responses to change in posture or vitamin C supplementation in sickle cell anaemia subjects. Pathophysiology 15(1): 25–30.

Kato, G. J., Wang, Z., Machado, R. F., Blackwelder, W. C., Taylor, J. G. 6th, Hazen, S. L. (2009). Endogenous nitric oxide synthase inhibitors in sickle cell disease: Abnormal levels and correlations with pulmonary hypertension, desaturation, haemolysis, organ dysfunction and death. Br J Haematol. 145: 506–13.

Kawchak, D. A., Schall, J. I., Zemel, B. S., Ohene-Frempong, K., Stallings, V. A. (2007). Adequacy of dietary intake declines with age in children with sickle cell disease. J Am Diet Assoc. 107: 843–8.

Kehinde, M. O., Ogungbemi, S. I., Anigbogu, C. N., Jaja, S. I. (2015). L-arginine supplementation enhances antioxidant activity and erythrocyte integrity in SCA subjects. Pathophysiology 22: 137–42. https://doi.org/0.1016/j.pathophys.2015.05.001

Khan, S. A., Damanhouri, G., Ali, A., Khan, S. A., Khan, A., Bakillah, A. (2016). Precipitating factors and targeted therapies in combating the perils of sickle cell disease: A special nutritional consideration. Nutrit Metabol. 13: 50. https://doi.org/10.1186/s12986-016-0109-7

King, J. C., Cousins, R. J. (2006). Zinc. In: Shils, M. E., Shike, M., Ross, A. C., Caballero, B., Cousins, R. J., editors. Modern nutrition in health and disease. 10th ed. Lippincott Williams and Wilkins. p. 271–85.

Klings, E. S., Farber, H. W. (2001). Role of free radicals in the pathogenesis of acute chest syndrome in sickle cell disease. Respir Res. 2: 280–5.

Lee, M. T., Kattan. M., Fennoy, I., Arpadi, S. M., Miller, R. L., Cremers, S. (2018). Randomised phase 2 trial of monthly vitamin D to prevent respiratory complications in children with sickle cell disease. Blood Adv. 2(9): 969–78. https://doi.org/10.1182/bloodadvances.2017013979

Lemanek, K. L., Brown, R. T., Armstrong, F. D., Hood, C., Pegelow, C., Woods, G. (2002). Dysfunctional eating patterns and symptoms of pica in children and adolescents with sickle cell disease. Clin Pediatr (Phila). 41: 493–500.

Lesourd, B. M., Mazari, L. (1997). Immune responses during recovery from protein-energy malnutrition. Clin Nutrit. 16(Supplement 1): 37–46. https://doi.org/10.1016/s0261-5614(97)80047-7

Lindenbaum, J. (1977). Folic acid requirement in situations of increased need. In: Workshop on Human Folate Requirements, ed. Folic acid: Biochemistry and physiology in relation to the human nutrition requirement. National Academy of Sciences. 256–76.

Martyres, D. J., Vijenthira, A., Barrowman, N., Harris-Janz, S., Chretien, C., Klaassen, R. J. (2016). Nutrient insufficiencies/deficiencies in children with sickle cell disease and its association with increased disease severity. Pediatr Blood Cancer. 63(6): 1060–4.

Minniti, C. P. (2018). L-glutamine and the dawn of combination therapy for sickle cell disease. New Engl J Med. 379(3): 292–4. https://doi.org/10.1056/NEJMe1800976

Mohanty, D., Mukherjee, M. B., Colah, R. B., Wadia, M., Ghosh, K., Chottray, G. P. (2008). Iron deficiency anaemia in sickle cell disorders in India. Indian J Med Res. 127(4):366–9.

Morris, C. R. (2014). Alterations of the arginine metabolome in sickle cell disease. A growing rationale for arginine therapy. Hematol Oncol Clin N Am. 28: 301–21. https://doi.org/10.1016/j.hoc.2013.11.008

Morris, C. R., Morris, S. M., Hagar, W., Warmerdam, J. V., Claster, S., Kepka-Lenhart, D. (2003). Arginine therapy: A new treatment for pulmonary hypertension in sickle cell disease? Am J Respir Crit Care. 168: 63–9. https://doi.org/10.1164/rccm.200208-967OC.

Nelson, M. C., Zemel, B. S., Kawchak, D. A., Barden, E. M., Frongillo, E. A. Jr., Coburn, S. P. (2002). Vitamin B6 status of children with sickle cell disease. J Pediatr Hematol Oncol. 24(6): 463–9.

Ohnishi, S. T., Ohnishi, T., Ogunmola, G. B. (2000). Sickle cell anaemia: A potential nutritional approach for a molecular disease. Nutrition 16(5): 330–8.

Okeahialam, T. C, Obi, G. O. (1982). Iron deficiency in sickle cell anaemia in Nigerian children. Ann Trop Pediatr. 2: 89–92.

Okochi, V. I., Okpurzor, J. (2005). Micronutrients as therapeutic tools in the management of sickle cell disease, malaria and diabetes. Afr J Biotechnol. 4: 1568–79.

Okpala, I., Ibegbulam, O., Duru, A., Ocheni, S., Emodi, I., Ikefuna, A. (2011). Pilot study of omega-3 fatty acid supplements in sickle cell disease. APMIS. 119: 442–8.

Oladipo, O. O., Temiye, E. O., Ezeaka, V. C., Obomanu, P. (2005). Serum magnesium, phosphate and calcium in Nigerian children with sickle cell disease. West Afr J Med. 24: 120–3.

Osunkwo, I., Ziegler, T. R., Alvarez, J., McCracken, C., Cherry, K., Osunkwo, C. E. (2012). High dose vitamin D therapy for chronic pain in children and adolescents with sickle cell disease: Results of a randomised double blind pilot study. Br J Haematol. 159: 211–5. https://doi.org/10.1111/bjh.12019

Pace, B. S., Liu, L., Li, B., Makala, L. H. (2015). Cell signalling pathways involved in drug-mediated foetal haemoglobin induction: Strategies to treat sickle cell disease. Exp Biol Med (Maywood). 240: 1050–64.

Prasad, A. S. (1997). Malnutrition in sickle cell disease patients. Am J Clin Nutrit. 66: 423–4.

Prasad, A. S., Cossack, Z. T. (1984). Zinc supplementation and growth in sickle cell disease. Ann Intern Med. 100: 367–371.

Rao, N. J., Sur, A. M. (1981). Iron deficiency in sickle cell disease. Acta Paediatr Scand. 69: 963–8.

Reed, J. D., Redding-Lallinger, R., Orringer, E. P. (1987). Nutrition and sickle cell disease. Am JHaematol. 24: 441–5. https://doi.org/10.1002/ajh.2830240416

Serjeant, G. R., Galloway, R. E., Gueri, M. C. (1970). Oral zinc sulphate in sickle-cell ulcers. The Lancet. 2: 891–3.

Singhal, A., Parker, S., Linsell, L., Serjeant. (2002). Energy intake and resting metabolic rate in preschool Jamaican children with homozygous sickle cell disease. Am J Clin Nutr. 75(6): 1093–7. https://doi.org/10.1093/ajcn/75.6.1093.

Stevens, M. C., Maude, G. H., Beckford, M., Grandison, Y., Mason, K., Taylor, B. (1986). Alpha thalassemia and the haematology of homozygous sickle cell disease in childhood. Blood 67: 411–4.

Talano, J. A., Cairo, M. S. (2015). Hematopoietic stem cell transplantation for sickle cell disease: State of the science. Eur J Haematol. 94: 391–9.

Taylor, S. C., Shacks, S. J., Mitchell, R. A., Banks, A. (1995). Serum interleukin-6 levels in the steady state of sickle cell disease. J Interferon Cytokine Res. 15: 1061–4.

Tomer, A., Kasey, S., Connor, W. E., Clark, S., Harker, L. A., Eckman, J. (2001). Reduction of pain episodes and prothrombotic activity in sickle cell disease by dietary n-3 fatty acids. Thromb Haemost. 85(6): 966–74.

Umeakunne, K., Hibbert, J. M. (2019). Nutrition in sickle cell disease: Recent insights. Nutrit Dietary Suppl. 11: 9–17. https://doi.org/10.2147/NDS.S168257

Vichinsky, E., Kleman, K., Embury, S., Lubin, B. (1981). The diagnosis of iron deficiency anaemia in sickle cell disease. Blood 58(5): 963–8.

Williams-Hooker, R., Hankins, J., Ringwald-Smith, K., Stockton, M., Shurley, T. A. (2013). Evaluation of hydration status, sodium and fluid intake in children with sickle cell anaemia. J Blood Disord Transf. 4(3): 1–4. https://doi.org/10.4172/2155-9864.1000143

Williams, R., Olivi, S., Li, C. S., Storm, M., Cremer, L., Mackert, P., Wang, W. (2004). Oral glutamine supplementation decreases resting energy expenditure in children and adolescents with sickle cell anaemia. J Paediatr Hematol Oncol. 26: 619–25. https://doi.org/10.1097/01.mph.0000140651.65591.b8

Zemel, B. S., Kawchak, D. A., Fung, E. B., Ohene-Frempong, K., Stallings, V. A. (2002). Effect of zinc supplementation on growth and body composition in children with sickle cell disease. Am J Clin Nutrit. 75: 300–7.

Zemel, B. S., Kawchak, D. A., Ohene-Frempong, K. W. A. K., Schall, J. I., Stallings, V. A. (2007). Effects of delayed pubertal development, nutritional status, and disease severity on longitudinal patterns of growth failure in children with sickle cell disease. Paediatr Res. 61(5, Part 1): 607–13.

14 Hydroxyurea in the Management of Sickle Cell Disease in Africa

Léon Tshilolo

Introduction

In 2010, the WHO Regional Office for Africa edited a document entitled "*Sickle-cell disease: a strategy for the WHO African Region*" (AFR/RC60/8), which offered a comprehensive situation analysis and roadmap for implementing priority interventions (WHO-AFRO, 2010). Among those priorities, new born and early diagnosis (in under 5 children) were implemented in some sub-Saharan African (SSA) countries as pilot studies meanwhile anti-pneumococcus and anti-haemophilus influenzae vaccines have been introduced and coupled to penicillin-prophylaxis and malaria prophylaxis. All these approaches contributed to the reduction of mortality of sickle cell disease (SCD) in these areas (Therrell et al., 2020; Tshilolo et al., 2008).

Pain and organ complications have not been reduced in most of the SSA countries because of less availability of opioids and drugs such as hydroxycarbamide or Voxeletor, which two molecules with a proved impact on vaso-occlusive pain and complications in SCD and that improve and extent the quality of life of SCD patients (Montalembert et al., 2021; Thein & Howard, 2018).

Basic management approaches for patients with SCD include penicillin prophylaxis beginning in infancy, anti-inflammatory and opioid therapy to address pain, maintenance of HU therapy when indicated and chronic blood transfusions for patients with or at risk for major complications. Access to these resources in Africa is limited by availability and affordability.

Based on a large use over more than 30 years, in adults and children (from nine months in the USA and two years in Europe), Hydroxycarbamide or HU has emerged as the primary disease-modifying therapy for SCD with salutary laboratory and clinical effects, including reduction in both mortality and mortality (Montalembert et al., 2021; Yawn et al., 2014).

HU is included in the WHO List of Essential Medicines for the treatment of sickle haemoglobinopathies (WHO, Geneva, 2019).

But only few African physicians used HU because there is a reluctance to use HU partially related to fears about potential side effects of this medication, especially in terms of fertility and carcinogenicity.

Clinical trials conducted in Africa demonstrated the safe and effective use of HU for SCD in children in low-resource settings (John et al., 2020; Nnebe-Agumadu et al.,

DOI: 10.4324/9781003463931-15

2021; Opoka et al., 2017; Tshilolo et al., 2019). However, the lack of robust data from clinical trials, long-term studies and patient-reported outcome studies from this region is a major knowledge gap leading to sub-optimal HU treatment in patients with SCD

Pharmacology

Hydoxycarbamide is a non-alkalyting antineoplastic agent that is used in a wide spectrum of conditions including oncology, heamatology, virology, rheumatology and dermatology (Moftah & Eswayah, 2022 Timson et al., 1975).

Pharmacocinetics and Properties of HU (Figure 14.1)

The pharmacokinetic profile of HU shows excellent oral bioavailability and a volume of distribution comparable with total body water, together with a high tendency to bind serum proteins. Hepatic and renal metabolic pathways constitute the eliminatory mechanisms that transform the parent compound into several end products, with urea being the principal metabolite. Pharmacodynamically, HU shows a strong correlation between therapeutic-toxic responses and blood concentration (Gwilt & Tracewell, 1998).

HU inhibits enzyme ribonucleotide reductase that incorporates thymine in DNA. With inhibition, an interruption in the DNA synthesis of erythroid precursors cells occurs at later stages of differentiation. This temporary interruption of DNA synthesis will restore the erythropoiesis due to haematopoietic stress and consequently a recruitment of young cells of the erythroid lineage with capacity to synthetise fetal haemoglobin (HbF) (Kaufman, 1992; Santos & Nogueira Maia, 2011).

By the effect of inhibition of ribonucleotide reductase, HU lowers the leucocyte and platelets counts in patients with SCD. Absolute neutrophil count of 2,000 per ml and/or platelets count of 80,000 per ml is typically used as a yardstick to determine the maximum tolerated dose (MTD) for individual patients (Owusu-Ansah et al., 2016; Tshilolo et al., 2008; Ware et al., 2016).

Anti-inflammatory activity of HU has been well described in animal models and in humans (Moftah & Eswayah, 2022; Owusu-Ansah et al., 2016).

The anti-inflammatory effect of HU as a potential therapeutic choice for the treatment of rheumatoid arthritis and in myelofibrosis-related arthritis was reported to be effective (Moftah & Eswayah, 2022).

HU was found to be able to reduce the serum levels of some pro-inflammatory cytokines like IL-6, IL-8 and TNF-α. In addition, several markers of intravascular haemolysis are reduced in patients with SCD on HU therapy suggesting that the drug targets inflammatory pathways that promote adhesion and haemolysis and both of the factors contribute in the pathophysiology of SCD (Owusu-Ansah et al., 2016; Zaram et al, 2020).

HU induces the increase of IL-10, an anti-inflammatory cytokine that usually is reduced in SCD patients. IL-10 induction may explain HU's beneficial effect in acute chest syndrome (ACS). Elsewhere, its capability to generate NO augments the overall ability to alleviate inflammation (Owusu-Ansah et al., 2016).

The Anti-viral activity of HU was reported to cover a wide array of viruses with a therapeutic effect against HIV, hepatitis C virus and; more recently, a hypothetical immune modulatory effect against Covid-19 (Moftah & Eswayah, 2022; Timson, 1975).

The Anti-malarial activity of HU is not only due to the increase of HbF that confers a relative resistance to Plasmodium but also to the effect of NO which protect against severe malaria in animals and humans (Anstey et al.,1996; Opoka et al., 2017). A recent paper (Olupot-Olupot et al., 2023) displayed that HU at MTD for children with SCA is associated with a significantly lower incidence of malaria infections; this association is greater at higher HU doses and is sustained over time. Potential mechanisms of action between HU and malaria remain incompletely defined, but treatment effects in children with SCA related to myelosuppression, reduced inflammation, iron chelation and antimalarial activity, in addition to general health improvement through higher Hb and HbF, could be important. Treatment-associated effects at MTD that target mild myelosuppression are especially salutary, and they justify using HU at MTD to achieve mild myelosuppression with ANC $<3.0 \times 10^6$/L (Olupot-Olupot et al., 2023).

The main effect of HU on SCD is due to its property of *HbF generation and NO endogen production.*

HU increases the production of gamma globin, which is incorporated largely into an asymmetric Hb tetramer (FS; α2γβS) that limits intra-erythrocytic HbS polymerisation and consequently sickling. Thus, there is greater survival of red cells, resulting in a reduction of vaso occlusive crisis (VOC) events (Owuso-Ansah et al., 2016; Santos & Nogueira Maia, 2011). Anyway, there is evidence that the beneficial effect of HU is not only limited to HbF increase, as many patients demonstrate clinical improvement before any significant increase in HbF level (Santos & Nogueira Maia, 2011).

HU has the ability to generate NO by pathways in which it can eventually transform itself into NO The importance of NO in the pathophysiology of SCD justified the use of potential donors, including HU, to supplement the deficit of NO due to its scavenging by heme (King, 2003; Moftah & Eswayah, 2022; Owusu-Ansah et al., 2016). Main properties of HU are synthetised in a diagram in Figure 14.1.

Actions and Mechanism in SCD

In addition to its evident effect on increase of HbF and NO production, the full mechanism of action of HU is not completely understood, but it also helps with red blood cell (RBC) hydration and decreases neutrophils and platelets, which also helps to improve blood flow and decrease sickling.

Platelets and neutrophils in SCD have an activated phenotype that promotes expression of multiple adhesion molecules (VLA-4, Mac-1 I-CAM, VCAM-1, E and P-selectin, etc.) and enhances expression of multiple surface receptors that promote aggregation of platelets and increased secretion of inflammatory mediators such as IL-1β, IL-6. Neutrophil activation increases membrane exposure of phosphatidyl-serine (PS) on sickle red cells which promotes retention of the leucocytes in the lung. HU markedly inhibits this process in part by disrupting the neutrophil-mediated sickle erythrocytes PS exposure (Moftah & Eswayah, 2022; Owusu-Ansah et al., 2016).

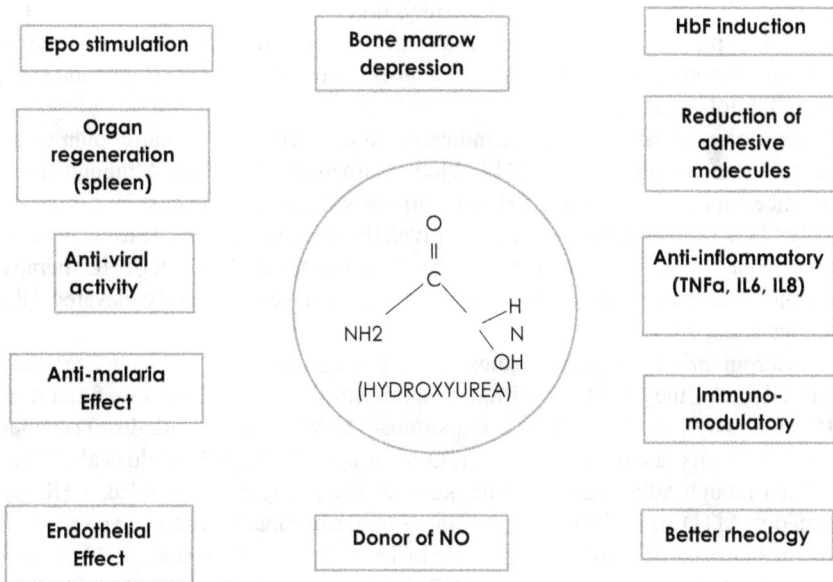

Figure 14.1 Main mechanism and effects of HU in sickle cell disease.

HU decreases the expression of adhesion receptors on RBCs and endothelial cells. In addition, it releases a nitric oxide moiety that not only decreases platelet and coagulation activation, but may also lessen endothelial injury through its vasodilatory effects.

HU reduces also the cardiopulmonary complications like ACS and PH, two major causes of mortality in adults with SCD. The Pediatric Hydroxyurea in Sickle Cell Anemia (BABY HUG) study enrolled 299 children aged 9–18 months between 2003 and 2007. The rate of ACS was significantly reduced in patients receiving HU (95% confidence interval, 0.15–0.87) (Wang et al., 2011).

Indications and Posology

Recent guidelines retain that HU will be prescribed to all SCD patients independently of the presence of acute or chronic complications.

According to a 2014 expert panel report sponsored by the National Heart, Lung, and Blood Institute on the evidence-based management of SCA, HU therapy should be offered to all children as young as nine months of age, regardless of symptoms (Lopez et al., 2010).

In contrast to the NIH and British recommendations, the European countries collaborating in ESCORT-HU still recommend not treating asymptomatic children or trying to reach the MTD (Montalembert et al., 2021; Nnebe-Agumadu et al., 2021; Tshilolo et al., 2019).

Globally, *the main indications of HU* concerns VOC, ACS, and other non-VOC complications like severe chronic anemia, conditional transcranial doppler velocities and overt cerebral vasculopathy, organopathy (e.g., nephropathy, retinopathy and pulmonary hypertension), priapism, contraindication to blood transfusion and unreported indications (Montalembert et al., 2021; Nnebe-Agumadu et al., 2021; Tshilolo et al., 2019).

Controversial data concern the indication in leg ulcers and the cardiopulmonary complications (Klings et al., 2014; Montalembert et al., 2021). Although direct evidence supporting the use of HU in patients with isolated Tricuspid Reflux Velocity (TRV) above 2.5 m/s is lacking, given the increased risk of death in patients with increased TRV and the potential benefit and relatively low risk of HU therapy, HU should also be considered in patients found to have persistently elevated TRV (Klings et al., 2014).

Posology of HU varies according to the place where the trials have been realised. Globally, they are three different approaches that vary from low fixed dose (10 mg/kg/day), moderate (15–20 mg/kg/dose) to MTD (25–35 mg/dose) (Ahmad et al., 2018; Montalembert et al., 2021; Ofakunrin et al., 2020; Tshilolo et al., 2019).

Even though a fixed dose (20 mg/kg) was classically recommended, a HU escalated to MTD (max 35 mg/kg) has more relevant impacts. The average MTD is around 25 mg/kg/day with an initial dose of 15 mg/kg/day (John et al., 2020; Nnebe-Agumadu et al., 2021; Opoka et al., 2017; Tshilolo et al., 2019; Ware et al., 2016).

Doses are adjusted according to weight and haematological parameters; schedule visits need to be organised with monitoring for clinical evolution and periodic surveillances of laboratory parameters.

Even though debates can exist about the best approach, some authors in Africa observed good results and efficacy of low-dose HU in the control of symptoms and complications of SCD. They found that it was equally effective, less toxic and ideal in resource-poor settings (Ahmad et al., 2018). The same authors in a cohort of 85 Nigerian SCA children, the minimum dosing used was 7.4 mg/kg/day while the highest dose was 30.4 mg/kg/day. Globally adverse events were observed in the same proportion but low-dose HU was less toxic. In Europe, the Agence Européenne des Médicaments, (*European Drug Administration*) (EMA) recommended an initial dose of 15 mg/kg/d and no systematic attempt to reach the MTD (Montalembert et al., 2021).

Generally, HU is administrated in a *unique daily dose*, but because of the less availability of different formulation, in some SSA countries, HU is administrated on alternating day regimen. Some authors (Maharaj et al., 2019) observed in a cohort of Afro-Caribbean children that then overall rates of painful crises were similar in those on a daily and on alternating day regimens of the drug in all settings.

Regular monitoring for side effects is essential and depends on the recommendation reported in different studies. In Europe, the recommendation was to monitor the Cell Blood Count (CBC) every two months and the percentage of HbF every six months (Montalembert et al., 2021). Based on our experience, routinely monitoring in SSA countries will concern the CBC every month in the first two quarters of treatment and every tree month later; HbF every 3–6 months and malaria test in the occasion of the collection of blood or in case of fever.

Biological and Clinical Efficacy

Most of the laboratory outcomes of long-term clinical importance for SCA patients are the increase of haemoglobin level and HbF and the decrease in leucocyte, neutrophil and reticulocyte counts.

HU therapy reduces the incidence of vaso-occlusive pain events, ACS, splenic sequestration, infections, malaria, transfusions, number of hospitalisation and death (John et al., 2020; Montalembert et al., 2021; Ofakunrin et al., 2020, Opoka et al., 2018; Thein & Howard, 2018; Tshilolo et al., 2019). It also ameliorates the chronic organ damages (Tshilolo et al., 2019; Ware et al., 2016).

In the Reach trial, the rates of infection also declined, including rates of non-malaria infection (142.5 vs. 90.0 events per 100 patient-years; incidence rate ratio, 0.62; 95% CI, 0.53–0.72) and severe infection of grade 3 or higher (28.9 vs. 8.0 events per 100 patient-years; incidence rate ratio, 0.28; 95% CI, 0.19–0.42) (Tshilolo et al., 2019).

About the impact on cardiopulmonary function, recent studies have reported that left ventricular dilation and hypertrophy improved significantly with HU treatment. Elsewhere, HU therapy was associated with a decrease in TR velocity in children with SCA. The authors postulated that reduction in haemolysis and improvement in anemia led to this improvement (Arushi et al., 2021; Klings et al., 2014).

Side Effects, Toxicity (Ahmad et al., 2018; John et al., 2020; Maharaj et al., 2019; Montalembert et al., 2021; Nnebe-Agumadu et al., 2021; Ofakunrin et al., 2020; Opoka et al., 2017; Santos & Nogueira Maia, 2011; Thein & Howard, 2018; Tshilolo et al., 2019; Ware et al., 2016)

Few side effects are described in patients submitted to HU for a long time: skin or mucosa discoloration, neutropenia, thrombocytopenia, reticulocytopenia, oligo or azoospermia. Most of these adverse events are transitory (John et al., 2021; Montalembert et al., 2021; Nnebe-Agumadu et al., 2021; Tshilolo et al., 2019).

Neutropenia was defined as an absolute neutrophil count (ANC) < 2,000/mm^3 and thrombocytopenia as an absolute number of platelets <150,000/mm^3 (Montalembert et al., 2021; Tshilolo et al., 2019). No infection was reported during the neutropenic episodes in most of the studies on use of HU in Africa (Ahmad et al., 2018; Ofakunrin et al., 2020; Tshilolo et al, 2019).

Other skin toxicities were observed predominantly in adults, being mostly dry skin and nail pigmentation and subtle hair loss (Ahmad et al., 2018; Moftah & Eswayah, 2022; Montalembert et al., 2021). These lesions are one of the reasons for the fear of use of HU, specifically in young ladies. Other commonly reported reactions consisted of mostly self-reported gastrointestinal (nausea, abdominal pain), nervous system (dizziness, headache), and general (fatigue) disorders, predominantly in adults. Some authors described an increase in appetite and physical activity (Ofakunrin et al., 2020).

Fertility and Teratogenicity

One of the reasons of fear of HU-use in Africa concerns the presumptive impact on fertility and teratogenicity. Fertility concerns males and teratogenicity pregnant women. It is important to highlight a such precision as some women are also reluctant to use of HU because of fear to be sterile.

HU most likely decreases spermatogenesis, but additional studies are needed to assess whether this effect is reversible. Preliminary evidence suggests that the effect of HU on spermatogenesis and sperm quality may be reversed when HU is stopped (Joseph et al., 2021).

About the impact of HU on pregnancy, no absolute data are known in humans. In the European experience, among 110 pregnancies exposed to HU (at least in the first quarter) no malformations were observed in neonates and no maternal mortality was reported (Montalembert et al., 2021)

The fear of development of a secondary cancer is not justified even though there have been very few cases of myelodysplastic syndrome or acute leukemia after HU administration to patients with SCD (Montalembert et al., 2021).

Furthermore, in vitro assays and rodent studies have not shown mutagenic activity and no case has been reported in the longest follow-up cohorts suggesting that these events could be simply related to SCD or aging of the population (Brunson et al., 2017).

Follow-up and Monitoring

Regular monitoring for side effects is essential and depends on the recommendation reported in different studies. In Europe, the recommendation was to monitor the CBC every two months and the percentage of HbF every six months (Montalembert et al., 2021). Based onour experience, routinely monitoring in SSA countries will concern the CBC every month in the first two quarters of treatment and every three month later; HbF every 3–6 months and malaria test in the occasion of the collection of blood or in case of fever.

Laboratory effects include a predictable rise in the haemoglobin concentration, HbF percentage and mean corpuscular volume along with a concurrent decrease in absolute reticulocyte count, total leukocyte count and absolute neutrophil count. These laboratory values, in addition to examination of the peripheral blood film for erythrocyte morphology, are used to escalate. Patients with MTD also can be used to monitor medication adherence. These laboratory effects have been demonstrated to be consistent and sustainable in both adults and children with SCA (John et al., 2020; Opoka et al., 2017; Tshilolo et al., 2019; Ware et al., 2016).

Conclusion

Most of the recent trials and studies on the use of HU in Africa (Ahmad et al., 2018; John et al., 2020; Klings et al., 2014; Ofakunrin et al., 2020; Opoka et al., 2017; Tshilolo et al., 2019) have concluded that it's use in Africa is feasible, safe and affordable and offers biological and clinical benefits with a strike impact in reducing the CVO events, number of hospitalisation, need of blood transfusion, malaria events, abnormal DTC values (Ahmad et al., 2018; John et al., 2020; Ofakunrin et al., 2020; Opoka et al., 2017; Tshilolo et al., 2019).

All these impacts contribute to reduce the social exclusion of SCA patients and offers more social integration and regular scholarship.

Because of the high cost of HU in most of the SSA countries, it seems reasonable to use low-HU dose in resource-poor settings because of the advantages and the efficacy in controlling symptoms and some complications (Strousse, 2015).

HU is the only widely used drug, which modifies disease pathogenesis. As many countries in SSA begin newborn screening programmes to identify children with sickle cell anemia, wider access to HU may provide a simple and inexpensive oral medication that can alter the disease course and prolong survival.

References

Ahmad, H. R., Faruk, J. A., Sobowale, A. M., Solomon, A., Mustapha, A. N., & Ogunrinde, O. G. (2018). The use of hydroxycarbamide in children with sickle cell anemia. *Sahel Medical Journal, 21*, 189–193.

Anstey, N. M., Weinberg, J. B., Hassanali, M. Y., Mwaikambo, E. D., Manyenga, D., Misukonis, M. A., Arnelle, D. R., Hollis, D., McDonald, M. I., & Granger, D. L. (1996). Nitric oxide in Tanzanian children with malaria: Inverse relationship between malaria severity and nitric oxide production/nitric oxide synthase type 2 expression. *The Journal of Experimental Medicine, 184*(2), 557–567.

Brunson, A., Keegan, T. H. M., Bang, H., Mahajan, A., Paulukonis, S., & Wun, T. (2017). Increased risk of leukemia among patients with sickle cell disease in California. *Blood, 130*, 1597–1599.

Dhar, A., Leung, T. M., Appiah-Kubi, A., Gruber, D., Aygun, B., Serigano, O., & Mitchell, E. (2021). Longitudinal analysis of cardiac abnormalities in pediatric patients with sickle cell anemia and effect of hydroxyurea therapy. *Blood Advances, 5*(21), 4406–4412. https://doi.org/10.1182/bloodadvances.2021005076

Gwilt, P. R., & Tracewell, W. G. (1998). Pharmacokinetics and pharmacodynamics of hydroxyurea. *Clinical Pharmacokinetics, 34*, 347–358.

John, C. C., Opoka, R. O., Latham, T. S., Hume, H. A., Nabaggala, C., Kasirye, P., Ndugwa, C. M., Lane, A., & Ware, R. E. (2020). Hydroxyurea dose escalation for sickle cell anemia in Sub-Saharan Africa. *The New England Journal of Medicine, 382*, 2524–2533.

Joseph, L., Jean, C., Manceau, S., Chalas, C., Arnaud, C., Kamdem, A., Pondarré, C., Habibi, A., Bernaudin, F., Allali, S., de Montalembert, M., Boutonnat-Faucher, B., Arlet, J.-B., Koehl, B., Cavazzana, M., Ribeil, J.-A., Lionnet, F., Berthaut, I., & Brousse, V. (2021). Effect of hydroxyurea exposure before puberty on sperm parameters in males with sickle cell disease. *Blood, 137*, 826–829.

Kaufman, R. E. (1992). Hydroxyurea: Specific therapy for sickle cell anemia? *Blood, 79*(10), 2503–2506.

King, S. B. (2003). The nitric oxide producing reactions of hydroxyurea. *Current Medicinal Chemistry, 10*, 437–452.

Klings, E. S., Machado, R. F., Barst, R. J., Morris, C. R., Mubarak, K. K., Gordeuk, V. R., Kato, G. J., Ataga, K. I., Simon Gibbs, J., Castro, O., Rosenzweig, E. B., Sood, N., Hsu, L., Wilson, K. C., Telen, M. J., Decastro, L. M., Krishnamurti, L., Steinberg, M. H., Badesch, D. B., Gladwin, M. T., & American Thoracic Society Ad Hoc Committee on Pulmonary Hypertension of Sickle Cell Disease. (2014). An official American Thoracic Society clinical practice guideline: Diagnosis, risk stratification, and management of pulmonary hypertension of sickle cell disease. *American Journal of Respiratory and Critical Care Medicine, 189*(6), 727–740.

Lopez, L., Colan, S. D., Frommelt, P. C., Ensing, G. J., Kendall, K., Younoszai, A. K., Lai, W. W., & Geva, T. (2010). Recommendations for quantification methods during the performance of a pediatric echocardiogram: A report from the Pediatric Measurements Writing Group of the American Society of Echocardiography Pediatric and Congenital Heart Disease Council. *Journal of the American Society of Echocardiography, 23*(5), 465–495, quiz 576–577.

Maharaj, K., Bodkyn, C., Greene, C., & Bahadursingh, S. (2019). Efecto de la Terapia con Hidroxiurea en los Eventos Clínicos Adversos y los Indices Haematológicos de Pacientes Paediátricos con Aanemia de Células Falciformes. *West Indian Medical Journal, 68*(2), 80–85.

Moftah, M. B., & Eswayah, A. (2022). Repurposing of hydroxyurea against covid-19: A promising immunomodulatory role. *Assay and Drug Development Technologies, 20*(1), 55–62.

Montalembert, M., Voskaridou, E., Oevermann, L., Cannas, G., Habibi, A., Loko, G., Joseph, L., Colombatti, R., Bartolucci, P., Brousse, V., Galactéros, F., & All ESCORT HU Investigators (2021). Real-life experience with hydroxyurea in patients with sickle cell disease: Results from the prospective ESCORT-HU cohort study. *Haematology, 96*(10), 1223–1231. https://doi.org/10.1002/ajh.26286

Nnebe-Agumadu, U., Adogah, A. I., Ifeanyi, E., James, E., Kumode, E., Nnodu, O., & Adekile, A. (2021). Hydroxyurea in children with sickle cell disease in a resource poor setting: Monitoring and effects of therapy. A practical perspective. *Pediatric Blood & Cancer, 68*, e28969. https://doi.org/10.1002/pbc.28969

Ofakunrin, A. O., Oguche, S., Adekola, K., Okpe, E. S., Afolaranmi, T. O., Diaku-Akinwumi, I. N., Zoakah, A. I., & Sagay, A. S. (2020). Effectiveness and safety of hydroxyurea in the treatment of sickle cell anemia in children in Jos, North Central Nigeria. *Journal of Tropical Pediatrics, 66*, 290–298.

Olupot-Olupot, P., Tomlinson, G., Williams, T. N., Tshilolo, L., Santos, B., Smart, L. R., McElhinney, K., Howard, T. A., Aygun, B., Stuber, S. E., Lane, A., Latham, T. S., Ware, R. E., & REACH Investigators. (2023). Hydroxyurea treatment is associated with lower malaria incidence in children with sickle cell anemia in sub-Saharan Africa. *Blood, 141*(12), 1402–1410.

Opoka, R. O., Ndugwa, C. M., Latham, T. S., Lane, A., Hume, H. A., Kasirye, P., Hodges, J. S., Ware, R. E., & John, C. C. (2017). Novel use of hydroxyurea in an African Region with malaria NOHARM: A trial for children with sickle cell anemia. *Blood, 130*(24), 2585–2593.

Owusu-Ansah, A., Ihunnah, C. A., Walker, A. L., & Ofori-Acquah, S. F. (2016). Inflammatory targets of therapy in sickle cell disease. *Translational Research, 167*, 281–297.

Santos, F. K., & Nogueira Maia, C. N. (2011). Patients with sickle cell disease taking hydroxyurea in the Hemocentro Regional de Montes Claro. *Revista Brasileira de Hematologia e Hemoterapia, 33*(2), 105–109.

Strousse, J. J. (2015). Is low hydroxyurea the solution to the global epidemic of sickle cell disease? *Pediatric Blood Cancer, 62*, 929–930.

Thein, S. L., & Howard, J. (2018). How I treat the older adult with sickle cell disease. *Blood, 132*(17), 1750–1760.

Therrell, B. L. Jr., Lloyd-Puryear, M. A., Ohene-Frempong, K., Ware, R. E., Padilla, C. D., Ambrose, E. E., Barkat, A., Ghazal, H., Kiyaga, C., Mvalo, T., Nnodu, O., Ouldim, K., Rahimy, M. C., Santos, B., Tshilolo, L., Yusuf, C., Zarbalian, G., Watson, M. S., & On behalf of the faculty and speakers at the First Pan African Workshop on Newborn Screening

(2020). Empowering newborn screening programs in African countries through establishment of an international collaborative effort. *Journal of Community Genetics, 11,* 253–268.

Timson, J. (1975). Hydroxyurea. *Mutation Research, 32,* 115–132.

Tshilolo, L., Kafando, E., Sawadogo, M., Cotton, F., Vertongen, F., Ferster, A., & Gulbis, B. (2008). Neonatal screening and clinical care programmes for sickle cell disorders in sub-Saharan Africa: Lessons from pilot studies. *Public Health, 122*(9), 933–941.

Tshilolo, L., Tomlinson, G., Williams, T. N., Santos, B., Olupot-Olupot, P., Lane, A., Aygun, B., Stuber, S. E., Latham, T. S., McGann, P. T., Ware, R. E., & REACH Investigators (2019). Hydroxyurea for children with sickle cell anemia in sub-Saharan Africa. *The New England Journal of Medicine, 380,* 121–131.

Wang, W. C., Ware, R. E., Miller, S. T., Iyer, R. V., Casella, J. F., Minniti, C. P., Rana, S., Thornburg, C. D., Rogers, Z. R., Kalpatthi, R. V., Barredo, J. C., Brown, R. C., Sarnaik, S. A., Howard, T. H., Wynn, L. W., Kutlar, A., Armstrong, F. D., Files, B. A., Goldsmith, J. C., Thompson, B. W., & BABY HUG investigators (2011). Hydroxycarbamide in very young children with sickle-cell anaemia: A multicentre, randomised, controlled trial (BABY HUG). *Lancet, 377*(9778), 1663–1672.

Ware, R. E., Davis, B. R., Schultz, W. H., Brown, R. C., Aygun, B., Sarnaik, S., Odame, I., Fuh, B., George, A., Owen, W., Luchtman-Jones, L., Rogers, Z. R., Hilliard, L., Gauger, C., Piccone, C., Lee, M. T., Kwiatkowski, J. L., Jackson, S., Miller, S. T., …, Adams, R. J. (2016). Hydroxycarbamide versus chronic transfusion for maintenance of transcranial Doppler flow velocities in children with sickle cell anaemia — TCD with transfusions changing to hydroxyurea (TWiTCH): A multicentre, open-label, phase 3, noninferiority trial. *Lancet, 387,* 661–670.

World Health Organization Model List of Essential Medicines: 21st list (2019). Geneva: World Health Organization. https://apps.who.int/iris/handle/10665/325771. License: CC BY-NC-SA 3.0 IGO.

World Health Organization Regional Committee for Africa. (2010). Sickle-cell disease: A strategy for the WHO African Region. Report of the Regional Director. Sixtieth session, Malabo, Equitorial Guinea.

Yawn, B. P., Buchanan, G. R., Afenyi-Annan, A. N., Ballas, S. K., Hassell, K. L., James, A. H., Jordan, L., Lanzkron, S. M., Lottenberg, R., Savage, W. J., Tanabe, P. J., Ware, R. E., Murad, M. H., Goldsmith, J. C., Ortiz, E., Fulwood, R., Horton, A., & John-Sowah, J. (2014). Management of sickle cell disease: Summary of the 2014 evidence-based report by expert panel members. *Journal of the American Medical Association, 312*(10), 1033–1048.

Zahran, A. M., Nafady, A., Saad, K., Hetta, H. F., Abdallah, A.-E. M., Abdel-Aziz, S. M., Embaby, M. M., Abo Elgheet, A. M., Darwish, S. F., Abo-Elela, M. G. M., Elhoufey, A., & Elsayh, K. I. (2020). Effect of hydroxyurea treatment on the inflammatory markers among children with sickle cell disease. *Clinical and Applied Thrombosis/Hemostasis, 26,* 1–7.

15 Niprisan and Other Homegrown Anti-Sickling Medications

Successes and Challenges

Oluseyi Oniyangi and Ugochi O. Ogu

Introduction

The increasing use of traditional herbal medications or phytomedicines has been reported all over the world, and more especially so for chronic conditions including sickle cell disease (SCD) (Busari & Mufutau, 2017; Lubega, Osingada, & Kasirye, 2021; Organization, 2013). The World Health Organization (WHO) estimates that up to 80% of people living in the low- and middle-income countries (LMIC) of the world utilize herbal medicines as their primary source of health care due to its acceptability, accessibility, affordability, local beliefs, and cultural practices (Organization, 2013). In other more developed areas of the world, the field of complementary and alternate medicine (CAM) as an alternative to orthodox medicine is also expanding, and the use of these traditional herbal medications or natural herbs is part of it (Organization, 2013). These herbal medications have been used by both adults and children with SCD (Lubega et al., 2021). The WHO defines herbal medicine as 'any plant-derived materials or products that contain either raw or processed ingredients from one or more plants with therapeutic or other human benefits' (Organization, 2013). Majority of these medications are in the form of phytomedicines, a term which is often used interchangeably with traditional or herbal medications, nutraceuticals, phytopharmaceuticals, phytonutrients, or phytotherapy (Organization, 2018). Phytomedicines have been found to be useful and efficacious by the people most affected by SCD, especially in the LMIC (Oniyangi & Cohall, 2020).

Extensive in vitro research has shown that these phytomedicines, among other functions have the ability to both prevent sickling of the red blood cell (RBC) in adverse conditions, as well as reverse the event when it has occurred (Ngozi Awa Imaga & Taiwo, 2017). This modality of action has earned them the appellation of anti-sickling agents, the prototype of which is Niprisan, a polyherbal drug of different parts of four herbs developed in Nigeria (Wambebe et al., 2001). While Niprisan has been extensively scientifically evaluated for its use in SCD, this is not so for other phytomedicines in use, many of which are unknown, untested scientifically, and unregulated in use, raising concerns about their safety and toxicity profiles (Organization, 2013, 2018; Wambebe et al., 2001).

DOI: 10.4324/9781003463931-16

These anti-sickling agents could be important for managing SCD, particularly in LMIC, where there is a mismatch of orthodox health care practitioner to patient ratio, expensive orthodox medications out of reach of majority, and very importantly the beliefs and cultural practices of the locale; and where the collaboration of orthodox and traditional medicines would be beneficial. This chapter focuses on the use of phytomedicines in SCD.

Definition of Phytomedicines

Traditional medicine as defined by the WHO is 'the sum total of the knowledge, skill, and practices based on the theories, beliefs, and experiences indigenous to different cultures, whether explicable or not, used in the maintenance of health as well as in the prevention, diagnosis, improvement or treatment of physical and mental illness' (Organization, 2013). This includes the use of phytomedicines/ herbal medicines. There are various definitions of the terms herbal medicine or phytomedicines, many of which include herbs, herbal materials, herbal preparations, and/or finished herbal products and essential oils that contain as active ingredients, parts of plants, plant materials, extracts/fractions of these, or combinations thereof in a form suitable for administration to patients (Organization, 2019). These combinations are quite often complex mixtures of compounds from different herbs in variable concentrations with therapeutic and healing properties (Organization, 2013, 2018). Thus, a herbal medicine or a phytopharmaceutical preparation can be defined as 'a medicine derived exclusively from a whole plant or parts of plants and manufactured in a crude form or as a purified pharmaceutical formulation' (Srivastava, Srivastava, Pandey, Khanna, & Pant, 2019). A phytomedicine may thus be more simply defined as 'a medicine derived from plants in their original state and standardized for use in a dosage regimen' (Oniyangi & Cohall, 2020).

History of Phytomedicine Use for SCD

Prior to the coming of orthodox medicine, or the first publication of SCD by Herrick in 1910, it is obvious that the disorder must have been identified in the areas of the world where it occurs. This is due to the local names given to SCD in the areas of the world it occurs, which suggest that the variability in the natural course of SCD had been known, particularly the painful crises and the high morbidity and mortality associated with it. Examples of these names are *abiku, ogbanje and sankara-miji* among the Yoruba, Igbo and Hausa people respectively of Nigeria, *Ene mewu: Okyena me wu, onye kye ba* in Ghana and *Kulaja Pandu/Anuvamshika Pandu* in Indian ayurvedic texts, and they suggest children destined to die and be reborn in families, or have recurrent acute painful episodes of ill-health (Ameh, Tarfa, & Ebeshi, 2012; Dennis-Antwi, Culley, Hiles, & Dyson, 2011; Mishra & Pandya, 2019). Traditional herbal medicines, the oldest form of health care known to man, have been the mainstay of treatment for ill health in these areas for many centuries. It can therefore be assumed that these herbal medicines have been used for people with SCD for many centuries, prior to the coming of orthodox medicine.

Furthermore, many medicines such as quinine for treatment of malaria used in orthodox treatment today are derived directly from these traditional medications. However, documentation of the use of herbal medicines for SCD is scarce, as the requisite information was often passed down orally in generations of traditional healers, particularly in Sub-Saharan Africa (SSA), which has the largest burden of the disease globally. However, Indian traditional medicine – Ayurveda – is documented in classic texts which contain detailed observations of diseases as well as remedies for the conditions, and it is likely that these include ailments with signs and symptoms of SCD (Bhatt, 2010; Mishra & Pandya, 2019).

Some of the earliest documentation of the use of herbal medicines for SCD comes from Ibadan and Ile Ife, Nigeria in the 1970s, with reports on the beneficial effects of *Fagara Zanthyloides* in reducing painful crises in SCD (Ameh et al., 2012). Others were in the form of case reports and case series on the use of herbal medicines for SCD. This was followed by the extensive in vivo research into the composition of and identification of active ingredients of herbal medicines for SCD and very importantly the modes of action (Ameh et al., 2012; Ngozi Awa Imaga & Taiwo, 2017; Okoh, Alli, Tolvanen, & Nwegbu, 2019). This was later followed on by the laboratory use of the extracts of promising phytomedicines in experiments involving transgenic mice and then by the limited in vitro clinical trials of phytomedicines use in SCD, some of which are yet to be completed. (Ameh et al., 2012; Oniyangi & Cohall, 2020). There have also been systematic reviews with and without meta-analysis on the subject (Okoh et al., 2019; Oniyangi & Cohall, 2020). Furthermore, there has been research into the molecular activities of these phytomedicines as well as into their potential epigenetic effects (Okoh et al., 2019). The literature is vast and extensive, as well as all encompassing. We can only make an attempt at summarizing what is available.

Herbal Medicines Used for SCD

There are documentations of hundreds of herbal medicines currently in use for SCD (Ngozi Awa Imaga & Taiwo, 2017; Okoh et al., 2019; Organization, 2013). These include those from Nigeria, Ghana, Niger, Cameroon, Uganda, Democratic republic of Congo (DRC) and Tanzania in SSA, India and Brazil to name a few. Majority of these have not been standardized for use or subjected to modern scientific evaluation (Oniyangi & Cohall, 2020). Efficacy and toxicity studies in humans are also limited (Organization, 2013). There is therefore the possibility that some knowledge may be lost, and some of the plants for the herbal medication go extinct on account of this.

Research into herbal medicines used for SCD has been extensive and has identified a multitude from SSA and the Indian subcontinent among others. These include *Fagara Xanthyloides* (local name – Ori ata), commonly used as a chewing stick for cleaning the teeth among the Yoruba people in South-west Nigeria, clove (*Eugenia caryophyllata,* local name 'kanunfari' among the Hausa people of West Africa); *Piper guineense* (local names 'eche' in Idoma or 'akwa-ose' in Igbo languages of Middle belt and South-east Nigeria, respectively), and *Sorghum bicolor* (the leaf stalk yields an extract that looks like blood). Others include *Cajanus Cajun*, grains of paradise *Aframomum melegueta*, *Pterocarpus osun*, unripe pawpaw *(papaya) Carica papaya fruit and leaves*, Garlic cloves *Allium sativum*; *Hymenocardia acida and Khaya senegalensis* bark or leaves. These all grow commonly in SSA and are often eaten as foods or used as spices, and some are also constituents of common Ayurvedic herbal medicines (Ameh et al., 2012; Amujoyegbe, Idu, Agbedahunsi, & Erhabor, 2016; Ilagouma, Amadou, Issaka, & Ikhiri, 2019; Imaga, 2013; Mrinalini, Snehal, Shubham, Ayesha, & Subhash, 2021; Okoh et al., 2019). Yogaraj and Laxadi guguly are two Ayurvedic medicines, as are *Plumbago zeylanica* (local name: Mitrak mool) and Maricha *Piper nigrum* (Mishra & Pandya, 2019; Srivastava et al., 2019). *Pfaffia paniculata* (local name: Brazilian Ginseng) is used for SCD by the South American tribes of Brazil (Araújo, Bydlowski, & Mendoza, 2009). It is interesting to note that although these plants grow in different parts of the world, they have been used for similar purposes where present.

Some of these herbal medicines have been standardized for use as phytomedicines, combined in various ways and marketed in tablets, capsule or powder form such as Niprisan, Ciklavit (*Cajanus cajan*), Dioscovite, *Carica papaya* L., Jobelyn (*Sorghum bicolor*), Ajawaron (*Cissus populnea*) and Pfaffia paniculata (Akinsulie, Temiye, Akanmu, Lesi, & Whyte, 2005; Araújo et al., 2009; Ngozi Awa Imaga & Taiwo, 2017; Wambebe et al., 2001). The prototype of these phytomedicines used for SCD is Niprisan, a multiherbal preparation of different parts of four plants – *Piper guineenses* seeds, *Pterocarpus osun* stem, *Eugenia caryophyllum* fruit and *Sorghum bicolor* leaves (Wambebe et al., 2001). Niprisan, initially called Nicosan, is a 'homegrown' efficacious medication for SCD developed at the Nigerian Institute for Pharmaceutical Research and development (NIPRID).

Photographs of some of these plants and herbs used in phytomedicines for SCD are shown in Figure 15.1.

Composition of Phytomedicines

Research into the pharmacology of phytomedicines has shown that they contain certain substances or naturally occurring compounds called phytochemicals that are the active components responsible for their actions (Organization, 2018). These phytochemicals: saponins (made up of triterpene glycosides and sterols); flavonoids (comprise various polyphenolic compounds), and their subgroups isoflavones, quercetins, catechins and anthrocyanins; glycosides (comprise molecules in which sugar bound to other non-sugar functional groups); tannins and other phenolic/polyphenolic compounds (organic compounds containing multiple phenol rings); alkaloids (basic organic compounds containing at least one Nitrogen atom) such as piperine and terpenoids (naturally occurring organic compounds derived from 5-carbon compound isoprene) and derivatives – terpenes and diterprenes, carotenoids or tetratrepenoids (Chung, Wong, Wei, Huang, & Lin, 1998; Dey et al., 2020; Mugford & Osbourn, 2013; Okoh et al., 2019; Panche, Diwan, & Chandra, 2016; Rasouli, Farzaei, & Khodarahmi, 2017).

Fagara xanthyloides stick and plant (wild lime, prickly ash bush)

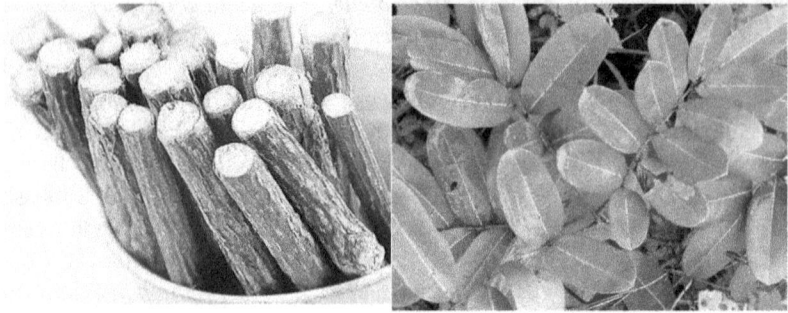

Eugenia caryophyllata (cloves) seeds

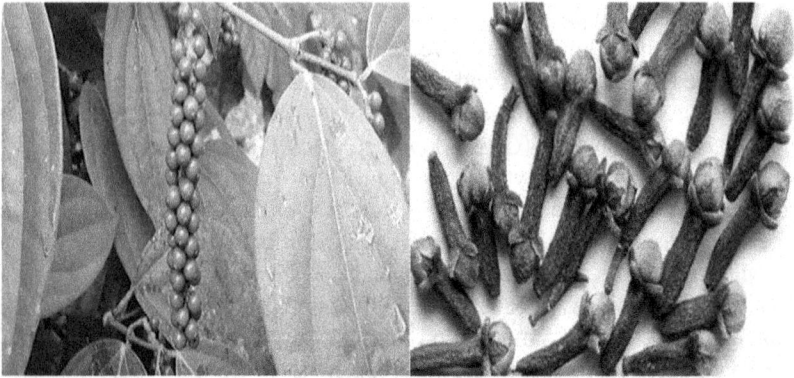

Sorghum bicolor seeds

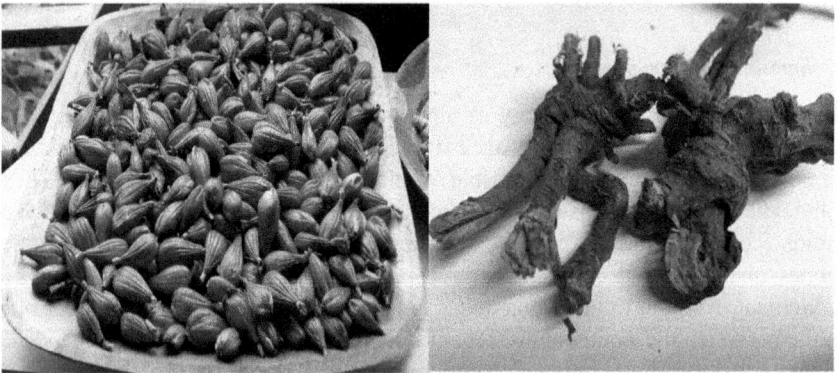

Figure 15.1 Plants and herbs used in phytomedicines for SCD.

Other phytochemicals are the amino acids – both essential ones such as tryptophan and non-essential ones such as phenylalanine and tyrosine; Quinone (aromatic organic compounds) derivatives such as anthraquinones and enzymes such as papain (cysteinie protease enzyme found in papaya); vanilloids (compounds such as capsaicin with a vinyl group) and cannabinoids (Dey et al., 2020).

Phytochemicals are found in different parts of the plants including the roots (*Fagara zanthoxyloides*, *Pfaffia paniculata*, *plumbargo zeylanica*), stem (*Khaya senegalensis*, *Pterocarpus osun*), bark (*Acacia Xanthoploea* (*Fabaceae*), leaf (*Hymenocardia acidai, soghum bicolor*), seeds *(Cajanus cajan, Piper guineeneses)*, bulbs (garlic *Eugenia caryophyllata*) and fruit (*Carica papaya*). They are used singly and in combination and prepared in various ways as medicines. It appears that all parts of the plants are useful in the preparation of these phytomedicines (Ilagouma et al., 2019; Okoh et al., 2019). There are various forms of preparations of these phytochemicals which include decoction, maceration, spray, infusions, and powder form (Ilagouma et al., 2019; Organization, 2018).

Phytomedicine Use in SCD – How They Work

Phytomedicines are used in SCD to manage the condition, by treating and preventing the severe painful crises associated with the disease, preventing and managing infections, improving nutrition and immunity as well as preventing and managing anemia (Ameh et al., 2012). These management goals are reached through the use of different medicinal plants, singly and in combination via various modes of administration. The beneficial effects of these plant medicines occur through the activities of the phytochemicals contained within them and are often complementary and/or synergistic (Okoh et al., 2019). Through extensive in vitro research, the phytochemicals have been shown to have analgesic, antioxidant, hematinic, anti-inflammatory, anti-adhesion and anti-infective properties, as well as improvement of the immune system and general metabolism (Okoh et al., 2019).

The plant polyphenols which include flavonoids (and their subgroups) and hydroxybenzoic acid have been shown to have anti-oxidative, anti-inflammatory, and anti-mutagenic effects. The flavonoids have potent antioxidant activity (Okoh et al., 2019; Rasouli et al., 2017). They are also anti-hemolytic, maintain RBC membrane integrity, and inhibit hemoglobin polymerization and platelet aggregation (Okoh et al., 2019). In addition to these, the tannins have antimicrobial, anti-mutagenic and anti-cancer properties (Mugford & Osbourn, 2013). The glycosides and sterols such as saponins have anti-infective (antibacterial, antifungal and antiviral), anti-inflammatory and anti-mutagenic effects, and have also been shown to be antidiabetic (Ameh et al., 2012; Panche et al., 2016). The quinone derivatives are anti-oxidant and anti-hemolytic, while the proteins – globulins and amino acids, e.g. tryptophan, tyrosine especially the phenylalanine esters have the property of anti-sickling and reversing sickling as well as maintaining membrane stability (Okoh et al., 2019). The enzyme papain has been shown to have antioxidant properties and in combination with proteins such as phenylalanine is anti-sickling (Okoh et al., 2019).

Similar effects are produced by the alkaloids (Dey et al., 2020; Okoh et al., 2019). The tarpenoids have potent analgesic effects, as do the cannabinoids, e.g. β-Caryophyllene and vanilloids, e.g. capsaicin (Ameh et al., 2012; Dey et al., 2020; Okoh et al., 2019). Furthermore, phytochemicals rich in arginine such as pumpkin seed, soy bean, and peanuts improve nutrition and arginine metabolism (Okoh et al., 2019).

The activities of these phytomedicines in SCD have been obtained following detailed research, and follow on from the pathophysiology of the disease, shown below in an illustration that simplifies the process, from an article by Sundd, Gladwin, an Novelli (2019)

Mechanisms of Action of Phytomedicines in SCD

Several phytomedicines have been found to have beneficial effects on the course and outcome of SCD. Research into the mechanisms of action of these medications have largely come about from in vitro studies, with limited in vivo work in transgenic mice and humans. The mechanism of action of some of the phytomedicines are known, while in others this is not so. The activities of these phytomedicines in SCD have been obtained following detailed research, and follow on from the pathophysiology of the disease, shown below in a simple illustration in Figure 15.2 (Sundd et al., 2019).

The basic pathophysiologic mechanisms in SCD are an interplay in a vicious cycle of the following processes following erythrocyte injury: Hb S polymerization, hemolysis, adhesion mediated aso-occlusion, endothelial dysfunction, activation of sterile inflammatory pathways, and reduced nitric oxide bioavailability (Sundd et al., 2019). The phytomedicines have been found to have effect in almost all pathophysiologic mechanisms in SCD. The net effects of these herbal medicines are most often associated with an anti-sickling activity of the RBCs. Phytomedicines in SCD have been found to both prevent sickling process, as well as reverse the event once it has occurred. This is done via various mechanisms, either singly or synergistically. This effect is brought about by the phytochemicals present in these plants.

Anti-sickling mechanisms: Phytomedicines have been shown to affect their actions through some of these anti-sickling mechanisms:

• **Prevention and reversal of Hb S polymerization**: Polymerization can be prevented through five possible ways – block intermolecular contacts in the sickle Hb fiber, induce Hb F production, increase Hb S oxygen affinity, improve Hb S solubility by reducing concentration of 2,3-diphosphoglycerate (2,3-DPG) in the sickle red cell, and reduce intracellular sickle Hb concentration (Eaton & Bunn, 2017). Phytomedicines have been shown to have the ability to both prevent Hb S polymerization, as well as return the process to normal even when it has occurred. This is one of the mechanisms of action of Niprisan®, a freeze-dried extract of Piper guineenses seeds, *Pterocarpus osun* stem, *Eugenia caryophyllum* fruit and Sorghum bicolor leaves; as well as the extract of the seeds of

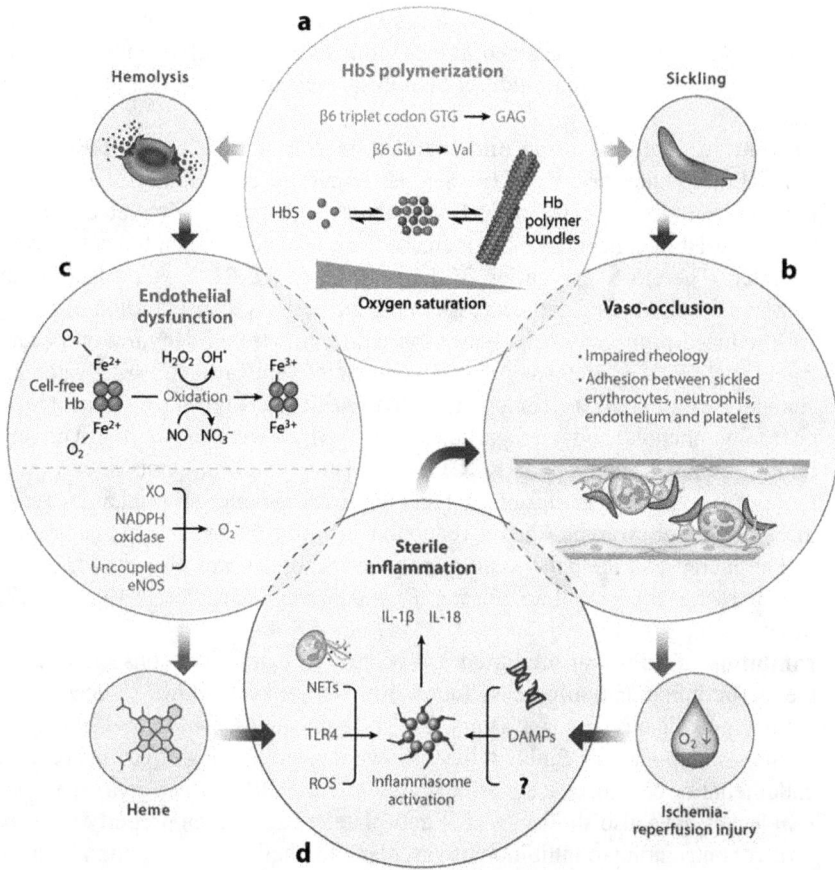

Figure 15.2 Pathophysiology of SCD.

Source: Reproduced with permission of authors (Snudd P, et al, 2019).

Cajanus cajan (a major constituent of Ciklavit®), both phytomedicines from Nigeria (Akinsulie et al., 2005; Wambebe et al., 2001).

- **RBC membrane stabilizing effect**: These drugs have also been shown to have membrane stabilizing effects, which further prevents RBC polymerization and thus hemolysis. *Zanthoxylum zanthoxyloides* (*Fagara*, orin-ata) roots, Cajanus cajan and *Carica papaya* leaf extracts have all been shown in vitro to have this property (Okoh et al., 2019).
- **Improved deformability of RBCs**: The extract of the powdered root of *Pfaffia paniculata* is a sodium ionophore which has shown improvement of deformability in vitro, as did the extract of *Raphiostylis beninensis* stems (Mozar et al., 2015; Oniyangi & Cohall, 2020).

- **Prevention of hemolysis**: The aqueous extract of *Lonchocarpus cyanescens* and *Pfaffia paniculata* roots and a methanolic extract of *Raphiostylis beninensis* stems have shown inhibition of hemolysis (Mozar et al., 2015; Oniyangi & Cohall, 2020).
- **Prevention of dehydration and increase in cell volume of the RBC**: The intracellular concentration of Hb S is an important determinant of RBC polymerization (Eaton & Bunn, 2017). When the RBCs are dehydrated, the intracellular Hb S concentration is increased and vice versa when the cell is well hydrated. Therefore, prevention of dehydration of the RBC would lead to an increase in cell volume and decrease in the intracellular concentration of Hb S, with reduced propensity to polymer formation. Sickle cell dehydration occurs from loss of K^+, Cl^-, and water through two major pathways – Ca^{2+}-activated K^+ channel (IK1 or Gardos channel). The phytomedicines – green tea extract (GTE or tea polyphenols) and aged garlic extract (AGE) – were shown to effectively inhibit the K-Cl cotransport (KCC) mechanisms (Ohnishi, Ohnishi, & Ogunmola, 2001). In vivo studies of Niprisan in transgenic mice showed an increase in hydrated cell volume, thus a reduction in intracellular HbS concentration and an increase in the delay time to polymerization, as was also shown by the root extract of the Brazillian ginseng, *Pfaffia paniculate* (Eaton & Bunn, 2017; Mozar et al., 2015).
- **Inhibition of adhesion mediated** aso-occlusion: One of the consequences of the sterile inflammation process found in SCD has been shown to occur with the phytomedicines (Eaton & Bunn, 2017). Amino acids, especially L-phenylalanine, a component of Ciklavit, have shown this anti-gelling effect, preventing endothelial or cell surface adhesions (Ameh et al., 2012). *Pelargonium xasperum* leaves have also shown specific anti-platelet aggregation property in vitro, further contributing to inhibition of vascular endothelial damage and inflammatory process (Okoh et al., 2019).
- **Anti-oxidant properties**: Nitric oxide generation and/or arginase inhibition as a mechanism for vasodilation, prevention of endothelial dysfunction, production of free oxygen radicals, improvement in RBC oxidation, and prevention of aso-occlusion have been reported by some phytomedicines (Eaton & Bunn, 2017). This anti-oxidant effect is another mechanism of action of Niprisan® mediated by *Pterocarpus osun* stem and *Sorghum bicolor* leaves (Wambebe et al., 2001). Extracts of *Plumbago zeylanica* and *Zanthoxylum zanthoxyloides root as well as Carica papaya* leaf also have this property.
- **Hb F inducers**: Hemoglobin F inducers have been shown to increase the amount of Hb F available in RBCs. This increase in Hb F concentration in the RBC tends to have a protective effect against the deleterious actions of Hb S, and decrease or prevent polymerization, as well as reducing the severity of the phenotypic expression of SCD (Bianchi, Zuccato, Lampronti, Borgatti, & Gambari, 2009). This is one of the mechanisms of action of the drug hydroxyurea, a standard of care in SCD as discussed in another chapter. Although there is extensive literature on novel therapies involving Hb F inducers

in SCD, there is still limited information on this with phytomedicines. Several phytomedicines induce fetal hemoglobin through different mechanisms such as increased erythroid differentiation to Hb F lines (*Bergaptene* from *A. marmelos*), epigenetics (*Angelicin* in *A. arcangelica*), and increased Hb F production (*Rapamycin* and *Mithramycin* from Strept hygroscopius found in the soil, and Streptomyces specie, respectively) (Bianchi et al., 2009; Ng & Ko, 2014). Ciklavit was reported in vitro laboratory experiments to induce the production of Hb F, as did *Pfaffia paniculata*, Gum arabic, broccoli sprout homogenate, an extract of labdane diterpene from *Curcuma comosa*, and leaves of *Terminalia catappa* – the Indian almond used in Nigerian herbal medicine for SCD (Ameh et al., 2012).

- **The anti-sickling mechanism of action of some phytomedicines remains unknown** such as the seeds of *Wrightia tinctoria* (Oniyangi & Cohall, 2020).

Effects of Phytomedicines on Epigenetics in SCD

Epigenetics refers to how behaviors and environment can cause changes that affect genetic manifestations (Wei, Huang, Yang, & Kang, 2017). This is done without change to the actual sequence or structure of DNA molecules, but rather to the gene expression. This includes the production of proteins or specialized enzymes that may reversibly chemically modify DNA bases (e.g. DNA methylation), histone production or RNA interference (RNAi) (Holoch & Moazed, 2015; Wei et al., 2017). In addition, Single Nucleotide Polymorphisms (SNP) which contribute to genetic variability have been shown to occur in SCD (Okoh et al., 2019). These processes may be contributory to the variability of expression of SCD, in which the same genetic mutation responsible for SCD exhibits varying phenotypic or clinical presentations and varying manifestations of disease severity.

Phytomedicines have been shown to contribute to epigenetic changes in SCD through the following epigenetic mechanism (Okoh et al., 2019).

Histone methylation and deacetylation: *Sulforaphane*, a phytochemical isolated from broccoli sprouts and other cruciferous vegetables, has been shown to upregulate the production of the nuclear factor – erythroid-derived factor 2 NRF2, which regulates the expression of antioxidants thereby protecting the cells from the effects of inflammation in sickle cell crises. Flavonoids and many other phytomedicines containing Vitamin C may also have this effect (Okoh et al., 2019). Other herbal medications have been shown in vitro to regulate the availability of hepcidin in SCD via this mechanism. Hepcidin is essential for iron metabolism and could either prevent iron overload from blood transfusions or increase the iron in RBCs preventing anemia.

DNA demethylation: Flavonoids have been shown to down regulate the expression of the gene (e.g. at the CpGs site on DNA strands) that turns off the production of Hb F. This could lead to reactivation of fetal globin genes to produce Hb F. This therefore increases the presence of Hb F with its multiple beneficial effects in SCD (Okoh et al., 2019).

Effects of Phytomedicines on Pain Control in SCD

Pain is one of the most significant clinical features of SCD, and the major reason why health care is sought. Phytomedicines are important in the control of pain in SCD. Opioids such as cannabis and their derivatives, which have been used for centuries for pain control are still in use as such today. The pathophysiological mechanisms of aso-occlusion and ischemia-reperfusion injury, inflammation, endothelial damage/vasculopathy, organ damage, and neuropathy may all cause pain in SCD (Sundd et al., 2019). The mechanisms of analgesia by phytomedicines, apart from the anti-sickling effect of the drugs, are due in part to their direct effect on specific pain receptors in the body.

Apart from the opioids and derivatives which have been discussed elsewhere in the book, other phytomedicines containing the cannabinoids and vanilloids have potent analgesic properties. B-*Caryophyllene*, present in *P. Guineense* and *E. caryophyllata* components of Niprisan, are cannabinoids similar in action to *Cannabis sativa*, the oldest known pharmacologically active form of Cannabis (Ameh et al., 2012). *Capsaicin and piperine* also present in *P. Guineense* and *E. caryophyllata are vanilloids. Isomeric divanilloylquinic acids* are also present in *Fagara zanthoxyloides* (Ameh et al., 2012).

Effects of Phytomedicines on Nutrition

Poor nutritional status in SCD is associated with impaired growth and deficient immune functions. Nutritional research in SCD has identified macro (protein, carbohydrate, lipids) and micronutrient deficiencies as being contributory to the clinical outcomes of the disease, including disease severity. Deficiencies of ascorbic acid (Vitamin C), alpha-tocopherol (Vitamin E), Vitamin A, Vitamin B group (2, 6, 12), Vitamin D, Vitamin E, and retinol have been reported in SCD. Folic acid, iron, calcium, zinc, and magnesium are other micronutrient deficiencies reported in SCD (Alabi, Adegboyega, Olawoyin, & Babatunde, 2022). Apart from being associated with poor growth, impaired or delayed development and occurrence of infections, these nutritional deficiencies are linked to painful crises associated with sickling and aso-occlusion, activation of sterile inflammation pathways, increased oxidative stress, and diminished arginine and nitric oxide bioavailability (Alabi et al., 2022; Imaga, 2013; Okoh et al., 2019). Therapies targeted at correcting these deficiencies have shown improvement in clinical outcomes. These could be achieved using phytomedicines. The phytomedicines are from medicinal plants which are often eaten as part of the dietary intake of affected children with SCD, such as foods containing naturally occurring phytochemicals rich in polyphenols such as flavonoids, vanilloids, arginase and other constituents of phytomedicines (Alabi et al., 2022; Imaga, 2013; Okoh et al., 2019). Nutritional supplementation with folate, protein, energy rich foods, and polyunsaturated fatty acids such as Omega 3 as well as micronutrients Vitamins A, B12, C, D, E, zinc, magnesium, and iron have all been associated with promoting healthy growth in children and preventing acute and chronic complications of the disease (Imaga, 2013).

Phytomedicines and Immune Response

Phytomedicines may boost the immune response through epigenetic mechanisms. This could include the effects on genes targeting the production of such proteins that increase interleukins (IL 2) production, and others that affect the pathways of senescence of the thymus gland and its functions (Okoh et al., 2019). Combinations of the phytochemicals found in phytomedicine compositions such as *Alchornia cordifolia leaf, Allium sativum rhizome, Annona senegalensi* leaf have been shown to have this effect (Okoh et al., 2019). Saponins such as occurs in *Tetracera alnifolia* and *Trema orientalis* leaf and bark have antimicrobial properties that enhance the natural resistance to infections, as well the restorative functions of the body (Chung et al., 1998). As stated above, nutritional deficiencies are also associated with diminished immune responses.

Uses of Phytomedicines in Clinical Practice

Similar to the goals of management with orthodox medications, phytomedicines are used in SCD to manage and control symptoms (both acute and long term) of the disease and to prevent and/or limit the occurrence of crises most especially those associated with pain (Ameh et al., 2012). Scientific evaluation into the efficacy of the phytomedicines in clinical practice has shown they have many beneficial effects in SCD. One of the earliest documentations (over half a century ago – since the 1970s) of herbal medicines to manage SCD is the use of *Zanthoxyllum (Fagara) zanthoxyloides*, called ori-ata locally and used as a chewing stick by the Yoruba people of South-west Nigeria. With its anti-sickling, membrane stabilizing and analgesic effect, it has been found useful in the prevention and treatment of acute and chronic painful crises in SCD, reducing both the frequency and severity of painful episodes (Ameh et al., 2012).

Phytomedicines have been used to manage and control signs and symptoms of SCD, both in steady state and with complications including (Ameh et al., 2012; Imaga, 2013):

- Management and prevention of painful crises
- Management and prevention of anemia
- Management and prevention of dehydration
- Prevention and management of infection
- Treatment of complications – specific phytotherapy, wound care with antiseptic herbs
- Nutritional supplementation

Much of the scientific evidence for the use of phytomedicines in SCD has come from the limited randomized controlled clinical trials available on the subject (albeit with varying degrees of quality of evidence). A Cochrane systematic review on the subject identified three of such trials for evaluation (Oniyangi & Cohall, 2020). Despite the limitations inherent in the design of these trials, they have yielded useful information on the effects of the phytomedicines in SCD. Thus, they have been found useful in reducing the duration, frequency, and severity of painful crises, including priapism and acute chest syndromes (*Niprisan, Ciklavit* and *Pffafia painiculata*). Other reported findings were an increase in the hemoglobin concentration of participants (although *Ciklavit* trial reported a fall in the Packed Cell Volumes), decreased episodes of blood transfusions, and an improved quality of life across board. The phytomedicine *Pffafia painiculata* was also useful in the reduction of episodes of jaundice, thromboembolism and although not significantly different from the placebo group – leg ulcers.

Adverse Effects

There is limited information on the adverse effects of phytomedicines used for SCD. They appear to be relatively safe drugs. However, as discussed above, the evidence for the adverse effects of these drugs is spare, and much more research is required in this regard. Reported adverse events are few and include vomiting and diarrhea, easy tiredness with Ciklavit, non-itching macular rashes three to four days after starting treatment, which disappeared a few days later, and headache with Niprisan. The evaluations of the liver and kidney function tests remained normal with the phytomedicines, although there was a non-significant decrease in Packed Cell Volume reported with Ciklavit (Oniyangi & Cohall, 2020).

Review of the Literature on Phytomedicines for SCD

Several phytomedicines have been used, few with literature behind them. We will discuss the three phytomedicines which have been most researched: Niprisan®, Ciklavit® and Pfaffia Paniculata.

Niprisan®

Niprisan is a phytomedicine formulated from freeze-dried extract of four plants: *Piper guineenses seeds*, *Pterocarpus osun* stem, *Eugenia caryophyllum* fruit and *Sorghum bicolor* leaves (Nathan, Tripathi, Wu, & Belanger, 2009; Wambebe et al., 2001). It was developed in Nigeria by the National Institute for Pharmaceutical Research and Development (NIPRD), based on indigenous medicinal plants used by traditional healers for the management of SCD. In 1992, Niprisan was brought to the attention of NIPRD by a traditional health practitioner and local reverend, Late Paul O. Ogunyale, who was a master's degree holder and claimed to be using Niprisan to treat his congregation members affected by SCD (Perampaladas et al., 2010). A memorandum of understanding was developed between the Late Reverend Ogunyale, and the NIPRD, which enabled the NIPRD access to the herbal recipe used by Reverend Ogunyale to treat people with SCD (Perampaladas et al., 2010; Wambebe, 2018). The goal behind this collaboration was to further research and develop the herbal recipe scientifically.

Initial animal studies in rats demonstrated favorable short-term toxicity profile (Awodogan et al., 1996). In vitro studies conducted by NIPRD revealed that under low oxygen tension, Niprisan protected RBC samples from sickle cell patients from sickling, as well as reverse already sickled RBCs in a dose-dependent manner (Gamaniel et al., 1998). These data provided some evidence on the potential efficacy of Niprisan and prompted further research. An in vitro study using blood from subjects with homozygous SCD at steady state established Niprisan as a potent anti-sickling agent (Iyamu, Turner, & Asakura, 2002). Results showed that a concentration of 0.05 mg/ml was needed to inhibit 50% of erythrocyte sickling and caused a sixfold prolongation in delay time for deoxy-Hb S polymerization compared to untreated samples. Furthermore, solubility of deoxy-Hb S significantly increased in the presence of Niprisan. Analysis revealed a slight shift in oxygen affinity to the left without any apparent change in the Hill coefficient, suggesting direct interaction with Hb molecules (Iyamu et al., 2002). Further studies were carried out on transgenic sickle mice to evaluate survival under severe acute hypoxic conditions (Iyamu, Turner, & Asakura, 2003). Results revealed prolonged survival in Niprisan treated mice, from 10 minutes in untreated mice to 60 minutes in mice treated with the highest tested dose of Niprisan. Percentage of sickled cells in venous blood samples decreased in treated vs untreated mice, in a dose-dependent manner. On histological examination, lung alveolar capillaries of untreated mice showed entrapment of large numbers of sickled cells which improved with increased doses of Niprisan (Iyamu et al., 2003). Based on the above in vitro and in vivo findings, phase I, IIA, and IIB clinical trials were eventually completed.

A phase I clinical trial using Niprisan capsules (500 mg for adults, 250 mg for children) was carried out to assess safety of Niprisan in healthy volunteers (Wambebe, 2018). Twenty volunteers with AA genotype, all staff of NIPRD, were enrolled in the study conducted between March and July 1994. None of the subjects experienced any side effects (Wambebe, 2018).

From August 1994 to February 1997, a phase IIA trial was conducted. Results showed decreased frequency and severity of pain crises, decreased hospitalizations, and decreased incidence of anemia and jaundice, without evidence of adverse effect on the kidney and liver (Wambebe, 2018). In addition, they reported increased appetite, weight gain, and increased school attendance. These positive findings led to the development of a phase IIB trial.

Published in 2001, the phase IIB randomized placebo-controlled double-blinded cross-over trial reported outcome on 82 subjects with SCD who received once-daily oral dose of Niprisan at a dose of 12 mg/kg, or placebo to evaluate the safety and efficacy of Niprisan in patients with SCD (Wambebe et al., 2001). The study started with a four-month pretrial period from April 1997, and actual trial from August 1997 to August 1998, with crossover at six months into the actual trial. Before the pretrial period, subjects were randomized into two groups: Groups A and B, and during actual trial, one group initially received Niprisan and the other received placebo, with crossover at six months, and each subject serving as their own control. Inclusion criteria included subjects aged 2–45 years of age, with Hb SS and at least three VOCs in the prior year. Health diaries were provided for self-assessment of health status. About 83% of subjects were 19 years old or below. Results showed that Niprisan significantly reduced frequency of SCD crisis associated with severe pain compared to placebo (mean value of 7.9 vs 22.1 in Group A for first six months of study, 4.1 vs 6.9 in Group B after crossover, $p < 0.01$) (Wambebe et al., 2001). Using the health diary, subjects on Niprisan rated their health below average less times than those on placebo. Though this was not statistically significant in Group A (mean of 12.2 vs 31.3, $p > 0.05$), it became significant after crossover in Group B (mean of 8.7 vs 18.7, $p < 0.01$) (Wambebe et al., 2001). Adverse events included macular non-pruritic rash that resolved 3–4 days after onset in two subjects taking Niprisan and headaches in six subjects on Niprisan and two subjects on placebo (Wambebe et al., 2001). Renal and liver profiles did not reveal any toxicity (Wambebe et al., 2001).

Following success of the clinical trials, a multipurpose pilot-scale extraction facility was established at NIPRD, made possible by a grant from the UN Development Programme (UNDP), with partnership of the UN Industrial Development Organization (UNIDO) (Wambebe, 2018). By 1998, Niprisan was patented in 46 countries, via a grant from the UNDP (Wambebe, 2018).

Eventually, the company Xechem International Inc. (the United States) was granted the exclusive license for commercial production and global marketing of Niprisan (Nathan et al., 2009; Wambebe, 2018). Xechem set up a manufacturing facility at Abuja, Nigeria, for the commercial production of Niprisan on a global scale. This collaboration marked a first if its kind, where the rights of a medicine fully developed in Africa by indigenous scientists were transferred to a western country/continent to enable upscaled production and global marketing. A commemorative ceremony to mark this milestone took place on July 18, 2002 (Wambebe, 2018). Niprisan was granted orphan drug status by the US Food and Drug Administration (FDA) in 2003 and the European Medicines Agency (EMA) in 2004 (Perampaladas et al., 2010; Wambebe, 2018). In July 2006, the National Agency for Food and Drug Administration and Control (NAFDAC) approved Niprisan (brand name Nicosan), for sale in Nigeria, with an official launch attended by the then Nigerian President Olusegun Obasanjo showing governmental support for the initiative (Perampaladas et al., 2010).

However, due to internal conflicts and financial difficulties, Xechem International filed for bankruptcy in the United States in late 2008 and had its license for Niprisan revoked by the Nigerian government in early 2009 (Hassan & Scott, 2008; Perampaladas et al., 2010; Wambebe, 2018). This led to closing down of its factory in Nigeria and cessation of drug production (Ndhlovu, 2010). It is reported that the Nigerian government took over production through NIPRD but the plan fell through and production stopped in 2015 (Edward-Ekpu, 2019). Since the patent expired in 2017, an Illinois pharmaceutical company, Xickle currently sells its own version of Niprisan (Xickle RBC-Plus) at US$99 for a month's supply (Edward-Ekpu, 2019)

In 2016, results of an open-label, phase IB dose-escalation study of SCD 101 (Niprisan) were reported. The study enrolled 26 subjects with Hb SS and Hb S/beta0 thalassemia, aged 18–55, with primary endpoint of safety of SCD-101 dosed orally (550 mg, 1100 mg, 2200 mg and 4400 mg BID) for 28 days (Swift et al., 2016). Results revealed the drug was safe and well tolerated, without dose reductions or interruptions due to drug-related effects, and without significant change changes in renal/hepatic profiles or markers of hemolysis. It was reported that a repeat cohort study at a higher dose (2,750-mg TID) was ongoing, as well as planned crossover and multisite phase II studies, but results are yet to be reported (Swift et al., 2016). Systematic reviews conducted over the years, most recently in 2020, concluded that Niprisan appeared to be safe and effective in reducing severe painful crises in SCD and encouraged further trials to assess and validate its role in managing people with SCD (Oniyangi & Cohall, 2020).

The story of Niprisan highlights the multi-factorial challenges that can impede successful development, manufacturing, and global scaling of a novel drug with potential benefits to a specific disease population in low-middle income countries. Perampaladas et al. detailed key strategies to foster collaboration among policymakers, entrepreneurs, and domestic innovators in SSA and the developing world, which include supporting business-friendly environments, brokering benefit-sharing agreements with traditional medical healers, expanding incentives for local innovation, improving standardization and quality control, foster partnerships to fill gaps in knowledge and technical expertise, and engaging skilled entrepreneurial leaders (Perampaladas et al., 2010).

Ciklavit®

Ciklavit is a plant extract preparation derived from Cajanus cajan, an edible bean, locally available in Nigeria (Akinsulie et al., 2005; Iweala, Uhegbu, & Ogu, 2009). The anti-sickling property of the extract has been attributed to the amino acid phenylalanine, predicted to be responsible for about 70% of the extract's anti-sickling potency, as well as hydroxybenzoic acid (Akojie & Fung, 1992; Ekeke & Shode, 1990). Prior studies have shown effectiveness of Cajanus cajan in reversing sickle cells (Akojie & Fung, 1992; Draman-Donou, Sangaré-Bamba, Drogon, Fofie, & Sawadogo, 2020; Ekeke & Shode, 1985; Iwu, Igboko, Onwubiko, & Ndu, 1988; Ogoda Onah, Akubue, & Okide, 2002).

In 2005, results of a single-blind placebo-controlled study to assess the properties of Cajanus cajan extract were reported. The study randomized 100 subjects with sickle cell anemia at steady state into treatment and placebo. Treatment consisted of 10-ml aliquot of extract that contained 49 mg of protein with phenylalanine as its major component (26.3%). Inclusion criteria included homozygous SCD confirmed on electrophoresis, in steady state for two weeks prior to enrolment, ages 1–15 years. Subjects with crises, evidence of organ failure, febrile illness in the two weeks preceding enrolment were excluded. Results revealed decreased number of painful episodes pre-study vs during study (total episodes 207–109, p = 0.03 in treatment group vs 191–164 in placebo, p = 0.01). It was concluded that Cajanus cajan may reduce painful crises in sickle cell anemia (Akinsulie et al., 2005). No further larger-scale studies have been reported but Ciklavit is currently available for purchase via several websites.

Pfaffia paniculata

Pfaffia paniculata, also known as Brazilian ginseng, is a perennial wild plant of the Amaranthaceae family that grows in South America (Araújo et al., 2009; Ballas, 2000). It's powdered root extract has been historically used by South American Indians to cure a variety of ailments (Ballas, 2000). An in vitro study published in 2000 was carried out to investigate the effect of Pfaffia paniculata on hydration status of sickle erythrocytes (Ballas, 2000). Washed RBCs from 9 subjects with SCD and 11 controls were exposed to an in vitro concentration of 50 mg/ml of Pfaffia to mimic a similar in vivo concentration achieved with the marketed dosage of 500 mg three times daily. Red cell indices, cation content, and deformability studies were carried out. Results revealed improved deformability of sickle cells and increase in their sodium content and mean corpuscular volume (MCV). The group proposed that Pfaffia paniculata improved rheological properties of sickle erythrocytes, most likely as a sodium ionophore (Ballas, 2000). Another study published in 2015 supported findings of improved red cell deformability in SCD (Mozar et al., 2015).

In 2009, results of another in vitro study verifying the anti-sickling properties of Pfaffia paniculata were published. This was a double-blinded randomized controlled trial comparing the safety and efficacy of *Pfaffia paniculate* to placebo in children with SCD in an outpatient setting in Brazil (Oniyangi & Cohall, 2020). Thirty children with SCD were randomized and enrolled to receive either treatment (two capsules containing the powder extract of Pfaffia paniculata – 500 mg each capsule every eight hours) or placebo for three months. Red blood cells were incubated with pfaffia paniculata, and red cell indices were obtained from peripheral blood immediately before and two and three months after the beginning of the treatment. Results revealed decrease in sickle cells, erythroblast and reticulocytes in blood as well as increase in hemoglobin and hematocrit levels. The authors concluded that Pfaffia paniculata extract possessed anti-sickling properties and can lead to improvement in sickle cell symptoms (Araújo et al., 2009). No further larger-scale studies have been reported but Pfaffia paniculata remains widely available for purchase, as a herbal supplement.

Conclusion/Future of Phytomedicines in SCD

In conclusion, there is still a lot to be uncovered in the utility of phytomedicines for SCD. There seems to be a lot of untapped potential in the application of phytomedicine to SCD, especially in a region like SSA, where access to the current preventative and curative treatments is largely inaccessible. Niprisan remains a prime example of what has been done well and the much-needed areas for improvement – a drug that was developed locally, is now being sold internationally at a price the local benefactors cannot afford. Fostering collaboration among traditional medical healers, physicians and physician scientists, policymakers, investors, and innovators could lead to the discovery and development of phytomedicines with scientifically proven efficacy in SCD. Local production and distribution will go a long way to reduce costs associated with the medicine, as well as costs to consumers. It is imperative that this collaboration continues to be expanded upon, in the long-term interest of patients living with SCD in SSA. This represents a critical avenue for sustainable and holistic care for people living with SCD, the importance, and consequences of which cannot be over-emphasized.

References

Akinsulie, A. O., Temiye, E. O., Akanmu, A. S., Lesi, F. E., & Whyte, C. O. (2005). Clinical evaluation of extract of Cajanus cajan (Ciklavit) in sickle cell anaemia. *J Trop Pediatr*, *51*(4), 200–205. https://doi.org/10.1093/tropej/fmh097

Akojie, F. O., & Fung, L. W. (1992). Antisickling activity of hydroxybenzoic acids in Cajanus cajan. *Planta Med*, *58*(4), 317–320. https://doi.org/10.1055/s-2006-961475

Alabi, O. J., Adegboyega, F. N., Olawoyin, D. S., & Babatunde, O. A. (2022). Functional foods: Promising therapeutics for Nigerian children with sickle cell diseases. *Heliyon*, *8*(6), e09630. https://doi.org/10.1016/j.heliyon.2022.e09630

Ameh, S. J., Tarfa, F. D., & Ebeshi, B. U. (2012). Traditional herbal management of sickle cell anemia: Lessons from Nigeria. *Anemia*, 607436. https://doi.org/10.1155/2012/607436

Amujoyegbe, O. O., Idu, M., Agbedahunsi, J. M., & Erhabor, J. O. (2016). Ethnomedicinal survey of medicinal plants used in the management of sickle cell disorder in Southern Nigeria. *J Ethnopharmacol*, *185*, 347–360. https://doi.org/10.1016/j.jep.2016.03.042

Araújo, J. T., Bydlowski, S., & Mendoza, T. R. T. (2009). Pfaffia paniculata extract improves hydratation of eritrocytes in vitro and sickle cell disease symptoms. *Revista Brasileira de Medicina*, *66*, 386–389.

Awodogan, A., Wambebe, C., Gamaniel, K., Okogun, J., Orisadipe, A., & Akah, P. (1996). Acute and short-term toxicity of NIPRISAN in rats I: Biochemical study. *J Pharmacol Res Dev*, *1*, 39–45.

Ballas, S. K. (2000). Hydration of sickle erythrocytes using a herbal extract (Pfaffia paniculata) in vitro. *Br J Haematol*, *111*(1), 359–362. https://doi.org/10.1046/j.1365-2141.2000.02276.x

Bhatt, A. (2010). Evolution of clinical research: A history before and beyond james lind. *Perspect Clin Res*, *1*(1), 6–10.

Bianchi, N., Zuccato, C., Lampronti, I., Borgatti, M., & Gambari, R. (2009). Fetal hemoglobin inducers from the natural world: A novel approach for identification of drugs for the treatment of {beta}-thalassemia and sickle-cell anemia. *Evid Based Complement Alternat Med*, *6*(2), 141–151. https://doi.org/10.1093/ecam/nem139

Busari, A. A., & Mufutau, M. A. (2017). High prevalence of complementary and alternative medicine use among patients with sickle cell disease in a tertiary hospital in Lagos, South West, Nigeria. *BMC Complement Altern Med*, *17*(1), 299. https://doi.org/10.1186/s12906-017-1812-2

Chung, K. T., Wong, T. Y., Wei, C. I., Huang, Y. W., & Lin, Y. (1998). Tannins and human health: A review. *Crit Rev Food Sci Nutr*, *38*(6), 421–464. https://doi.org/10.1080/10408699891274273

Dennis-Antwi, J. A., Culley, L., Hiles, D. R., & Dyson, S. M. (2011). 'I can die today, I can die tomorrow': Lay perceptions of sickle cell disease in Kumasi, Ghana at a point of transition. *Ethn Health*, *16*(4–5), 465–481. https://doi.org/10.1080/13557858.2010.531249

Dey, P., Kundu, A., Kumar, A., Gupta, M., Lee, B. M., Bhakta, T., … Kim, H. S. (2020). Analysis of alkaloids (indole alkaloids, isoquinoline alkaloids, tropane alkaloids). *Recent Adv Nat Products Anal*, 505–567. https://doi.org/10.1016/B978-0-12-816455-6.00015-9

242 *Oluseyi Oniyangi and Ugochi O. Ogu*

Draman-Donou, E. N., Sangaré-Bamba, M., Drogon, E., Fofie, Y., & Sawadogo, D. (2020). Evaluation and comparison of anti-sickling activities of macerated seeds of Cajanus cajan and phenylalanine. *Int J Adv Res.* **8** (Feb). 872–876 (ISSN 2320-5407). www.journalijar. com

Eaton, W. A., & Bunn, H. F. (2017). Treating sickle cell disease by targeting HbS polymerization. *Blood*, *129*(20), 2719–2726. https://doi.org/10.1182/blood-2017-02-765891

Edward-Ekpu, U. (2019). Nigerian scientists patented a sickle cell drug using a traditional herbal remedy—then it all fell apart. Retrieved from https://qz.com/africa/1547079/nigerian-scientists-patented-a-sickle-cell-drug-using-a-traditional-herbal-remedy-then-it-all-fell-apart

Ekeke, G. I., & Shode, F. O. (1985). The reversion of sickled cells by Cajanus cajan. *Planta Med*, *51*(6), 504–507. https://doi.org/10.1055/s-2007-969576

Ekeke, G. I., & Shode, F. O. (1990). Phenylalanine is the predominant antisickling agent in Cajanus cajan seed extract. *Planta Med*, *56*(1), 41–43. https://doi.org/10.1055/s-2006-960880

Gamaniel, K., Amos, S., Akah, P., Samuel, B., Kapu, S., Olusola, A., … Wambebe, C. (1998). Pharmacological profile of NIPRD 94/002/1-0: A novel herbal antisickling agent. *J Pharmaceut Res Dev*, *3*(2), 89–94.

Hassan, A., & Scott, C. (2008). Sickle cell drug mired in controversy. *SciDev. net-Enterprise.* Retrieved from https://www.scidev.net/global/news/sickle-cell-drug-mired-in-controversy/

Holoch, D., & Moazed, D. (2015). RNA-mediated epigenetic regulation of gene expression. *Nat Rev Genet*, *16*(2), 71–84. https://doi.org/10.1038/nrg3863

Ilagouma, A. T., Amadou, I., Issaka, H., & Ikhiri, K. (2019). Preliminary study to identify anti-sickle cell plants in Nigers traditional pharmacopoeia and their phytochemicals. *J Med Plants Res*, *13*(19), 509–517.

Imaga, N. A. (2013). Phytomedicines and nutraceuticals: Alternative therapeutics for sickle cell anemia. *Sci World J*, 269659. https://doi.org/10.1155/2013/269659

Imaga, N. A., & Taiwo, O. (2017). Different therapeutic interventions and mechanisms of action of antisickling agents currently in use in sickle cell disease management. *EMJ Hematol.* 2017;5(1):113–117. DOI/10.33590/e

Iweala, E. E., Uhegbu, F. O., & Ogu, G. N. (2009). Preliminary in vitro antisickilng properties of crude juice extracts of Persia Americana, Citrus sinensis, Carica papaya and Ciklavit®. *Afr J Tradit Complement Altern Med*, *7*(2), 113–117. https://doi.org/10.4314/ajtcam.v7i2.50867

Iwu, M. M., Igboko, A. O., Onwubiko, H., & Ndu, U. E. (1988). Effect of cajaminose from Cajanus cajan on gelation and oxygen affinity of sickle cell haemoglobin. *J Ethnopharmacol*, *23*(1), 99–104. https://doi.org/10.1016/0378-8741(88)90118-3

Iyamu, E. W., Turner, E. A., & Asakura, T. (2002). In vitro effects of NIPRISAN (Nix-0699): A naturally occurring, potent antisickling agent. *Br J Haematol*, *118*(1), 337–343. https://doi.org/10.1046/j.1365-2141.2002.03593.x

Iyamu, E. W., Turner, E. A., & Asakura, T. (2003). Niprisan (Nix-0699) improves the survival rates of transgenic sickle cell mice under acute severe hypoxic conditions. *Br J Haematol*, *122*(6), 1001–1008. https://doi.org/10.1046/j.1365-2141.2003.04536.x

Lubega, M., Osingada, C. P., & Kasirye, P. (2021). Use of herbal medicine by caregivers in the management of children with sickle cell disease in Mulago National Referral Hospital – Uganda. *Pan Afr Med J*, *39*, 163. https://doi.org/10.11604/pamj.2021.39.163.20740

Mishra, G., & Pandya, D. (2019). A revised ayurvedic approach to sickle cell disease. *Int Ayurvedic Med J*, 2019, 55–58.

Mozar, A., Charlot, K., Sandor, B., Rabaï, M., Lemonne, N., Billaud, M., ... Ballas, S. K. (2015). Pfaffia paniculata extract improves red blood cell deformability in sickle cell patients. *Clin Hemorheol Microcirc*, *62*(4), 327–333. https://doi.org/10.3233/ch-151972

Mrinalini, B., Snehal, K., Shubham, B., Ayesha, S., & Subhash, P. (2021). Dominance of herbal medicines in treating sickel cell anemia. *Int J Ayurveda Pharma Res*, *9*(2). https://doi.org/10.47070/ijapr.v9i2.1816

Mugford, S. T., & Osbourn, A. (2013). Saponin synthesis and function. In T. J. Bach & M. Rohmer (Eds.), *Isoprenoid synthesis in plants and microorganisms: New concepts and experimental approaches* (pp. 405–424). Springer New York.

Nathan, S., Tripathi, P., Wu, Q., & Belanger, F. C. (2009). Nicosan: Phytomedicinal treatment for sickle cell disease. In *African Natural plant products: New discoveries and challenges in chemistry and quality* (Vol. 1021, pp. 263–276): American Chemical Society.

Ndhlovu, D.-F. (2010). Funding woes afflict African herbal therapy institute. *Nature*. https://doi.org/10.1038/news.2010.602

Ng, N. Y., & Ko, C. H. (2014). Natural remedies for the treatment of beta-thalassemia and sickle cell anemia – current status and perspectives in fetal hemoglobin reactivation. *Int Sch Res Notices*, 123257. https://doi.org/10.1155/2014/123257

Ogoda Onah, J., Akubue, P. I., & Okide, G. B. (2002). The kinetics of reversal of pre-sickled erythrocytes by the aqueous extract of Cajanus cajan seeds. *Phytother Res*, *16*(8), 748–750. https://doi.org/10.1002/ptr.1026

Ohnishi, S. T., Ohnishi, T., & Ogunmola, G. B. (2001). Green tea extract and aged garlic extract inhibit anion transport and sickle cell dehydration in vitro. *Blood Cells Mol Dis*, *27*(1), 148–157. https://doi.org/10.1006/bcmd.2000.0368

Okoh, P. M., Alli, A. L., Tolvanen, E. E. M., & Nwegbu, M. M. (2019). Herbal drug use in sickle cell disease management; Trends and perspectives in Sub-Saharan Africa – A systematic review. *Current Drug Discovery Technol*, *16*(4), 372–385. https://doi.org/10.2174/1570163815666181002101611

Oniyangi, O., & Cohall, D. H. (2020). Phytomedicines (medicines derived from plants) for sickle cell disease. *Cochrane Database Syst Rev*, *9*(9), Cd004448. https://doi.org/10.1002/14651858.CD004448.pub7

Organization, W. H. (2013). *WHO traditional medicine strategy: 2014–2023*. World Health Organization.

Organization, W. H. (2018). WHO guidelines on good herbal processing practices for herbal medicines. *WHO Technical Report Series* (1010).

Organization, W. H. (2019). *WHO global report on traditional and complementary medicine 2019*. World Health Organization.

Panche, A. N., Diwan, A. D., & Chandra, S. R. (2016). Flavonoids: An overview. *J Nutr Sci*, *5*, e47. https://doi.org/10.1017/jns.2016.41

Perampaladas, K., Masum, H., Kapoor, A., Shah, R., Daar, A. S., & Singer, P. A. (2010). The road to commercialization in Africa: Lessons from developing the sickle-cell drug Niprisan. *BMC Int Health Hum Rights*, *10*(Suppl 1), S11. https://doi.org/10.1186/1472-698x-10-s1-s11

Rasouli, H., Farzaei, M. H., & Khodarahmi, R. (2017). Polyphenols and their benefits: A review. *Int J Food Prop*, *20*(sup2), 1700–1741. https://doi.org/10.1080/10942912.2017.1354017

Srivastava, A., Srivastava, P., Pandey, A., Khanna, V. K., & Pant, A. B. (2019). Chapter 24 - phytomedicine: A potential alternative medicine in controlling neurological disorders. In M. S. Ahmad Khan, I. Ahmad, & D. Chattopadhyay (Eds.), *New look to phytomedicine* (pp. 625–655). Academic Press.

Sundd, P., Gladwin, M. T., & Novelli, E. M. (2019). Pathophysiology of sickle cell disease. *Annu Rev Pathol*, *14*, 263–292. https://doi.org/10.1146/annurev-pathmechdis-012418-012838

Swift, R., Abdulmalik, O., Chen, Q., Asakura, T., Gustafson, K., Simon, J. E., ... Gillette, P. N. (2016). SCD-101: A new anti-sickling drug reduces pain and fatigue and improves red blood cell shape in peripheral blood of patients with sickle cell disease. *Blood*, *128*(22), 121. https://doi.org/10.1182/blood.V128.22.121.121

Wambebe, C. (2018). The story of niprisan: A clinically effective phytomedicine for the management of sickle cell disorder. In *African indigenous medical knowledge and human health* (pp. 151–164). CRC Press.

Wambebe, C., Khamofu, H., Momoh, J. A., Ekpeyong, M., Audu, B. S., Njoku, O. S., ... Ogunyale, O. (2001). Double-blind, placebo-controlled, randomised cross-over clinical trial of NIPRISAN in patients with sickle cell disorder. *Phytomedicine*, *8*(4), 252–261. https://doi.org/10.1078/0944-7113-00040

Wei, J.-W., Huang, K., Yang, C., & Kang, C.-S. (2017). Non-coding RNAs as regulators in epigenetics (review). *Oncol Rep*, *37*(1), 3–9. https://doi.org/10.3892/or.2016.5236

16 Investigational Therapies and Advances in Science for SCD

A Glimmer of Hope

Dunia Hatabah and Miguel Abboud

Pathophysiology of SCD Disease

To better understand sickle cell disease (SCD) treatment, it is important to understand its pathophysiology. A better understanding of the mechanisms of disease will, hopefully, lead to the development of targeted approaches to treatment which has hitherto been focused on effective but nonspecific supportive and preventive therapies (Figure 16.1). SCD is caused by a single nucleotide mutation substituting glutamine for valine at position 6 in the β-globin chain, forming sickle hemoglobin, HbS (Goldstein, Konigsberg, & Hill, 1963). Under states of low oxygen tension, HbS polymerizes causing the cells to develop the characteristic sickle shape. Sickling of the erythrocyte leads to injury of the membrane, cellular dehydration, and eventually, premature clearance. Clinically, repetitive HbS polymerization (sickling) manifests in chronic hemolytic anemia and recurrent episodic vaso-occlusive events the hallmark of which are painful crises and cumulative organ damage.

The pathophysiology of SCD is that of a multicellular paradigm that is not limited to the sickled red blood cells (RBCs) but also involves other cell types in almost every organ of the body (Figure 16.2). Polymerization of HbS triggers a conformational change in the RBC rendering it less flexible and more adhesive. The rigid RBCs are then more easily sequestered in the microcirculation causing episodic and sustained vaso-occlusion. In addition to mechanical sequestration, chemical adhesion plays a significant role in vaso-occlusion. Chemical adhesion is a consequence of endothelial dysfunction from free Hb released from hemolyzed RBCs and depleted nitric oxide (NO) (Zhang et al., 2016). Endothelial dysfunction creates the inflammatory milieu of SCD which in turn leads to the recruitment of neutrophils and platelets. This is confirmed by the fact that patients with higher neutrophil count usually have more severe disease (Miller et al., 2000). Neutrophils are central agents in vaso-occlusion as they interact with both the endothelium and RBCs. This aspect of the pathophysiology has gained significant relevance as adhesion is mediated by molecules such as P- and E-selectin which are now targets for novel therapeutic agents. Platelets are also activated forming aggregates with monocytes, neutrophils, and erythrocytes in a P-selectin-dependent manner (Zhang et al., 2016). The constant interaction between RBC and endothelium creates an inflammatory state and promotes a hypercoagulable state. This is

DOI: 10.4324/9781003463931-17

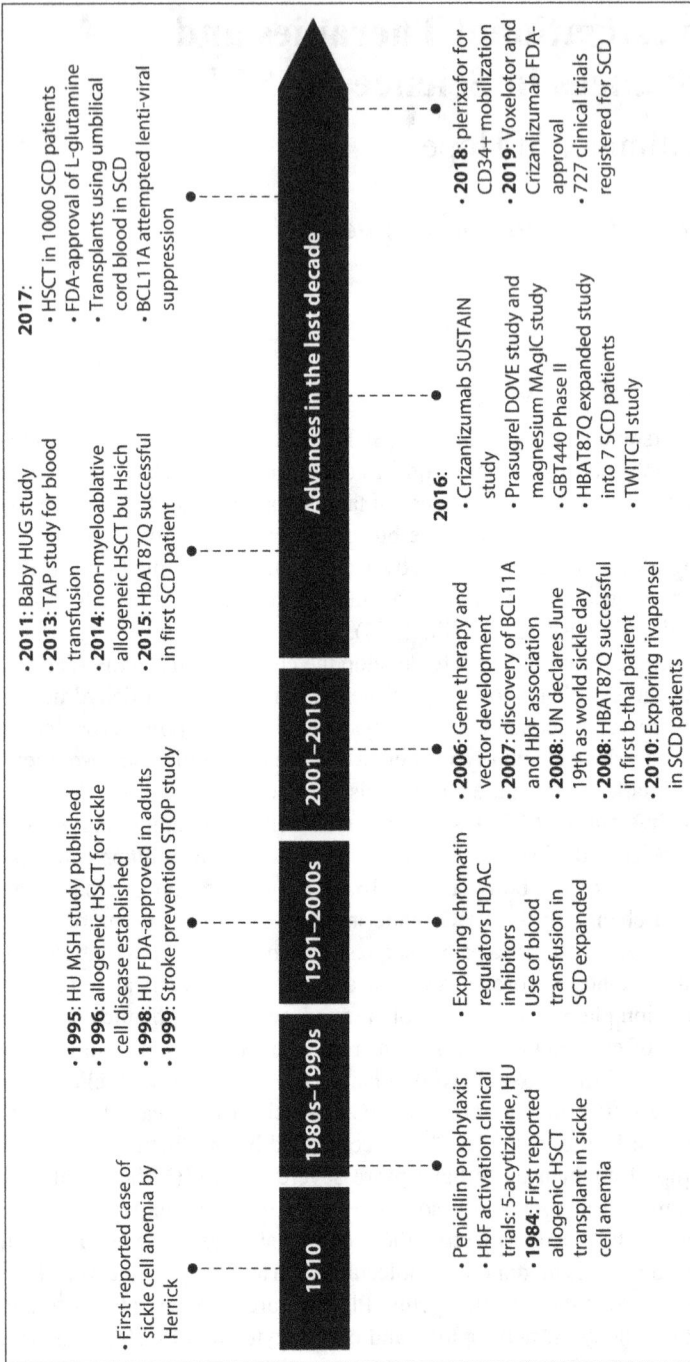

Figure 16.1 Timeline of sickle cell disease historic events (Salinas Cisneros & Thein, 2020).

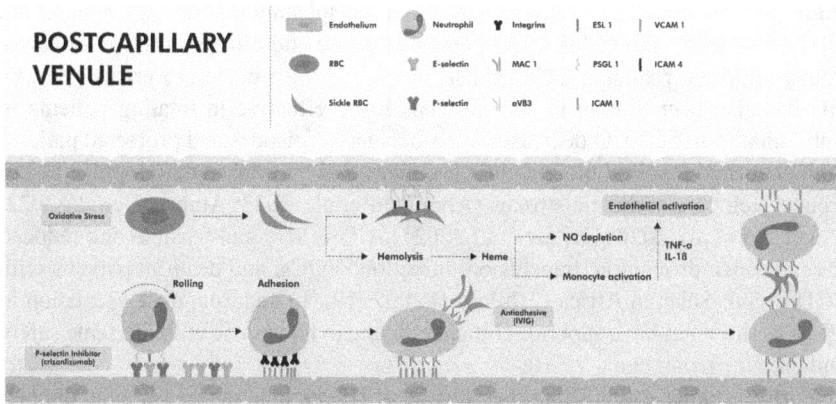

Figure 16.2 Pathophysiology of sickle cell disease.

evidenced by increased levels of tissue factor and coagulation factors, and clinically in the increased incidence of venous and arterial thrombotic events in SCD patients (Brunson et al., 2017).

Targeting the downstream sequelae of HbS polymerization has gained momentum in clinical trials of many potential therapeutic agents; however, none have yet proven to be as effective as "anti-sickling" approaches that act via induction of HbF. Increasing HbF concentrations delays the time to HbS polymerization by diluting HbS, in addition, the γ-chains of HbF have a direct inhibitory effect on polymerization (Eaton & Bunn, 2017). This is evidenced in patients with co-existing SCD and hereditary persistence of HbF who typically have a benign clinical course (Serjeant, Serjeant, & Mason, 1977). Even modest elevations in HbF are associated with a decreased severity of SCD and increased overall survival (Platt et al., 1994).

Insight into the pathophysiology of SCD has paved the way for targeted treatment which can be summarized into four categories: (1) HbF induction and anti-sickling (2), inhibition of vaso-occlusion, (3) inflammation, and (4) gene therapy.

HbF Induction and Anti-sickling

Hydroxyurea (HU) is an antineoplastic drug that inhibits ribonucleotide reductase, a pathway involved in pyrimidine metabolism. The specific mechanism of action for HU is not well established. However, HU has exhibited significant improvement in morbidity and mortality in SCD patients. This is due to several attributed mechanisms including HbF induction and increased concentration, increased NO availability, increased red cell volume, and reduced interaction between RBCs and the endothelium.

In 1998 the randomized Multi-Center Study of Hydroxyurea (MSH) demonstrated that HU significantly reduced painful crises, acute chest syndrome, and hospital admissions in adults with SCD (Charache et al., 1996). In 2011 the BABY HUG trial was designed to determine whether HU in young children aged 9–17 months can safely prevent end-organ damage namely in the spleen and kidneys (Wang et al., 2011). The study showed that HU possesses a safe and efficient profile for use in young children, reducing ACS, transfusions, and vaso-occlusive crises (VOCs). HU has also been shown in several trials to be effective in treating patients in Sub-Saharan Africa. HU decreased vaso-occlusive episodes and protected patients with abnormal cerebral blood velocities, measured by transcranial doppler TCDs, from developing ischemic strokes (Abdullahi et al., 2023; Ambrose et al., 2022; Galadanci et al., 2020; Heitzer et al., 2021). HU is safe and feasible and reduced the incidence of malaria, transfusion, infection, VOCs, and death in patients with SCD in Sub-Saharan Africa (Tshilolo et al., 2019). In addition, dose escalation in HU was shown to have superior clinical efficacy to fixed dose with the same safety and efficacy (John et al., 2020).

Further studies establishing the efficacy of HU include the transcranial doppler with Transfusion switching to Hydroxyurea study (TWiTCH) which showed that HU is comparable to blood transfusion in primary stroke prevention (Ware et al., 2016). HU increases HbF concentrations equally in RBCs referred to as F-cells and some studies have shown its impact on HbF induction decreases over time (Salinas Cisneros & Thein, 2020). Several other treatments to increase HbF (including pharmacologic agents as well as gene-editing techniques) are currently undergoing clinical trials. Some of these treatments will be discussed in a later section and the other promising therapies are outlined in Table 16.1.

Voxelotor (oxbryta) is a unique Food and Drug administration (FDA)-approved anti-sickling agent. In 2019 it received FDA approval for the treatment of SCD in patients >12 years of age. Voxelotor binds the α-chain of HbS causing allosteric modification and an increase in Hb-O$_2$ affinity (Howard et al., 2021). This in turn inhibits sickling and destruction of erythrocytes which improves Hb level and decreases markers of hemolysis. The HOPE trial showed improvements in Hb level and hemolytic markers but there was no statistically significant reduction in VOCs or acute chest syndrome (ACS) (Howard et al., 2021). However, it has been theorized that Voxelotor may benefit SCD patients with a hemolytic phenotype as

Table 16.1 Treatment for HbF induction.

Drug	Target	Mechanism
Panobinostat	Pan histone deacetylase (HDAC)	In vitro analysis of HDAC inhibition has shown to increase levels γ-globin. *(ClinicalTrials. gov Identifier: NCT01245179).*
Decitabine	DNMT1	Inhibition of DNMT1 which is involved in shutting down γ-globin chain production after birth is associated with increased levels of HbF when given orally with tetrahydrouridine. *(ClinicalTrials.gov Identifier: NCT01685515).*

opposed to those with a vaso-occlusive phenotype. Patients with a hemolytic phenotype usually have limited options to improve their anemia symptoms if they have not responded to HU or the patients cannot tolerate HU, including blood transfusions and their associated complications. Voxelotor can be a good option for these patients as it can increase their Hb levels (Oksenberg et al., 2016) with or without HU. In 2021, Voxelotor received FDA approval for the treatment of SCD in patients ≥4 years. At the present time, the phase 2 HOPE -KIDS 1 trial is studying Voxelotor in children aged 6 months to 18 years (NCT02850406).

A next generation HbS polymerization inhibitor GBT 021601 is currently being investigated in a phase 2/3 study. Compared to voxelotor, GBT021601 may result in greater Hb occupancies at lower dosages, which may lessen treatment burden and enhance clinical outcomes. Saraf et al have reported on the preliminary safety and efficacy of oral GBT021601 in adults with SCD (Saraf et al., 2023). GBT021601 was well tolerated with an increase in mean Hb levels, without an associated increase in pain episodes (Saraf et al., 2023).

Inhibiting Vaso-occlusion

Painful crisis is the hallmark of SCD, with VOCs being the principal cause of emergency department visits (Brousseau et al., 2010). It has been postulated that adherence of sickled erythrocytes to the dysfunctional endothelium accompanied by platelets and leukocytes is a driver of vaso-occlusion. Continuous production of reactive oxygen species (ROS) with subsequent oxidative stress contributes to the ongoing inflammation and endothelial dysfunction that promote vaso-occlusion in SCD. An abundant redox cofactor in RBCs is nicotinamide adenine dinucleotide (NAD) and its reduced form NADH+ that play an important role in maintaining redox balance (Morris et al., 2017). Glutamine is the amino acid precursor of NAD, and its uptake is greatly increased in sickled RBCs as compared to controls (Niihara et al., 1995). Studies have shown that the oral administration of L-glutamine is associated with clinical improvement and an increase in NAD redox ratio in the RBCs (Niihara et al., 1998). Furthermore, treatment of sickled RBCs of five SCD patients with L-glutamine has decreased the adhesion of sickled cells to human umbilical vein endothelial cells compared to control SCD patients treated with placebo (Niihara et al., 2005). SCD severity was shown to correlate with erythrocyte adherence (Hebbel et al., 1980). In 2018 a phase 3 trial tested the efficacy of L-glutamine and showed that over 48 weeks the median number of pain crises was lower in patients receiving oral L-glutamine with or without HU as compared to placebo with or without HU (Niihara et al., 2018). L-glutamine is now an FDA-approved therapy for patients with SCD.

As the endothelium has become increasingly recognized as an important contributor to the activation of adhesion molecules leading to vaso-occlusion, novel therapies have emerged targeting adhesion molecules (Figure 16.3). In 2019 Crizanlizumab (Adakveo) was approved by the FDA for the treatment of SCD. Crizanlizumab is a monoclonal antibody targeting P-selectin. Crizanlizumab was shown to decrease the annual rate of VOCs, time to first VOC, and hospitalization

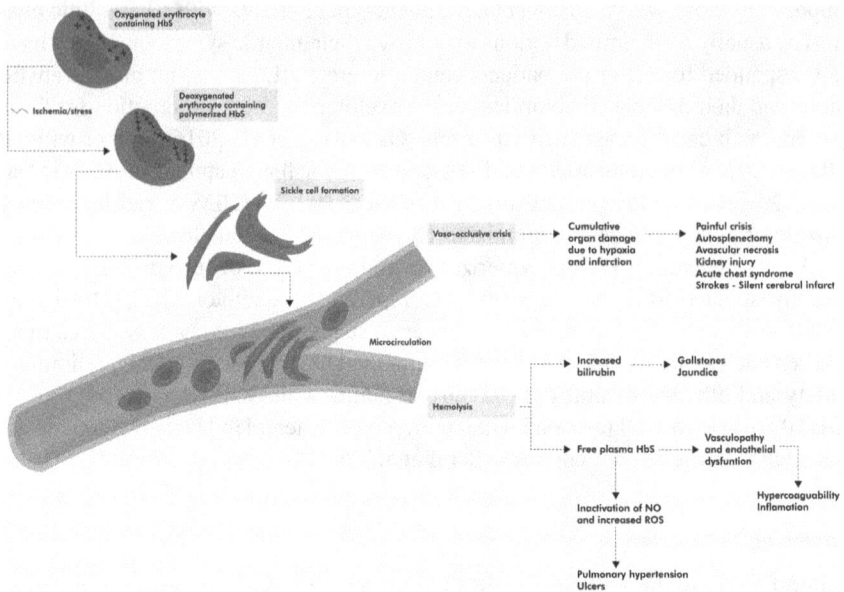

Figure 16.3 Pathophysiology of vaso-occlusion in sickle cell disease.

due to VOCs in several clinical trials (Ataga et al., 2017; Kutlar et al., 2019). Despite approval that continues in the US a recent trial failed to demonstrate superiority of crizanlizumab over placebo in decreasing the rate of VOCs in patients with SCD ≥ 12 years old (Abboud et al., 2023). Preliminary data from the SPARTAN trial exploring the efficacy of crizanlizumab in patients with priapism has shown that patients with SCD-related priapism treated with crizanlizumab over a 26-week period had roughly half as many priapic events when compared to baseline (Idowu et al., 2023).

Studies of other anti-adherence agents including sevuparin (heparinoid), rivapansel (pan-selectin inhibitor), and poloxamer (nonionic block polymer surfactant) unfortunately have failed to demonstrate any impact of these agents in shortening the duration of a painful crisis once started. It thus seems that anti-adhesive agents may be more useful in preventing VOCs from developing rather than treating VOC (Biemond et al., 2021; Casella et al., 2021; Telen et al., 2016). Their impact on end-organ dysfunction remains to be demonstrated.

Other promising therapies targeting vaso-occlusion include arginine (Morris et al., 2005). Arginine metabolism in SCD differs between adults and children. Adults are arginine deficient at a steady state whereas children are arginine sufficient (Morris, 2014; Morris et al., 2005). However, arginine levels drop in both adults and children during VOCs and ACS. Arginine is the obligate substrate of NO and arginine dysregulation leads to depletion of NO which contributes to the oxidative stress already established in SCD patients (Morris, 2014). NO is an important regulator of vascular health; states of deficient NO are associated with increased platelet aggregation and inflammation. Arginine deficiency in the population is complex; however, it can be restored by arginine supplementation known as the "arginine paradox" (Morris, 2014). Oral administration of arginine in adult SCD patients at baseline has shown a paradoxical decrease in NO synthesis as compared to controls that showed an increase in synthesis (Morris et al., 2000). However, in SCD patients with VOCs, intravenous arginine dramatically increased NO synthesis in a dose-dependent manner (Morris et al., 2013). Multiple phase 2 trials have demonstrated the efficacy and safety of arginine in VOCs (Morris et al., 2013; Onalo, Cilliers, & Cooper, 2021; Onalo, Cilliers, Cooper, & Morris, 2022; Onalo, Cooper, et al., 2021; Reyes et al., 2022). In Nigeria oral arginine therapy improved pain control in children with SCD-VOC with reduction in time-to-crisis resolution, length of hospital stay and analgesic requirement in children receiving arginine compared to placebo (Onalo et al., 2021). Oral arginine has also shown to improve cardiopulmonary hemodynamics by decreasing tricuspid regurgitant velocity (a marker of pulmonary hypertension) and improving blood pressure parameters in children with SCD-VOC compared to placebo (Onalo et al., 2022). A phase 3 trial of intravenous arginine in children with SCD is currently underway (Rees et al., 2023).

Inflammation

It has been previously mentioned that SCD is an inflammatory state, targeting inflammation should impact SCD complications. SCD patients are trapped in a vicious cycle of continuous inflammation characterized by constitutional activation of platelets, neutrophils, coagulation factors, monocytes, and endothelium.

Inhibiting platelets was theorized to decrease inflammation, as platelet activation contributes to increasing leukocyte activation and RBC adhesion. Prasugrel, ticagrelor, and clopidogrel are all platelet inhibitors studied to assess this theory. Unfortunately, clinical trials using these drugs have yielded negative results with no decrease in the incidence of VOC (Conran & Rees, 2017; Heeney et al., 2015; Kanter et al., 2019). Statins and intravenous immunoglobulins (IVIG) also have an anti-inflammatory effect and early studies are promising. Clinical trials investigating the roles of statins have shown a decrease in inflammatory and adhesive factors such as C-reactive protein, E-selectin, and I-CAM1. Simvastatin specifically has decreased pain crises and inflammation markers when used in conjunction with HU (Hoppe et al., 2017). A clinical trial assessing Simvastatin's effectiveness on central nervous vasculature is currently underway (ClinicalTrials.gov Identifier: NCT03599609).

Murine studies have shown that administration of IVIG in sickle cell mice rapidly reversed acute VOCs through neutrophil adhesion inhibition (Chang et al., 2008). These studies laid down a solid base for clinical trials, a phase I human clinical trial of IVIG vs placebo demonstrated a decrease in Mac-1 in the low-dose IVIG patients (Manwani et al., 2015). A phase II trial is currently underway to determine the safety and effectiveness of IVIG in the treatment of VOCs in SCD patients (ClinicalTrials.gov Identifier: NCT01757418).

Stem Cell Transplantation and Gene Therapy

Curative therapies were first described in an eight-year-old girl with SCD who underwent a hematopoietic stem cell transplant (HSCT) (Johnson et al., 1984). The patient had developed acute myeloblastic leukemia (AML) and underwent HSCT which cured both her SCD and AML. Since then, many trials have shown the positive impact of matched sibling donor transplantation in both children and selected adults with SCD. While fully myeloablative regimens are preferred in children with matched sibling donors, less intensive regimens are being investigated in adults. It is of interest to note that patients with SCD do not need to maintain 100% myeloid donor chimerism, 20% myeloid donor chimerism has been shown to cure SCD (Fitzhugh et al., 2017).

Allogenic HSCT is being extensively studied with more than 35 clinical trials currently registered. HSCT provides a new source of erythropoiesis and can also reverse organ dysfunction. Allogenic HSCT is safest and most effective with a matched sibling donor (MSD). Patients can undergo bone marrow conditioning with either reduced-intensity chemotherapy or myeloablative chemotherapy (Gluckman et al., 2017). This is the preferred approach for children. Using these regimens has been proven to be safest in patients less than 15 years with the best results obtained in patients below 5 years of age, with an MSD and no contraindications to transplant. Studies have shown that patients 16 years or older were associated with a greater risk of graft-versus-host disease (GVHD) and worse overall survival (Gluckman et al., 2017). This is because adult patients have more extensive cumulative organ damage rendering conditioning to be too toxic. In adults, Hsieh et al. demonstrated that a non-myeloablative regimen that includes alemtuzumab, low dose total body radiation, and post-transplant sirolimus was safe and effective for MSD transplantation of older patients with many co-morbidities (Hsieh et al., 2009).

Major limitations of HSCT include toxicity, cost, and the fact that only about 18% of patients have an MSD. To date, results with matched unrelated bone marrow donors or cord blood have been poor with a high incidence of GVHD. Many studies are now underway utilizing haploidentical family donors, with promising results. Broadly there are two approaches to haploidentical transplants one utilizing alpha and beta T-cell depletion and the other utilizing post-transplant cyclophosphamide. Initial studies have shown promising results with both techniques and the best modality is yet to be determined. Despite the advances, all HSCT procedures generate higher risks for GVHD, graft rejection, morbidity, and mortality, and finding donors is a major limitation (Angelucci et al., 2014; Bolaños-Meade et al., 2012; Fitzhugh et al., 2014; Saraf et al., 2018). Overcoming these limitations can be achieved with autologous HSCT where the patients' own stem cells are harvested, genetically engineered, and reinserted into the host.

Genetically modified autologous cells abrogate the need for a matched donor, and since there is no foreign cellular introduction immunosuppression and GVHD are no longer risks (Esrick & Bauer, 2018). Albeit its advantages autologous HSCT remains a challenge in SCD patients, and the reasons are twofold. First, the collection of stem cells includes the harvesting of CD34$^+$ cells which are of suboptimal quantity and quality in SCD patients. This leads to the need for multiple harvesting procedures which increases the risk of an acute pain crisis with every harvest. Secondly, the procedure in which these cells are harvested entails the use of granulocyte-colony stimulating factor (G-CSF). G-CSF is contraindicated in SCD patients as it increases white cell count posing an increased risk for ACS, VOCs, and even death (Salinas Cisneros & Thein, 2020).

Plerixafor is an agent that assists with the harvesting of CD34+ cells with a safer profile in SCD patients. Plerixafor stimulates the release of CD34+ cells from the bone marrow without the associated increase in white cell count. Furthermore, the harvested cells have shown to be of great quality and quantity eliminating the risk of pain crisis due to multiple harvesting techniques (Boulad et al., 2018; Esrick et al., 2018). Once these cells have been harvested genetic alterations of SCD can be edited through several methods.

The genetic defect in SCD can be altered through either gene addition or gene editing. Gene addition utilizes a lentivirus as a vector to deliver therapeutic genes. This involves autologous hematopoietic transplant of stem cells treated ex vivo with gene therapy. HbA^{T87Q} is an anti-sickling adult HbA analogue with a modified β-globin gene (Pawliuk et al., 2001; Takekoshi, Oh, Westerman, London, & Leboulch, 1995). The modified β-globin gene is transduced into autologous hematopoietic stem cells with the BB305 lentiviral vector, resulting in the production of HbA^{T87Q}. HbA^{T87Q} has 99.9% homology with adult Hb with similar oxygen-carrying capacity, and similar oxygen-Hb dissociation curves (Kanter et al., 2021). In 2017 Ribeil at al reported the successful treatment with lentiviral gene therapy in a patient with SCD with complete clinical remission and amelioration of the biologic hallmarks of the disease (Ribeil et al., 2017). On December 8th, 2024, FDA granted approval of Lyfgenia (lovotibeglogene autotemcel) to Bluebird Bio Inc (U.S. Food & Drug Administration, 2023). Lyfgenia is a cell-based gene therapy for the treatment of patients with SCD 12 years and older utilizing a lentiviral vector for genetic modification of allogenic stem cells. Data from a recent clinical trial of Lyfgenia in patients with SCD demonstrated sustained HbA^{T87Q} levels with almost complete resolution of VOCs up to 18 months post treatment (Kanter et al., 2023). Patients underwent stem cell mobilization with plerixafor, where their cells were genetically modified to produce HbA^{T87Q}. This was followed with busulfan myeloablative conditioning after which patients received the drug product awaiting engraftment and reconstitution with antisickling Hb. Safety profile was consistent with known adverse events of myeloablative conditioning and underlying SCD, no insertional oncogenesis or malignancies were detected. In previous clinical trials of Lyfgenia utilizing different manufacturing and transplantation techniques two patients developed hematologic malignancies (Goyal et al., 2021; Hsieh et al., 2020). Lyfgenia is a potentially curative and transformative therapy, however, it is prescribed with a black box warning, we believe follow up should be in all patients undergoing gene therapy who require high dose chemotherapy therapy such as busulfan.

As for gene editing, the technique cluster regularly interspaced short palindromic repeat (CRISPR) associated caspase 9 (Cas9) has gained the most popularity. CRISPR-Cas9 causes a double-strand break in a genome, followed by repair, resulting in either knockout or gene disruption. CRISPR-Cas 9 induces HbF by

Table 16.2 Current and upcoming studies of gene therapy in SCD (Kanter & Falcon, 2021).

Study name	*LentiGlobin	DREPAGLOBE	*CLIMB	PRECIZN-1	Genetic silencing of BCL11A	MOMENTUM	CEDAR
Type of gene therapy	Gene addition	Gene addition	Gene editing	Gene editing	Gene silencing	Gene addition	Gene correction
Editing tool	NA	NA	CRISPR-Cas9 RNP	Zinc finger	ShRNA	NA	HiFi CRISPR-Cas9 RNP
Vector (y/n)	BB305 LVV	DROBE 1 LVV	None	None	BCH-BB694 LVV that encodes a microRNA-adapted shRNA	γG16D LVV	Nonintegrating AAV6 donor DNA repair template
Genetic target (y/n)	NA	NA	Erythroid lineage-specific enhancer of the BCL11A gene	11A (BCL11A) locus (erythroid enhancer)	BCL11A mRNA	NA	Sickle mutation (adenosine > thymine [A—>T]
Drug product	LentiGlobin BB305	DREPAGLOBE	CTX001	BIVV003	BCH-BB694	ARU-1801	GPH101
Protein product	HbA^{T87Q}	βAS3, an antisickling β-globin protein (AS3) containing 3 amino acid substitutions in the wild-type HBB	HbF	HbF	HbF	HbF^{G16D}	HbA

* FDA approved (U.S. Food & Drug Administration, 2023).

causing erythrocyte-specific BCL11A gene disruption. Manifestations of SCD appear once HbF begins to wane, hence genetic studies have focused on understanding hemoglobin switching from HbF to HbA or pathologic HbS and others. BCL11A is a zinc finger protein ubiquitously expressed in human tissues that has been recognized as a repressor of HbF specifically in knockout mice erythroid cells. CRISPR-Cas 9 edits a specific enhancer region in the BCL11A gene leading to reduced expression of BCL11A and increased expression of γ-globin, reactivating HbF production. The alteration aims to recapitulate the phenotype of hereditary persistence of HbF (Traxler et al., 2016; Wienert et al., 2018). Preliminary results of this procedure showed a decrease in VOCs in patients with SCD (Esrick et al., 2019; Frangoul et al., 2021). On December 8th, 2024, the FDA also granted approval for Casgevy (exagamglogene autotemcel) to Vertex Pharmaceuticals Inc. (U.S. Food & Drug Administration, 2023). With this approval, Casgevy becomes the first FDA-approved treatment to make use of the novel genome editing technology CRISPR/Cas9. The CLIMB SCD-121 is a phase 3 trial of a single infusion of exagamglogene autotemcel in patients with SCD. Results show early and sustained increases in Hb and HbF, and achieved primary endpoint of VOC elimination in 95% of patients, and secondary endpoint of VOC-related inpatient hospitalization elimination in 100% of patients, and improved quality of life (Frangoul et al., 2023). Patients underwent a similar process as patients receiving Lyfgenia, except for stem cell treatment with CRISPR-Cas 9 instead of a lentiviral vector. Safety profile was consistent with known adverse events of autologous HSCT and myeloablative conditioning with no reported malignancies.

While these treatments are a step in the right direction and have great potential however the elevated price tag will render them inaccessible to the majority of patients with SCD who live in low and middle-resource settings. Therefore, it is important to make these treatments available and affordable for so that people everywhere with SCD have the option of gene therapy.

New Therapies in Low- and Middle-Resource Country Settings

The future of therapies for SCD is promising with new targeted therapies emerging every day. These are potentially disease-modifying agents that will have an impact on pain and end-organ dysfunction. However, to date, the main modalities that have improved survival and quality of life have been newborn screening, penicillin prophylaxis, prompt attention to fever, transcranial doppler screening for stroke prevention, use of HU, and access to safe transfusions (Figure 16.1). Though highly effective and relatively inexpensive these modalities are only accessible to a few patients in low- and middle-resource countries where most people with SCD live. With the recent FDA approval of gene therapy, the disparity in treatment access is expected to grow. Thus, major efforts are needed to sensitize patients, health care providers, and policymakers so that access to care is assured for all patients with SCD, starting with effective newborn screening and follow-up programs. Only then can the new therapies have an additive and significant impact on most patients.

References

Abboud, M. R., Cançado, R. D., De Montalembert, M., Smith, W. R., Rimawi, H., Voska-ridou, E., ... Adomakoh, Y. D. (2023). Efficacy, safety, and biomarker analysis of 5 Mg and 7.5 Mg doses of crizanlizumab in patients with sickle cell disease: Primary analyses from the phase III STAND study. *Blood, 142*(Supplement 1), 272. https://doi.org/10.1182/blood-2023-185429.

Abdullahi, S. U., Sunusi, S., Abba, M. S., Sani, S., Inuwa, H. A., Gambo, S., ... Kassim, A. A. (2023). Hydroxyurea for secondary stroke prevention in children with sickle cell anemia in Nigeria: A randomized controlled trial. *Blood, The Journal of the American Society of Hematology, 141*(8), 825–834.

Ambrose, E. E., Latham, T., Songoro, P., Charles, M., Lane, A., Stuber, S. E., ... Smart, L. R. (2022). Hydroxyurea with dose-escalation to reduce primary stroke risk in children with sickle cell anemia in tanzania: Primary results of the sphere trial. *Blood, 140*(Supplement 1), 447–448.

Angelucci, E., Matthes-Martin, S., Baronciani, D., Bernaudin, F., Bonanomi, S., Cappellini, M. D., ... Peters, C. (2014). Hematopoietic stem cell transplantation in thalassemia major and sickle cell disease: Indications and management recommendations from an international expert panel. *Haematologica, 99*(5), 811–820. https://doi.org/10.3324/haematol.2013.099747

Ataga, K. I., Kutlar, A., Kanter, J., Liles, D., Cancado, R., Friedrisch, J., ... Gordeuk, V. R. (2017). Crizanlizumab for the prevention of pain crises in sickle cell disease. *New England Journal of Medicine, 376*(5), 429–439.

Biemond, B. J., Tombak, A., Kilinc, Y., Al-Khabori, M., Abboud, M., Nafea, M., ... Kowalski, J. (2021). Sevuparin for the treatment of acute pain crisis in patients with sickle cell disease: A multicentre, randomised, double-blind, placebo-controlled, phase 2 trial. *The Lancet Haematology, 8*(5), e334–e343.

Bolaños-Meade, J., Fuchs, E. J., Luznik, L., Lanzkron, S. M., Gamper, C. J., Jones, R. J., & Brodsky, R. A. (2012). HLA-haploidentical bone marrow transplantation with post-transplant cyclophosphamide expands the donor pool for patients with sickle cell disease. *Blood, 120*(22), 4285–4291. https://doi.org/10.1182/blood-2012-07-438408

Boulad, F., Shore, T., van Besien, K., Minniti, C., Barbu-Stevanovic, M., Fedus, S. W., ... Shi, P. A. (2018). Safety and efficacy of plerixafor dose escalation for the mobilization of CD34(+) hematopoietic progenitor cells in patients with sickle cell disease: Interim results. *Haematologica, 103*(5), 770–777. https://doi.org/10.3324/haematol.2017.187047

Brousseau, D. C., Owens, P. L., Mosso, A. L., Panepinto, J. A., & Steiner, C. A. (2010). Acute care utilization and rehospitalizations for sickle cell disease. *JAMA, 303*(13), 1288–1294. https://doi.org/10.1001/jama.2010.378

Brunson, A., Lei, A., Rosenberg, A. S., White, R. H., Keegan, T., & Wun, T. (2017). Increased incidence of VTE in sickle cell disease patients: Risk factors, recurrence and impact on mortality. *British Journal of Haematology, 178*(2), 319–326. https://doi.org/10.1111/bjh.14655

Casella, J. F., Barton, B. A., Kanter, J., Black, L. V., Majumdar, S., Inati, A., ... Kilinc, Y. (2021). Effect of poloxamer 188 vs placebo on painful vaso-occlusive episodes in children and adults with sickle cell disease: A randomized clinical trial. *JAMA, 325*(15), 1513–1523.

Chang, J., Shi, P. A., Chiang, E. Y., & Frenette, P. S. (2008). Intravenous immunoglobulins reverse acute vaso-occlusive crises in sickle cell mice through rapid inhibition of neutrophil adhesion. *Blood, 111*(2), 915–923. https://doi.org/10.1182/blood-2007-04-084061

Charache, S., Barton, F. B., Moore, R. D., Terrin, M. L., Steinberg, M. H., Dover, G. J., … Orringer, E. P. (1996). Hydroxyurea and sickle cell anemia. Clinical utility of a myelosuppressive "switching" agent. The multicenter study of hydroxyurea in sickle cell anemia. *Medicine (Baltimore)*, 75(6), 300–326. https://doi.org/10.1097/00005792-199611000-00002

Conran, N., & Rees, D. C. (2017). Prasugrel hydrochloride for the treatment of sickle cell disease. *Expert Opinion on Investigational Drugs*, 26(7), 865–872. Retrieved from http://europepmc.org/abstract/MED/28562105; https://doi.org/10.1080/13543784.2017.1335710

Eaton, W. A., & Bunn, H. F. (2017). Treating sickle cell disease by targeting HbS polymerization. *Blood*, 129(20), 2719–2726. https://doi.org/10.1182/blood-2017-02-765891

Esrick, E. B., Achebe, M., Armant, M., Bartolucci, P., Ciuculescu, M. F., Daley, H., … Williams, D. A. (2019). Validation of BCL11A as therapeutic target in sickle cell disease: Results from the adult cohort of a pilot/feasibility gene therapy trial inducing sustained expression of fetal hemoglobin using post-transcriptional gene silencing. *Blood*, 134(Supplement 2), LBA-5-LBA-5. https://doi.org/10.1182/blood-2019-132745

Esrick, E. B., & Bauer, D. E. (2018). Genetic therapies for sickle cell disease. *Seminars in Hematology*, 55(2), 76–86. https://doi.org/10.1053/j.seminhematol.2018.04.014

Esrick, E. B., Manis, J. P., Daley, H., Baricordi, C., Trébéden-Negre, H., Pierciey, F. J., … Biffi, A. (2018). Successful hematopoietic stem cell mobilization and apheresis collection using plerixafor alone in sickle cell patients. *Blood Advances*, 2(19), 2505–2512. https://doi.org/10.1182/bloodadvances.2018016725

Fitzhugh, C. D., Abraham, A. A., Tisdale, J. F., & Hsieh, M. M. (2014). Hematopoietic stem cell transplantation for patients with sickle cell disease: Progress and future directions. *Hematology/Oncology Clinics of North America*, 28(6), 1171–1185. https://doi.org/10.1016/j.hoc.2014.08.014

Fitzhugh, C. D., Cordes, S., Taylor, T., Coles, W., Roskom, K., Link, M., … Tisdale, J. F. (2017). At least 20% donor myeloid chimerism is necessary to reverse the sickle phenotype after allogeneic HSCT. *Blood*, 130(17), 1946–1948. https://doi.org/10.1182/blood-2017-03-772392

Frangoul, H., Altshuler, D., Cappellini, M. D., Chen, Y. S., Domm, J., Eustace, B. K., … Corbacioglu, S. (2021). CRISPR-Cas9 gene editing for sickle cell disease and β-thalassemia. *New England Journal of Medicine*, 384(3), 252–260. https://doi.org/10.1056/NEJMoa2031054

Frangoul, H., Locatelli, F., Sharma, A., Bhatia, M., Mapara, M., Molinari, L., … Grupp, S. (2023). Exagamglogene autotemcel for severe sickle cell disease. *Blood*, 142(Supplement 1), 1052. https://doi.org/10.1182/blood-2023-190139

Galadanci, N. A., Abdullahi, S. U., Abubakar, S. A., Jibir, B. W., Aminu, H., Tijjani, A., … Borodo, A. M. (2020). Moderate fixed-dose hydroxyurea for primary prevention of strokes in Nigerian children with sickle cell disease: final results of the SPIN trial. *American Journal of Hematology*, 95(9), E247.

Gluckman, E., Cappelli, B., Bernaudin, F., Labopin, M., Volt, F., Carreras, J., … Eapen, M. (2017). Sickle cell disease: An international survey of results of HLA-identical sibling hematopoietic stem cell transplantation. *Blood*, 129(11), 1548–1556. https://doi.org/10.1182/blood-2016-10-745711

Goldstein, J., Konigsberg, W., & Hill, R. J. (1963). The structure of human hemoglobin. VI. The sequence of amino acids in the tryptic peptides of the beta chain. *Journal of Biological Chemistry*, 238, 2016–2027.

Goyal, S., Tisdale, J., Schmidt, M., Kanter, J., Jaroscak, J., Whitney, D., … Bonner, M. (2021). Acute myeloid leukemia case after gene therapy for sickle cell disease. *New England Journal of Medicine*, 386(2), 138–147. https://doi.org/10.1056/NEJMoa2109167

Hebbel, R. P., Boogaerts, M. A., Eaton, J. W., & Steinberg, M. H. (1980). Erythrocyte adherence to endothelium in sickle-cell anemia: A possible determinant of disease severity. *New England Journal of Medicine, 302*(18), 992–995.

Heeney, M. M., Hoppe, C. C., Abboud, M. R., Inusa, B., Kanter, J., Ogutu, B., ... Rees, D. C. (2015). A multinational trial of Prasugrel for sickle cell vaso-occlusive events. *New England Journal of Medicine, 374*(7), 625–635. https://doi.org/10.1056/NEJMoa1512021

Heitzer, A. M., Longoria, J., Okhomina, V., Wang, W. C., Raches, D., Potter, B., ... King, A. A. (2021). Hydroxyurea treatment and neurocognitive functioning in sickle cell disease from school age to young adulthood. *British Journal of Haematology, 195*(2), 256–266

Hoppe, C., Jacob, E., Styles, L., Kuypers, F., Larkin, S., & Vichinsky, E. (2017). Simvastatin reduces vaso-occlusive pain in sickle cell anaemia: A pilot efficacy trial. *British Journal of Haematology, 177*(4), 620–629. https://doi.org/10.1111/bjh.14580

Howard, J., Ataga, K. I., Brown, R. C., Achebe, M., Nduba, V., El-Beshlawy, A., ... Vichinsky, E. (2021). Voxelotor in adolescents and adults with sickle cell disease (HOPE): long-term follow-up results of an international, randomised, double-blind, placebo-controlled, phase 3 trial. *Lancet Haematology, 8*(5), e323–e333. https://doi.org/10.1016/s2352-3026(21)00059-4

Hsieh, M. M., Bonner, M., Pierciey Jr., F. J., Uchida, N., Rottman, J., Demopoulos, L., ... Thompson, A. A. (2020). Myelodysplastic syndrome unrelated to lentiviral vector in a patient treated with gene therapy for sickle cell disease. *Blood Advances, 4*(9), 2058–2063.

Hsieh, M. M., Kang, E. M., Fitzhugh, C. D., Link, M. B., Bolan, C. D., Kurlander, R., ... Tisdale, J. F. (2009). Allogeneic hematopoietic stem-cell transplantation for sickle cell disease. *New England Journal of Medicine, 361*(24), 2309–2317. https://doi.org/10.1056/NEJMoa0904971

Idowu, M., DeBaun, M. R., Burnett, A., Darbari, D. S., Adam, S., Anderson, A. R., ... El Rassi, F. (2023). Primary analysis of spartan: A phase 2 trial to assess the efficacy and safety of crizanlizumab in patients with sickle cell disease related priapism. *Blood, 142*(Supplement 1), 146. https://doi.org/10.1182/blood-2023-179042

John, C. C., Opoka, R. O., Latham, T. S., Hume, H. A., Nabaggala, C., Kasirye, P., ... Ware, R. E. (2020). Hydroxyurea dose escalation for sickle cell anemia in Sub-Saharan Africa. *New England Journal of Medicine, 382*(26), 2524–2533. https://doi.org/10.1056/NEJMoa2000146

Johnson, F. L., Look, A. T., Gockerman, J., Ruggiero, M. R., Dalla-Pozza, L., & Billings III, F. T. (1984). Bone-marrow transplantation in a patient with sickle-cell anemia. *New England Journal of Medicine, 311*(12), 780–783.

Kanter, J., Abboud, M. R., Kaya, B., Nduba, V., Amilon, C., Gottfridsson, C., ... Leonsson-Zachrisson, M. (2019). Ticagrelor does not impact patient-reported pain in young adults with sickle cell disease: A multicentre, randomised phase IIb study. *British Journal of Haematology, 184*(2), 269–278. https://doi.org/10.1111/bjh.15646

Kanter, J., & Falcon, C. (2021). Gene therapy for sickle cell disease: where we are now? *Hematology, American Society of Hematology Education Program, 2021*(1), 174–180. https://doi.org/10.1182/hematology.2021000250

Kanter, J., Thompson, A. A., Kwiatkowski, J. L., Parikh, S., Mapara, M., Rifkin-Zenenberg, S., ... Tisdale, J. F. (2023). Efficacy, safety, and health-related quality of life (HRQOL) in patients with sickle cell disease (SCD) who have received lovotibeglogene autotemcel (Lovo-cel) gene therapy: Up to 60 Months of Follow-up. *Blood, 142*(Supplement 1), 1051. https://doi.org/10.1182/blood-2023-174229

Kanter, J., Walters, M. C., Krishnamurti, L., Mapara, M. Y., Kwiatkowski, J. L., Rifkin-Zenenberg, S., & Tisdale, J. F. (2021). Biologic and clinical efficacy of LentiGlobin for sickle cell disease. *New England Journal of Medicine, 386*(7), 617–628. https://doi.org/10.1056/NEJMoa2117175

Kutlar, A., Kanter, J., Liles, D. K., Alvarez, O. A., Cançado, R. D., Friedrisch, J. R., ... Zhu, Z. (2019). Effect of crizanlizumab on pain crises in subgroups of patients with sickle cell disease: A SUSTAIN study analysis. *American Journal of Hematology, 94*(1), 55–61.

Manwani, D., Chen, G., Carullo, V., Serban, S., Olowokure, O., Jang, J., ... Shi, P. A. (2015). Single-dose intravenous gammaglobulin can stabilize neutrophil Mac-1 activation in sickle cell pain crisis. *American Journal of Hematology, 90*(5), 381–385. https://doi.org/10.1002/ajh.23956

Miller, S. T., Sleeper, L. A., Pegelow, C. H., Enos, L. E., Wang, W. C., Weiner, S. J., ... Kinney, T. R. (2000). Prediction of adverse outcomes in children with sickle cell disease. *New England Journal of Medicine, 342*(2), 83–89. https://doi.org/10.1056/nejm200001133420203

Morris, C. R., Hamilton-Reeves, J., Martindale, R. G., Sarav, M., & Ochoa Gautier, J. B. (2017). Acquired amino acid deficiencies: A focus on arginine and glutamine. *Nutrition in Clinical Practice, 32*(1_suppl), 30s–47s. https://doi.org/10.1177/0884533617691250

Morris, C., Kuypers, F., Larkin, S., Sweeters, N., Simon, J., Vichinsky, E., & Styles, L. (2000). Arginine therapy: A novel strategy to induce nitric oxide production in sickle cell disease. SHORT REPORT. *British Journal of Hematology, 111*, 498–500. https://doi.org/10.1111/j.1365-2141.2000.02403.x

Morris, C. R. (2014). Alterations of the arginine metabolome in sickle cell disease: A growing rationale for arginine therapy. *Hematology/Oncology Clinics of North America, 28*(2), 301–321. https://doi.org/10.1016/j.hoc.2013.11.008

Morris, C. R., Kato, G. J., Poljakovic, M., Wang, X., Blackwelder, W. C., Sachdev, V., ... Gladwin, M. T. (2005). Dysregulated arginine metabolism, hemolysis-associated pulmonary hypertension, and mortality in sickle cell disease. *JAMA, 294*(1), 81–90.

Morris, C. R., Kuypers, F. A., Lavrisha, L., Ansari, M., Sweeters, N., Stewart, M., ... Vichinsky, E. P. (2013). A randomized, placebo-controlled trial of arginine therapy for the treatment of children with sickle cell disease hospitalized with vaso-occlusive pain episodes. *Haematologica, 98*(9), 1375–1382. https://doi.org/10.3324/haematol.2013.086637

Niihara, Y., Matsui, N. M., Shen, Y. M., Akiyama, D. A., Johnson, C. S., Sunga, M. A., ... Ho Cho, S. (2005). L-glutamine therapy reduces endothelial adhesion of sickle red blood cells to human umbilical vein endothelial cells. *BMC Hematology, 5*, 1–7.

Niihara, Y., Miller, S. T., Kanter, J., Lanzkron, S., Smith, W. R., Hsu, L. L., ... Vichinsky, E. P. (2018). A phase 3 trial of l-glutamine in sickle cell disease. *New England Journal of Medicine, 379*(3), 226–235. https://doi.org/10.1056/NEJMoa1715971

Niihara, Y., Zerez, C., Akiyama, D., & Tanaka, K. (1995). Increased red cell glutamate in sickle cell disease: Evidence that increased glutamine availability is a mechanism for increased total NAD. *Journal of Investigative Medicine, 43*, 131a.

Niihara, Y., Zerez, C. R., Akiyama, D. S., & Tanaka, K. R. (1998). Oral L-glutamine therapy for sickle cell anemia: I. Subjective clinical improvement and favorable change in red cell NAD redox potential. *American Journal of Hematology, 58*(2), 117–121.

Oksenberg, D., Dufu, K., Patel, M. P., Chuang, C., Li, Z., Xu, Q., ... Archer, D. R. (2016). GBT440 increases haemoglobin oxygen affinity, reduces sickling and prolongs RBC half-life in a murine model of sickle cell disease. *British Journal of Hematology, 175*(1), 141–153. https://doi.org/10.1111/bjh.14214

Onalo, R., Cilliers, A., Cooper, P., & Morris, C. R. (2022). Arginine therapy and cardio-pulmonary hemodynamics in hospitalized children with sickle cell anemia: A prospective, double-blinded, randomized placebo-controlled clinical trial. *American Journal of Respiratory and Critical Care Medicine*, *206*(1), 70–80. https://doi.org/10.1164/rccm.202108-1930OC

Onalo, R., Cooper, P., Cilliers, A., Vorster, B. C., Uche, N. A., Oluseyi, O. O., … Morris, C. R. (2021). Randomized control trial of oral arginine therapy for children with sickle cell anemia hospitalized for pain in Nigeria. *American Journal of Hematology*, *96*(1), 89–97. https://doi.org/10.1002/ajh.26028

Onalo, R., Cilliers, A., & Cooper, P. (2021). Impact of oral (L)-arginine supplementation on blood pressure dynamics in children with severe sickle cell vaso-occlusive crisis. *American Journal of Cardiovascular Disease*, *11*(1), 136–147. Retrieved from https://www.ncbi.nlm.nih.gov/pmc/articles/PMC8012291/pdf/ajcd0011-0136.pdf.

Pawliuk, R., Westerman, K. A., Fabry, M. E., Payen, E., Tighe, R., Bouhassira, E. E., … Eaves, C. J. (2001). Correction of sickle cell disease in transgenic mouse models by gene therapy. *Science*, *294*(5550), 2368–2371.

Platt, O. S., Brambilla, D. J., Rosse, W. F., Milner, P. F., Castro, O., Steinberg, M. H., & Klug, P. P. (1994). Mortality in sickle cell disease. Life expectancy and risk factors for early death. *New England Journal of Medicine*, *330*(23), 1639–1644. https://doi.org/10.1056/nejm199406093302303

Rees, C. A., Brousseau, D. C., Cohen, D. M., Villella, A., Dampier, C., Brown, K., … Morris, C. R. (2023). Sickle Cell Disease Treatment with Arginine Therapy (STArT): study protocol for a phase 3 randomized controlled trial. *Trials*, *24*(1), 538. https://doi.org/10.1186/s13063-023-07538-z

Reyes, L. Z., Figueroa, J., Leake, D., Khemani, K., Kumari, P., Bakshi, N., … Morris, C. R. (2022). Safety of intravenous arginine therapy in children with sickle cell disease hospitalized for vaso-occlusive pain: A randomized placebo-controlled trial in progress. *American Journal of Hematology*, *97*(1), E21–E24. Retrieved from https://www.ncbi.nlm.nih.gov/pmc/articles/PMC8722015/pdf/nihms-1752589.pdf; https://doi.org/10.1002/ajh.26396

Ribeil, J.-A., Hacein-Bey-Abina, S., Payen, E., Magnani, A., Semeraro, M., Magrin, E., … Cavazzana, M. (2017). Gene therapy in a patient with sickle cell disease. *New England Journal of Medicine*, *376*(9), 848–855. https://doi.org/10.1056/NEJMoa1609677

Salinas Cisneros, G., & Thein, S. L. (2020). Recent advances in the treatment of sickle cell disease. *Frontiers in Physiology*, *11*, 435. https://doi.org/10.3389/fphys.2020.00435

Saraf, S. L., Oh, A. L., Patel, P. R., Sweiss, K., Koshy, M., Campbell-Lee, S., … Rondelli, D. (2018). Haploidentical peripheral blood stem cell transplantation demonstrates stable engraftment in adults with sickle cell disease. *Biology of Blood and Marrow Transplantation*, *24*(8), 1759–1765. https://doi.org/10.1016/j.bbmt.2018.03.031

Saraf, S. L., Abdullahi, S. U., Akinsete, A. M., Fasola, F. A., Idowu, M., Pennington, S., … Lisbon, E. A. (2023). Preliminary results from a multicenter phase 2/3 study of next-generation HbS polymerization inhibitor GBT021601 for the treatment of patients with sickle cell disease. *Blood*, *142*(Supplement 1), 274. https://doi.org/10.1182/blood-2023-177781

Serjeant, G. R., Serjeant, B. E., & Mason, K. (1977). Heterocellular hereditary persistence of fetal haemoglobin and homozygous sickle-cell disease. *Lancet*, *1*(8015), 795–796. https://doi.org/10.1016/s0140-6736(77)92976-2

Takekoshi, K. J., Oh, Y. H., Westerman, K. W., London, I. M., & Leboulch, P. (1995). Retroviral transfer of a human beta-globin/delta-globin hybrid gene linked to beta locus control region hypersensitive site 2 aimed at the gene therapy of sickle cell disease. *Proceedings of the National Academy of Sciences*, *92*(7), 3014–3018.

Telen, M. J., Batchvarova, M., Shan, S., Bovee-Geurts, P. H., Zennadi, R., Leitgeb, A., & Lindgren, M. (2016). Sevuparin binds to multiple adhesive ligands and reduces sickle red blood cell-induced vaso-occlusion. *British Journal of Haematology, 175*(5), 935–948.

Traxler, E. A., Yao, Y., Wang, Y. D., Woodard, K. J., Kurita, R., Nakamura, Y., Weiss, M. J. (2016). A genome-editing strategy to treat β-hemoglobinopathies that recapitulates a mutation associated with a benign genetic condition. *Nature Medicine, 22*(9), 987–990. https://doi.org/10.1038/nm.4170

Tshilolo, L., Tomlinson, G., Williams, T. N., Santos, B., Olupot-Olupot, P., Lane, A., … Ware, R. E. (2019). Hydroxyurea for Children with Sickle Cell Anemia in Sub-Saharan Africa. *New England Journal of Medicine, 380*(2), 121–131. https://doi.org/10.1056/NEJMoa1813598

U.S. Food & Drug Administration. (2023). FDA Approves First Gene Therapies to Treat Patients with Sickle Cell Disease. https://www.fda.gov/news-events/press-announcements/fda-approves-first-gene-therapies-treat-patients-sickle-cell-disease?ipid=promo-link-block1

Wang, W. C., Ware, R. E., Miller, S. T., Iyer, R. V., Casella, J. F., Minniti, C. P., … Thompson, B. W. (2011). Hydroxycarbamide in very young children with sickle-cell anaemia: A multicentre, randomised, controlled trial (BABY HUG). *Lancet, 377*(9778), 1663–1672. https://doi.org/10.1016/s0140-6736(11)60355-3

Ware, R. E., Davis, B. R., Schultz, W. H., Brown, R. C., Aygun, B., Sarnaik, S., … Adams, R. J. (2016). Hydroxycarbamide versus chronic transfusion for maintenance of transcranial doppler flow velocities in children with sickle cell anaemia-TCD with transfusions changing to hydroxyurea (TWiTCH): A multicentre, open-label, phase 3, non-inferiority trial. *Lancet, 387*(10019), 661–670. https://doi.org/10.1016/s0140-6736(15)01041-7

Wienert, B., Martyn, G. E., Funnell, A. P. W., Quinlan, K. G. R., & Crossley, M. (2018). Wake-up sleepy gene: Reactivating fetal globin for β-hemoglobinopathies. *Trends in Genetics, 34*(12), 927–940. https://doi.org/10.1016/j.tig.2018.09.004

Zhang, D., Xu, C., Manwani, D., & Frenette, P. S. (2016). Neutrophils, platelets, and inflammatory pathways at the nexus of sickle cell disease pathophysiology. *Blood, 127*(7), 801–809. https://doi.org/10.1182/blood-2015-09-618538

17 Haematopoietic Cell Transplantation for Sickle Cell Disease

A Global Perspective

Sarita Rani Jaiswal and Suparno Chakrabarti

Introduction

Sickle cell disease (SCD) is the commonest inherited disorder of haemoglobi-nopathy worldwide (Weatherall, 2010). SCD is associated with an unpredictable clinical course with significant mortality and morbidity which ultimately leads to an enormous public health burden. While the exact data remains unknown, it is estimated that sub-Saharan Africa (SSA) accounts for over 80% of the global burden of SCD, with over quarter of a million children born each year with SCD (Piel et al., 2010; Williams, 2016). Much of our current knowledge on the natural history of SCD arises from studies originating from North America, where early diagnosis and supportive care in childhood have resulted in marked reduction in childhood deaths due to SCD, along with a significant improvement in overall lifespan over a period of four decades (Leikin et al., 1989; Perronne et al., 2002; Platt et al., 1994; Steinberg et al., 2003). However, the same is not the case with SSA, where lack of early diagnosis, increased childhood mortality and lack of documentation make an exact estimation nearly impossible (Williams, 2016).

Haematopoietic Cell Transplantation (HCT) in SCD

Even though hydroxyurea can reduce the disease severity in some patients with SCD and newer drugs such as crizanlizumab, voxeletor and L-glutamine might have a disease-modifying effect, an allogeneic haematopoietic cell transplantation (HCT) is the only time-tested curative treatment for SCD. The first HCT for SCD was performed in 1984 from a human leukocyte antigen (HLA) matched sibling donor (MSD) to treat Acute Myeloid Leukemia in a patient who also had SCD (Shah & Krishnamurti, 2021). This was associated with complete amelioration of symptoms related to SCD and raised the possibility of cure of SCD through HCT. However, consorted attempts to cure SCD with an allogeneic HCT began a decade later. Studies from the USA, Belgium and France showed, by the end of 1990s, that over 80% children with SCD can be effectively cured by an allogeneic HCT from an MSD, with a 10% risk each of mortality and graft-failure (Blume, Forman, & Appelbaum, 2008).

In this section, we are going to discuss the challenges of HCT for SCD, with respect to the available data on the outcome, based on donor availability,

DOI: 10.4324/9781003463931-18

patient age and geographical disparities, in light of the recent advances in modalities of HCT.

Principles and the Process of HCT

Allogeneic HCT is based on the principle of developing cellular tolerance between two genotypically non-identical individuals, where diseased haematopoietic stem cells (HSC) are replaced by normal healthy HSC. Pathbreaking canine experiments carried out by E.D. Thomas and colleagues in the 1960s established the basis for clinical HCT. Three principles evolved, which remain the pillars of HCT to date (Blume et al., 2008). The first was recognition HLA-compatibility between the donor and the patient as an absolute requirement. The second was treatment directed to the marrow and the immune system of the patient to allow engraftment, although a large component of it was initially directed as an anti-leukaemia treatment. This is called 'conditioning' or 'preparative-regimens'. The third was the use of immunosuppressive drugs post-transplant to prevent graft-versus-host disease (GVHD), a phenomenon where the alloreactive donor T cells attack the host organs resulting in mild to severe clinical manifestations which can sometimes be fatal.

Total body irradiation (TBI) at a single dose of 8Gy or above was found to cause irreversible myelosuppression as was busulfan (Bu) at 16 mg/kg. Such doses when employed with the conditioning treatment (CT) were termed myeloablative conditioning (MAC) (McPherson et al., 2011). However, it took some time to realise that the donor bone marrow (BM) graft infused following the CT was not merely replacing the host HSC, but incorporating a strong immunological effect, even in the absence of GVHD. This was termed as graft-versus-leukaemia/tumour (GVL/GVT) effect. This, along with preclinical studies demonstrating the ability to achieve engraftment in mice without MAC, led to the development of non-myeloablative conditioning (NMAC), where much lower doses of chemo-radiotherapy could be employed to achieve donor engraftment. This was a major paradigm shift in the field of HCT as hitherto only young and fit patients were deemed fit for a HCT. Introduction of NMAC widened the use of HCT amongst a wider spectrum of diseases and age groups, as we shall see in subsequent sections.

Allogeneic HCT is associated with certain unique complications, some of which stem from the toxicities of CT, some from the alloreactivity generated by the donor cells, while others stem from the severe immunodeficiency arising during the period following host immunoablation until recovery and maturation of donor-derived immune system. The recovery of innate immune system happens early by 30–60 days post-HCT, but the recovery of T and B cells are often protracted over several months and often years, opening the window for opportunistic viral infections such as Cytomegalovirus (CMV), Epstein Barr virus and Adenovirus amongst others (Zaia et al., 2009). Thus, the success of the process of HCT depends on a multitude of factors, some being modifiable and some not. The decision to proceed with a HCT, particularly for a disease, where life can be sustained meaningfully with supportive care, is dependent on the understanding and willingness of the parents and patients, and the wisdom and expertise of the physician.

HCT in Children and Young Adults with SCD

Development of HCT for SCD lagged other diseases by a decade or two in the West, due to various factors. The initial attempts involved diligent clinical trials led by researchers from France, the USA and Belgium. While HCT in the initial three decades saw a slow and steady development with matched sibling donor (MSD), the last decade saw some major strides in alternate donor HCT. In the following sections, we shall discuss the outcomes of HCT for SCD based on donor types.

MSD or MUD-HCT with MAC

Reports on more than 150 patients from the USA, Belgium, and France showed that an event-free survival (EFS) of 80–85% can be achieved in children with SCD with severe symptoms (Bernaudin et al., 2007; Dedeken et al., 2014; Vermylen et al., 1998; Walters et al., 1996). A decade later with a better understanding of the biology, the French group reported on 234 patients with median follow-up for 7.9 years showing a five-year EFS of 97.9% since the year 2000. EFS was not associated with age, but chronic graft-versus-host disease (cGVHD) was negatively associated with recipient's age more than 15 years and a lower (5–15 vs. 20 mg/kg) anti-thymocyte globulin (ATG) dose. At one year, 44% of patients had mixed chimerism (5–95% donor cells), but those prepared with ATG had no graft rejection. It is important to understand that no events related to SCD occurred in patients with mixed chimerism, even in those with 15–20% donor cells. However, events of haemolytic anemia were observed in patients with donor cells <50%. Amongst the younger patients (<30 years) with MSD and MAC, the EFS was 98% compared to 88% in patients receiving NMAC. However, NMAC could be helpful for fertility preservation especially in adult population (Bernaudin et al., 2020).

HCT with NMAC/RIC/Reduced Toxicity (RTC)

Following unsuccessful attempts at HCT with MAC in adults, HCT was not considered for older patients with SCD. Chakrabarti and colleagues in 2003 laid out the fundamentals of carrying out HCT in adults based on the following premises (Chakrabarti & Bareford, 2004). First, complete donor chimerism is not essential for the establishment of donor erythropoiesis as sickle erythroid lineage has an inherent competitive disadvantage. Second, mixed chimerism was shown to be stable in a subgroup of patients undergoing MAC-HCT for SCD. They reasoned that if NMAC based on fludarabine (Flu), alemtuzumab and cyclophosphamide (Cy) could be employed to achieve stable mixed chimerism as was shown in a patient with severe psoriasis, who had a NMAC-based allograft for lymphoma, cure of the sickle phenotype might be possible without any major risk of morbidity and mortality (Chakrabarti, Handa, Bryon, Griffiths, & Milligan, 2001). Subsequently, a group from the USA employed these principles in adult SCD patients with alemtuzumab, 3Gy TBI and sirolimus. All 30 patients transplanted on these protocols were alive at a median of two years with four losing the graft. None developed

GVHD (Hsieh et al., 2014). These results were a proof of the principles laid out by Chakrabarti et al., a decade earlier (Chakrabarti & Bareford, 2004).

Bhatia et al. has employed reduced toxicity MAC (RTC) from a matched sibling donor, in 18 patients, with a median age 8.9 years on 18 patients. Fifteen patients received sibling BM and three received sibling cord blood (CB) on the day of transplantation. Mean whole blood and erythroid donor chimerism was 91% and 88%, at days +100 and +365, respectively. Probability of grade II–IV acute GVHD (aGVHD) was 17%. Two-year EFS and overall survival (OS) were both 100%. Neurological, pulmonary and cardiovascular function were stable or improved at two years (Bhatia et al., 2014) (Table 17.1).

A retrospective survey was carried out from the European Group for Blood & Marrow Transplantation (EBMT), The Center for International Blood and Marrow Transplant Research (CIBMTR) and Eurocord registries on 1,000 patients undergoing an MSD-HCT for SCD until 2013. In this cohort, data on 846 children and 154 adults were analysed (Table 17.2). The OS and EFS were 92.9% and 91.4%. Graft failure (GF) was 2.3% and mortality was 7%. Outcome was better in younger patients (<16 years) and those transplanted after 2006. There was no impact of graft source [peripheral blood (PB) vs BM vs CB)], conditioning (MAC vs NMAC) or graft manipulation on the outcome. The study highlights an excellent outcome in younger children (OS – 95%, EFS – 93%, GVHD and EFS (GEFS) – 86%). At the same time, late deaths were observed in seven patients beyond five years. Thus, this survey reiterated the observations from individual studies that HCT from an MSD provided an excellent chance of leading a life free of SCD, if the procedure is carried out early (Gluckman et al., 2017).

Alternative Donor Transplantation

Unrelated Donor (URD) – Matched and Mismatched (Table 17.3)

A BMT-CTN Phase II study reported the outcome of URD-HCT in 29 children (<19 years) with alemtuzumab-Flu-melphalan (Mel) conditioning and calcineurin (CNI) methotrexate (Mtx) and methyl prednisone-based GVHD prophylaxis. Even though, 90% engrafted, EFS was 76% and 69% at one and two years, respectively, with the incidence of aGVHD of 28%. However, the major cause of morbidity and mortality was cGVHD (overall – 62%, extensive – 38%). In addition, the incidence of posterior reversible encephalopathy syndrome (PRES) was 34% in the first six months. This approach was clearly a suboptimal platform for URD-HCT for children with SCD (Kamani et al., 2012).

In a recent registry-based retrospective study, 71 patients from 20 EBMT centres, receiving MAC and CNI-Mtx/MMF as GVHD prophylaxis between 2005 and 2017, were reported. GF was 15% and both aGVHD and cGVHD were 23%. Even though overall OS and EFS were 88% and 62%, respectively, this was significantly impacted by HLA-matching between donor and the recipient (96% and 69% in 10/10 match vs 75% and 50% in 8–9/10 match) (Gluckman et al., 2020).

Table 17.1 Outcome of MSD-HCT in children with sickle cell disease.

References	Patients with SCD (Total)	Age-median (range in years)	Conditioning	Graft source +/-manipulation	Engraftment (%)	GVHD prophylaxis	Acute GVHD (%)	Chronic GVHD (%)	NRM (%)	DFS (%)/ GGRFS	OS (%)	Follow-up
Bernaudin et al. (2020)	234 MSD	8.4 (2.2–27.6)	rATG/Bu/Cy	BM 84% CB 12.8% CB + BM 1.2% PB 0.4%	97.4	CSA+–MMF	20.1	10.5	3.0	93.9	95	Five years
Bolanos-Meade et al. (2019)	17	6–31	Flu/Cy/TBI 4Gy/ATG	BM	94	PTCy/Siro/MMF	29	18	10.8	38	76 FDC 18 MDC	705 (355–943) days
Lucarelli et al. (2014)	40	2–17	Bu/Cy/rATG/Flu	BM	100	CsA/Mtx/Pred	17.5	5	5	91	92.5	1–10 years
Dedeken et al. (2014) Brussels (13)	50	1.7–15.3	Bu/Cy/ATG/Hu	BM 39 UC 3 BM + UC 7	92	CsA/Mtx or MMF(UCB)	15	20.5	20	85.6	94.1	0.4–21.3 years
Bhatia et al. (2014)	18	2.3–20.2	Bu/Flu/ALEM	BM15 CB 3	100	TAC/MMF	88	17	11	85	100	1,065 (135–2,731 days)
McPherson et al. (2011)	27	3.3–17.4	Bu/Cy/ATG	BM	100	CsA/Mtx	62	17	3.7	96	96	4.9 years
Strocchio et al. (2015) (61)	30	1.7–18.8	Bu/TT/Flu 160/Treo/TT/Flu/ATG	BM-22 CB -4 BM+CB 3 PBSC 1	93	CsA/Mtx or MMF	62	7	7	93	100	Seven years
King et al. (2015) (32)	43	3–20.3	ALEM/Flu/Mel	BM-22 CB 4 BM + CB 3 PBSC	97	CsA /or TAC	29	23	13.4	92.3	94.2	3.4 (0.7–11.8 years)

(Continued)

Table 17.1 (Continued)

References	Patients with SCD (Total)	Age-median (range in years)	Conditioning	Graft source +/- manipulation	Engraftment (%)	GVHD prophylaxis	Acute GVHD (%)	Chronic GVHD (%)	NRM (%)	DFS (%)/ GGRFS	OS (%)	Follow-up
Shenoy (2011) (51)	179	0.3–22	Bu/Cy/ATG/ALG/TLI/ALEM	Bu, Cy, ATG/ALG, TLI/ALEM	98	CsA	2–10	2–10	8–21	79–92	90–100	NA
Panepinto et al. (2007)	67	10	Bu/Cy	BM	86	Mtx/CsA Mtx/TAC/	10	22	15	85	97	Five years
Walters et al. (2010)												Thirteen years
(i) Belgium	36	1.7–23	Bu/Cy/ATG/TLI	BM	>95	CsA	4	14	15	85	94%	
(ii) France	19	–	Bu/Cy/ATG				1				68%	
(iii) Multicenter	60	4–38	Bu/Cy/ATG TLI				4				83%	
(iv) US vs. Other Europe	59	2.2–22	Bu/Cy/ATG				5				85%	
	16	3.3–15.9	Bu/Cy/ATG Cy/TBI				1				80%	
Shenoy et al. (2016) (38)	30 MUD	4–19	ALEM/Tu/Flu/Mel	BM	90	CNI/Mtx/MP	28	62	34	69	79	Twenty-six (12–62) months
Walters et al. (1996)	22	<16	Bu/Cy/ATGAM	BM	73	Cy/Mtx	9	9	27	73	91	10–51
Walters et al. (2000)	50	3–14	Bu/Cy/ATGAM/ALEM	BM	85	Cy/Mtx/Pred	11	7.6	16	84	94	38–95

Abbreviations: ALEM – Alemtuzumab; ALG – anti-lymphocyte globulin; ATG – anti-thymocyte globulin; ATGAM – horse anti-thymocyte globulin; BM – bone marrow; Bu- busulphan; CB – cord blood; CNIs – calcineurin inhibitors; CR – complete remission; CsA – Cyclosporine; Cy – cyclophosphamide; Flu – Fludarabine; GVHD – graft-versus-host disease; Gy – gray; HFD – halfmatched family donor; MAC – myeloablative conditioning; Mel – Melphalan; MMF – mycophenolate mofetil; mMUD – mismatched unrelated donor; Mtx – Methotrexate; MP – Methyl Prednisolone; MRD – matched related donor; MSD – matched sibling donor; NA – not available; NMA – non-myeloablative conditioning; NRM – non-relapse mortality; PB – peripheral blood; PBSC – peripheral blood stem cells; Plt – platelet; Pred – Prednisolone; PTCy – post-transplant cyclophosphamide; rATG – rabbit anti-thymocyte globulin; Rel – refractory; Rel relapsed; RIC – reduced intensity conditioning; Siro – Sirolimus; TAC – tacrolimus; TBI – total body irradiation; TCD – T-cell depletion; TLI – total lymphoid irradiation; TT – thiotepa; Treo – Treosulfan; UC – umbilical cord; UCB – umbilical cord blood.

Table 17.2 Outcome of MSD-HCT in adults with sickle cell disease.

References	Patients with SCD (total)	Age range (years)	Conditioning	Graft source +/-manipulation	Engraftment (%)	GVHD prophylaxis	Graft failure	Acute GVHD (%)	Chronic GVHD (%)	NRM (%)	EFS (%)	OS (%)	Follow-up (years)
Hsieh et al. (2014)	30	17–65	ALEM/TBI	PBSC	100	Siro	13	0	0	2.4	97.6	97	1.8–6
Kuentz et al. (2011)	15	16–27.5	Bu/Cy/rATG	PBSC	100	CsA/Mtx	0	8/15	2/15	7	92	93	3.4 (1–16.1 years)
Krishnamurti et al. (2015)	22 MSD+MUD	16–40	ATG/Flu/Bu	BM	100	CsA/TAC /Mtx	0	2/22	3/22	5	95	95	9.7 (1–31 months)
Pawlowska et al. (2017)	4	13–23	ATG/Bu	PBSC-1 BM-3	99.9–100	Cy/TAC/ MMF	43	25	75	0	100	100	5–11

Abbreviations: ALEM – Alemtuzumab; ALG – anti-lymphocyte globulin; ATG – anti-thymocyte globulin; ATGAM – horse anti-thymocyte globulin; BM – bone marrow; Bu – busulphan; CB – cord blood; CNIs – calcineurin inhibitors; CR – complete remission; CsA – Cyclosporine; Cy – cyclophosphamide; Flu – Fludarabine; GVHD – graft-versus-host disease; Gy – gray; HFD – half-matched family donor; MAC – myeloablative conditioning; Mel – Melphalan; MMF – mycophenolate mofetil; mMUD – mismatched unrelated donor; MUD – matched unrelated donor; Mtx – Methotrexate; MP – Methyl Prednisolone; MRD – matched related donor; MSD – matched sibling donor; NA – not available; NMA – non-myeloablative conditioning; NRM – non-relapse mortality; PB – peripheral blood; PBSC – peripheral blood stem cells; Plt – platelet; Pred – Prednisolone; PTCy – post-transplant cyclophosphamide; rATG – rabbit anti-thymocyte globulin; Ref – refractory; Rel – relapsed; RIC – reduced intensity conditioning; Siro – Sirolimus; TAC – tacrolimus; TBI – total body irradiation; TCD – T-cell depletion; TLI – total lymphoid irradiation; TT – thiotepa; Treo – Treosulfan; UC – umbilical cord; UCB – umbilical cord blood.

Table 17.3 Outcome of alternative donor HCT for children and young adults with sickle cell disease.

Ref	Patients with SCD (total)	Age range (years)	Conditioning	Graft source +/–manipulation	Engraftment (%)	GVHD prophylaxis	Graft failure	Acute GVHD (%)	Chronic GVHD (%)	EFS (%)	OS (%)	Follow-up (months)
Gluckman et al. (2020)	71	9.3	Treo/ Flu /TT (64%) Bu/Cy (12%)	BM 79% PB 21%	79	CsA + Mtx MMF + Siro CsA + MMF TAC +MMF	23	23	25	69+/–9 50+/–12	86+/–4 75+/–10	Three years
Eapen et al. (2019)	N = 910 MSD– 558 MUD111 Haplo137 MMUD– 104	<10= 408 10–17 = 265 18–29 = 161 30–49 = 76	MAC 478 NMA 181 RIC 251	BM 630 PB 177 UCB 102 TCD 11 CD34 sel 40	≤12 = 89% 13–49 = 86%	PTCy/Siro/ MMF52 PTCy/ Siro 21 PTCy/CNI/ MMF19 CNI/MMF 223 CNI/Mtx 419 CNI/Siro 5 CNI ONLY 52 Siro ONLY 68	MSD-32/557 MUD-29/104 Haplo-36/137 mMUD-29/104	N = 95/823 MSD- 32/513 MUD- 23/97 Haplo- 11/126 mMUD- 29/87	N = 910 MSD- 101/557 MUD- 37/111 Haplo- 22/137 mMUD- 30/104	MSD- 94.3 MUD- 85.6 Haplo- 73.7 mMUD- 72.1	MSD- 96.2 MUD- 86 Haplo- 90.5 mMUD- 84	N = 996 MSD-37 MUD-37 Haplo-25 mMUD-47
Krishnamurti et al. (2019)	22 17 MRD 5 MUD	17–36	Flu/Bu/ ATG	CD34 *10^6	100	Mtx/ CsA/TAC	4.5	18	14	82	91	36
Dedeken et al. (2014)	50	1.7–15.3	Bu/Cy	CB	92	CsA/Mtx	0	22	20	85.6	94.1	96

Abbreviations: ALEM – Alemtuzumab; ALG – anti-lymphocyte globulin; ATG – anti-thymocyte globulin; ATGAM – horse anti-thymocyte globulin; BM – bone marrow; Bu – busulphan; CB – cord blood; CNIs – calcineurin inhibitors; CR – complete remission; CsA – Cyclosporine; Cy – cyclophosphamide; Flu – Fludarabine; GVHD – graft-versus-host disease; Gy – gray; HFD – halfmatched family donor; MAC – myeloablative conditioning; Mel – Melphalan; MMF – mycophenolate mofetil; mMUD – mismatched unrelated donor; MUD – matched unrelated donor; Mtx – Methotrexate; MP – Methyl Prednisolone; MRD – matched related donor; MSD – matched sibling donor; NA – not available; NMA – non-myeloablative conditioning; NRM – non-relapse mortality; PB – peripheral blood; PBSC – peripheral blood stem cells; Plt – platelet; Pred – Prednisolone; PTCy – post-transplant cyclophosphamide; rATG– rabbit anti-thymocyte globulin; Ref – refractory; Rel – relapsed; RIC – reduced intensity conditioning; Siro – Sirolimus; TAC – tacrolimus; TBI – total body irradiation; TCD – T-cell depletion; TLI – total lymphoid irradiation; TT – thiotepa; Treo – Treosulfan; UC – umbilical cord; UCB – umbilical cord blood.

The above studies on URD suggest that the GVHD prophylaxis for URD-HCT remains suboptimal and GF is also a concern. However, the approaches adopted for HCT from haploidentical family donors as discussed in the next section might help improve the outcome after URD-HCT. Based on the current evidence, mismatched URD-HCT is not advisable for children with SCD.

Haploidentical Family Donor (HFD) (Table 17.4)

HLA mismatch is an unequivocal risk factor for both GF as well as GVHD. This has been amply demonstrated with URD-HCT. Early attempts at HLA-MM family donor or haploidentical family donor (HFD) transplantation with conventional approach were met with devastating results and were quickly abandoned (Chakrabarti & Jaiswal, 2021). Innovation of two major approaches in the 1990s and, subsequently, the first decade of the millennium have changed the landscape of alternate donor HCT. The first one involved ex vivo T-cell depletion (TCD) and the second was in vivo administration of high dose Cy on days +3 and +4 after cell infusion, popularly known as PTCy. Both approaches were aimed at elimination of alloreactive T cells which are directed to major mismatched HLA antigen and hence present at a higher frequency (Pawlowska et al., 2018).

Initial attempts at TCD involved immunomagnetic selection of CD34+ HSC, which resulted in less than 10^4 T and B cells in the graft (Aversa et al., 2005). Even though this was successful in achieving engraftment with megadose of CD34+cells and markedly reducing GVHD, a very high attrition was noted due to infection-related complications, attributable to poor immune reconstitution. Subsequent to this, selective depletion of TCRα/β and CD19 cells was associated with an impressive outcome and is currently the most widely used method for TCD in HFD-HCT (Gaziev et al., 2018).

PTCy, on the other hand, employs the unique attribute of Cy to eliminate alloreactive T cells from a T-cell replete graft, infused without prior immunosuppressive drugs. This leads to massive proliferation of alloreactive T cells from both host as well as the graft in the first 48–72 hours. Rapidly multiplying cells lack aldehyde dehydrogenase, which inactivates Cy, whereas quiescent cells including HSCs carry high amounts of this enzyme. Thus, exposure to high-dose Cy about 2–3 days after infusion of the graft can effectively kill proliferating alloreactive T cells, sparing HSCs and non-alloreactive T cells. This approach was associated with successful engraftment even with NMAC and acceptable rates of both aGVHD and cGVHD. The ease of delivering the PTCy protocol compared to technically challenging graft manipulation and the frugal cost made HFD-HCT possible across the globe (Luznik et al., 2008).

Both the approaches to HFD-HCT have been explored in SCD. The Johns Hopkins group employed the original NMAC protocol (Flu-Cy-2GyTBI) with PTCy in 12 patients with SCD. Even though the procedure was safe, the rate of GF was high at 43% (Bolanos-Meade et al., 2012). The same group achieved greater than 90% engraftment, when patients were conditioned with ATG and a higher dose of TBI (4Gy) (Bolanos-Meade et al., 2019). On the other hand, another group exploring the same approach witnessed GF in two out of the first three patients. Addition

Table 17.4 Outcome of a haploidentical HCT for children and young adults with sickle cell disease.

References	No of patients with SCD (total)	Age range (years)	Conditioning	GVHD prophylaxis	Engraftment (%)	Acute GVHD (%)	Chronic GVHD (%)	NRM (%)	GF/Relapse (%)	Overall survival (%)	Follow-up
Bolanos et al. (2012)	14	2–70	ATG/Flu/Cy	Cy/TAC/MMF	73	9	0	0	43	711 days	711 (224–1,981 days)
Gaziev et al. (2018)	7	2–17	Bu/TT/Cy/ATG	CsA/ MP	86	28	21	14	14	84	3.9 (0.5–5.2 years)
Dallas et al. (2013)	HFD-8 MSD-14	4–14	RIC-HFD MAC-MSD	PTCy	100	32 40	13 25	25	38	75 93	8–15 years
dela Fuente et al. (2019)	15	8–26	ATG/TT/Flu/ Cy/TBI	PTCy/Siro MMF	93	33	7	0	7	86	16.7 (6.5–30.8 months)
Jaiswal et al. (2020)	5	3–19	ATG/TT/Flu/Mel	PTCy/Siro COSBL	100	0	0	0	100	100	402 (366–1,642 days)
Kharya et al. (2021)	22	NA	ATG/TT/Flu/Cy/ TBI	PTCy/Siro MMF	100	20	NA	0	83	83	485 (198–802 days)

Abbreviations: ALEM – Alemtuzumab; ALG – anti-lymphocyte globulin; ATG – anti-thymocyte globulin; ATGAM – horse anti-thymocyte globulin; BM – bone marrow; Bu – busulphan; CB – cord blood; CNIs – calcineurin inhibitors; CR – complete remission; CsA – Cyclosporine; Cy – cyclophosphamide; Flu – Fludarabine; GVHD – graft-versus-host disease; Gy – gray; HFD-halfmatched family donor; MAC – myeloablative conditioning; Mel – Melphalan; MMF – mycophenolate mofetil; mMUD – mismatched unrelated donor; MUD – matched unrelated donor; Mtx – Methotrexate; MP – Methyl Prednisolone; MRD – matched related donor; MSD – matched sibling donor; NA – not available; NMA – non-myeloablative conditioning; NRM – non-relapse mortality; PB – peripheral blood; PBSC – peripheral blood stem cells; Plt – platelet; Pred – Prednisolone; PTCy – post-transplant cyclophosphamide; rATG – rabbit anti-thymocyte globulin; Ref – refractory; Rel – relapsed; RIC – reduced intensity conditioning; Siro – Sirolimus; TAC – tacrolimus; TBI – total body irradiation; TCD – T-cell depletion; TLI – total lymphoid irradiation; TT – thiotepa; Treo – Treosulfan; UC – umbilical cord; UCB – umbilical cord blood.

of thiotepa (TT) to this protocol resulted in sustained engraftment in the next 17 patients (de la Fuente et al., 2019). Yet, another group used only alemtuzumab and 4Gy TBI-based conditioning with sirolimus as GVHD prophylaxis as employed in MSD-HCT. This was associated with very high rates of GF until conventional PTCy was added to the regimen (King et al., 2015).

To reduce the incidence of GF, a group from India used pre-transplant immuno-suppressive therapy (PTIS). Conditioning was TT-based and GVHD prophylaxis consisted of PTCy, sirolimus, and mycophenolate mofetil (MMF) in 25 patients. GF was not seen in any of patients. Five patients developed acute grade II/IV GVHD (four classical acute, one late onset), and three had limited cGVHD. Out of 25 evaluable patients, 22 are alive and disease free, making an OS and disease-free survival (DFS) of 88% at 18 months (Kharya, Bakane, Agarwal, & Rauthan, 2021).

The approaches involving TCD also had mixed results. Foell et al. reported on 38 patients with advanced stage SCD. Twenty-five underwent HFD-HCT with TCD and 13 were transplanted from MSD with almost identical conditioning in both the groups. Engraftment was achieved in all with low incidence of GVHD. The OS was 88% in the HFD group and 100% in the MSD group (Foell, Klein-schmidt, Jakob, Troeger, & Corbacioglu, 2020).

T-Cell Co-stimulation Blockade (COSBL) and HFD-HCT

Alloreactivity following a HCT is primarily driven by the donor T cell, in response to HLA-disparate host tissue antigens. T-cell activation is a two-step process and binding of an alloantigen by TCR is the first step in T-cell activation. However, this alone is not enough to initiate T-cell activation. A second step is essential to complete this process which is called the 'co-stimulatory pathway' where CD 28 receptor on T cell recognise CD80 and CD86 ligands on antigen-presenting cells (APCs) (Figure 17.1A). Several hours following T-cell activation, an inhibitory receptor, cytotoxic T-lymphocyte-associated protein-4 (CTLA4), is induced or expressed on the T cell, which bind with CD80 and CD86 on APC with a greater affinity and inhibit T-cell activation and proliferation. If the T cells encounter the antigen but the co-stimulation does not take place, the activation of T cell is aborted and the T cell become anergic to the target antigens (Figure 17.1B).

A recombinant humanised construct of CTLA4 molecule with IgG1 (CTLA4Ig) was produced to block the co-stimulation pathway and was extensively studied in mice model for HCT and autoimmune diseases. It was approved for rheumatoid arthritis and other autoimmune diseases on December 23, 2005. Our group actively researched co-stimulation blocking pathway as a gateway to tolerance induction. Taking lead from pre-clinical studies by Kean and colleagues (Kean et al., 2002), our group explored its effect in combating alloreactivity in HFD-HCT (Jaiswal, Bhakuni, Aiyer et al., 2020; Jaiswal et al., 2017). Abatacept was first employed in a cohort with severe aplastic anaemia (SAA), at a dose of 10 mg/kg and employed on day −1, +5, +20 and 4 weekly thereafter until day+180 along with PTCy and sirolimus (Jaiswal et al., 2017). The incidence of aGVHD and cGVHD was 10% with EFS of 80%. Subsequently it was applied in HFD-HCT for SCD and thalassaemia

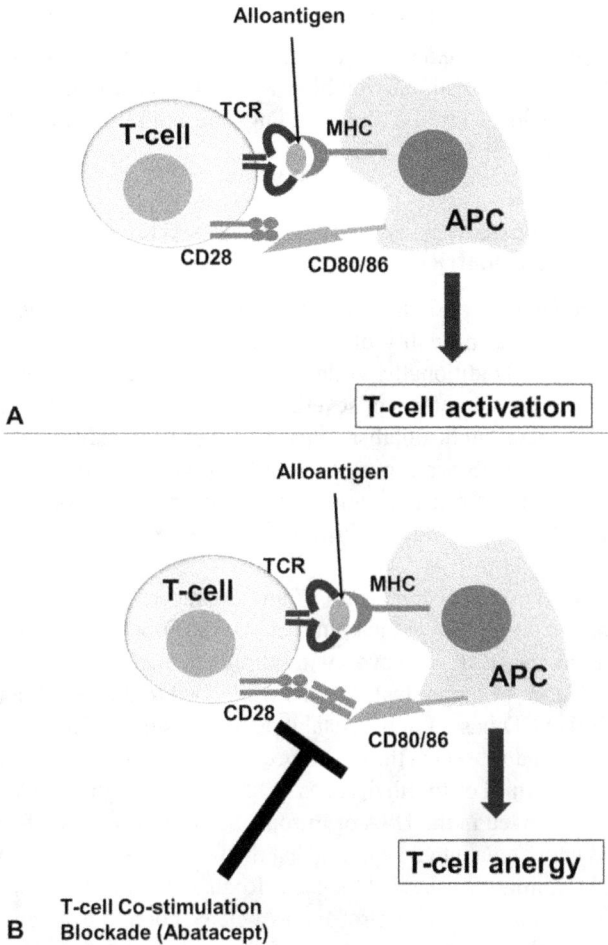

Figure 17.1 T-cell co-stimulation blockade (COSBL): (A) A pictorial illustration of primary co-stimulatory pathway mediated by ligation of CD28 receptor on T cell to CD80/CD86 receptors on antigen presenting cells (APC) resulting in T-cell activation. (B) The effect of co-stimulation blockade mediated by abatacept (CTLA4Ig) resulting in T-cell anergy.

as well, in the same schedule with an EFS of 90% (Jaiswal, Bhakuni, Aiyer et al., 2020). No aGVHD was documented and only one patient developed cGVHD. Unlike TCD there was no increase in incidence of opportunistic infections and mortality was also low, due to early and rapid proliferation of mature natural killer (NK) cell and memory T cells. Subsequent studies from the USA employed similar but shorter course of abatacept in URD-HCT. The study showed improved outcomes both in terms of GVHD and EFS (Shenoy et al., 2016).

Our group has explored the hitherto unexplained beneficial effect of abatacept on NK cells. They had used abatacept-primed donor lymphocyte infusions (DLI) in malignant diseases as early as D+7 post-HCT with rapid proliferation of NK cells and excellent anti leukaemic effect (Jaiswal et al., 2021; Jaiswal, Bhakuni, Joy et al., 2019). T cell co-stimulation blockade with abatacept might create a new paradigm in the field of HCT if these findings are born out in the large studies (Suparno Chakrabarti & Jaiswal, 2021).

Indications and Considerations for HCT in the Developed versus Developing Countries

HCT should be considered if it is clinically indicated for the benefit of patient to improve the long-term quality of life (QoL) in chronic diseases like SCD or Thalassemia Major. Traditionally, children with SCD are not recommended for HCT unless they have some form of severe complication for which they are requiring prolonged or recurrent hospitalisation and/or chronic transfusions (Table 17.5).

The best OS and EFS are reported in children younger than five years with MSD. Similarly, HCT from a younger donor (< or =12 years) showed better EFS in not only MSD HCT but all forms of alternative donor HCT (Eapen et al., 2019).

Initially, it was stroke (Walters et al., 1996) and recurrent vaso-occlusive crises (VOC) (Bernaudin et al., 2016; Panepinto et al., 2007), which accounted for bulk of the indications for HCT. However, with improvements in outcome of HCT for SCD, early evidence of organ dysfunctions was added to the list of potential indications for HCT. SCD has an unpredictable natural history. While majority of the children survive to adulthood in the developed countries, silent organ impairment is often evident in the third or fourth decades of life. Even though survival of children with SCD has improved in the USA or Europe, the same is not true for adults with SCD. There is enough data that supports that the fact that SCD-related organ damage starts early in infancy especially spleen (Rogers et al., 2011) or kidney (Ware et al., 2010), and even cerebral infarct and associated cognitive deficit manifesting at a later age. With increasing age, there is a progressive loss of FEV1 at 49cc/year, over 60% develop proteinuria and tricuspid regurgitant velocity (TRV) worsens progressively. Thus, progressive organ damage and dysfunction in adulthood result in a compromised health-related quality of life (HR-QOL) (Walters et al., 2010). While disease-modifying agents might improve some of the symptoms, the burden on the individual, family and healthcare system is not trivial. Hence, it is important to consider HCT with full understanding between parents or caregiver and the physician about the long-term pros and cons.

Many argue that if children can survive to adulthood with the best supportive care, they should not be subjected to a procedure which entails a risk of mortality and serious morbidity, however miniscule it might be. The paradox in this argument rests in the fact that the best results of HCT in SCD are obtained in those less than five years of age, and with each year added to the age, a 10% increase in hazard ratio for treatment failure (death or GF) is anticipated (Gluckman et al., 2017). Thus, majority of children face a great risk of both morbidity and mortality if transplanted in adulthood. In addition, there is no randomised controlled trial comparing

Table 17.5 Indication for HCT adults and young.

	Brain	Pulmonary	Painful crises	Cardiac	Renal
Age <15 years	Stroke or CNS event lasting longer than 24 hours	Recurrent acute chest syndrome Stage I or II sickle lung disease	Recurrent vaso-occlusive painful episodes or recurrent priapism	An echocardiographic finding of tricuspid valve regurgitant jet ≥ 2.7 m/s	Sickle nephropathy (glomerular filtration rate 30–50% of predicted normal)
Age 15–40 yrs	Clinically significant neurologic event (stroke) or any neurologic deficit lasting >24 hr	History of two or more episodes of acute chest syndrome in the two-yr period preceding HCT despite the institution of supportive care measures (i.e., asthma therapy and/or HU)	History of three or more severe pain crises per year in the two-year period preceding enrolment despite the institution of supportive care measures (i.e., a pain management pain and/or treatment with HU) Administration of regular RBC transfusion therapy, defined as receiving eight or more transfusions per year for one year to prevent vaso-occlusive clinical complications (i.e., pain, stroke, and acute chest syndrome)	An echocardiographic finding of tricuspid valve regurgitant jet ≥ 2.7 m/s	Sickle nephropathy (glomerular filtration rate 30–50% of predicted normal)

Abbreviations: CNS – central nervous system; HCT – haematopoietic cell transplantation; hr – hour; HU – hydroxyurea; RBC – red blood corpuscles; yr/yrs – year/years.

HCT in SCD and non-HCT treatment such as hydroxyurea, L-glutamine, voxeloter, crizalizumab, all of which need to be taken indefinitely.

Given the dilemma discussed above, one might argue in favour of an MSD-HCT in all children below the age of five years, provided they have an MFD. A recent analysis of the long-term follow-up on 218 children shows an OS of 95% and an EFS of 92% (Walters et al., 2016). Only 3% of the children who were cured of SCD were still on immuno-suppression therapy (IST) for cGVHD. Thus, the evidence is overwhelmingly in favour of an early HCT, not just in terms of survival, but mostly because of HR-QoL, where they are free of sickle-related symptoms and complications. While this debate might still be pertinent in the developed countries, the same scenario transposed in the context of SSA leaves little room for quandary, where the cost and availability of best supportive care for children with SCD remains a challenge for the healthcare system. Each year approximately 300,000 new-borns babies are born with SCD and 80% of those are in sSA (Piel et al., 2013). Thus, even though the data might be derived from the more developed countries, such a debate is redundant in sSA. The issue in sSA is not related to whether a child with MSD should be offered a HCT, but how could an MSD-HCT be offered in a resource-constrained setting?

Choosing the Right Donor

MSD is the donor of choice for HCT in patients with SCD with EFS in excess of 90% as the benchmark. The major obstacle to the development of an allogeneic transplantation in SCD is the lack of availability of HLA-MFDs. While choosing a donor, availability of HLA-matched sibling donor is the primary consideration for better results. However, only 18–20% patients with SCD are fortunate enough to have a matched donor in the family. Alternate donor is the only viable option for HCT. URD BM or peripheral blood transplantation has been developed as an effective alternative to MSD grafts for the treatment of haematologic malignancies, but its application in non-malignant disorders vis-à-vis SCD remains questionable as discussed above. The Pesaro group demonstrated that with extended haplotype matching, the outcome of URD transplantation in patients with thalassemia can be significantly improved. However, the major problem in developing a UD transplant programme is an underrepresentation of the ethnic groups with SCD in the national and international donor registries (Lucarelli et al., 1998).

HLA-haploidentical family donors are less explored in this context. However, as discussed above, the results of HFD-HCT have been encouraging in recent times with augmented RIC and/or augmented dose of TBI reducing the incidence of GF without increased regimen-related toxicity (RRT). GVHD and post-transplant haemophagocytic syndrome (PTHPS), which is quite unique to HFD-HCT in haemoglobinopathies, remain areas of major concern especially in non-Caucasian population (Jaiswal, Bhakuni, Aiyer et al., 2020).

The results of matched unrelated donor (MUD), mismatched unrelated donor (mMUD) or haploidentical donors (haplo) have been compared in a large data-based EBMT study on 910 patients with different conditioning intensity did not favour one alternative donor type over another (Eapen et al., 2019). Although experts' recommendation often tilts to MSD HCT being considered at an early age and alternate donor HCT can be considered in a clinical trial at a centre experienced in performing such type of HCT (Angelucci et al., 2014). Whilst multiple alternate donors available, apart from HLA additional factors to look for are ABO compatibility and CMV serostatus.

Our criteria for selection of donors are as follows if MSD is not available (Figure 17.2A):

a   MUD can be chosen only if 12/12 HLA matched (high resolution) is available otherwise, the donor should be permissible HLA-DP mismatched if 10/10 match is available.
b   MMUD is not acceptable.
c   Unrelated CB is only acceptable if Total Nucleated cell Count (TNC) is $>5 \times 10^7$/kg with 7–8/8 match in HLA-A, B, C and DRB1.
d   Haploidentical family donor should ideally be less than 40 years old. We have developed an algorithm for HFD based on abatacept-based HCT programme which is shown in the figure (Figure 17.2B) (Chakrabarti & Jaiswal, 2021).

Evaluation of the Patient Pre-HCT

Success of a HCT depends on proper evaluation of the patient and a correct choice of the donor. Patients should be evaluated for sickle-related organ damage prior to HCT as detailed below, with especial emphasis on central nervous system (CNS), lungs, heart, spleen, kidney and liver apart from other routine considerations (Shenoy, 2011).

The spleen function needs to be evaluated with liver-spleen nuclear medicine scan (Nickel et al., 2016) or RBC pit count. The renal function should be assessed by Glomerular filtration rate (GFR), specific gravity, albumin-creatinine ratio (Drawz et al., 2016). Magnetic resonance imaging (MRI) of brain is indicated to assess the neurological damage and transcranial doppler velocity for cranial blood flow velocity, dynamic spirometry and diffusion capacity for lungs and echocardiography for TRV predict the probability of further progression or reversibility. The estimation of donor-specific HLA antibodies (DSA) is a must for an alternate donor transplantation. All patients should be assessed for red-cell alloimmunisation prior to HCT (Chakrabarti & Jaiswal, 2021).

We encourage patients and families to consult a fertility specialist for consideration of options for fertility preservation if the patient has entered the pubertal age or for female in pre-pubertal age for ovary cryopreservation (Table 17.6).

Pre-Transplant Conditioning Immunosuppressive Therapy (pTIST)

Patients with acute leukaemia, who undergo an allogeneic HCT, have a much lower incidence of GF. This is primarily due to months of multi-agent chemotherapy they receive prior to HCT, lowering the HSC reserve as well as weakening the immune system. As a result, such patients often engraft with minimal

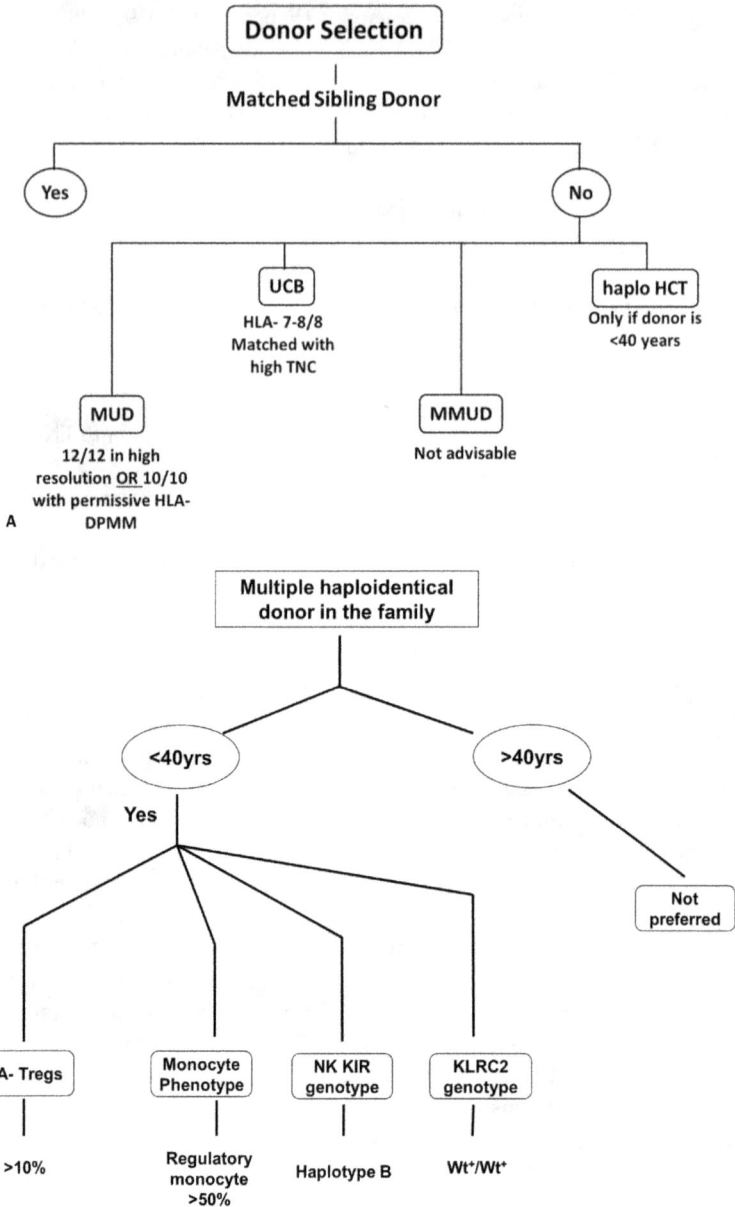

Figure 17.2 Donor selection criteria: (A) A flow chart of donor selection in patients with SCD eligible for HCT. (B) A flow chart of selection of haploidentical family donor when multiple donors are available. HCT – haematopoietic cell transplantation, HLA – human leukocyte antigen, KIR – killer immunoglubulin receptor, MM – mismatch, mMUD – mismatched unrelated donor, MUD – matched unrelated donor, NK – natural killer cells, TNC – Total Nucleated cell Count, UCB – umbilical cord blood.

Table 17.6 Pre-HCT recipient evaluation.

S.No.	Organs to screen	Organ-related complications	Tools to evaluate
1.	Brain	Stroke Cerebral blood flow velocity	Brain MRI/MR angiography. Transcranial doppler velocity
2.	Lung	Pulmonary hypertension Pulmonary function	Doppler transthoracic echocardiography for tricuspid regurgitant jet velocity (TRV) Serum LDH, NT-proBNP Dynamic spirometry and diffusion capacity (DL-CO)
3.	Heart	Cardiac-related problems Transfusional haemosiderosis	Doppler ultra sound Quantification of cardiac iron
4.	Spleen	Splenic function	Liver-spleen nuclear medicine scan, RBC pit count
5.	Renal	Renal function	GFR, Urine specific gravity, albumin creatinine ratio
6.	Liver	Severity of liver fibrosis Transfusional haemosiderosis	MR or USG elastography or/and liver biopsy Quantification of liver iron

conditioning. This was demonstrated in the exploratory NMAC study at Seattle, where only 2Gy TBI, CSA and MMF were given to the patients to achieve a successful engraftment (Gyurkocza & Sandmaier, 2014). True NMAC regimens are unlikely to succeed in conditions where patients are chemotherapy-naive. The RRT in class III thalassemia was found to be prohibitive in older children with major organ damage due to iron overload (Dallas et al., 2013). Hence, Lucarelli et al. introduced the concept of pre-conditioning immunosuppressive therapy (pTIST). In this protocol, patients are exposed to 8–12 weeks of myelosuppressive and immunosuppressive agents in moderation along with hyper transfusion to prevent the expansion of the thalassemia marrow activity prior to the conditioning. This allows successful engraftment with attenuation of MAC resulting in reduced RRT and improves EFS (Lucarelli, Isgro, Sodani, & Gaziev, 2012).

A similar concept was employed by several researchers prior to HFD-HCT for SCD and thalassemia. Researchers from Thailand used a fludarabine-based treatment for 2–3 cycles prior to conditioning and had shown impressive results of HFD-HCT in patients with thalassemia (Anurathapan et al., 2016). Another group from India employed similar pTIST in children with SCD with excellent outcomes (Kharya et al., 2021). Our group has employed COSBL with abatacept along with a B cell and plasma cell directed regimen for 12 weeks followed by HFD-HCT with 90% EFS (Jaiswal, Bhakuni, Aiyer et al., 2020; Jaiswal, Bhakuni, Bhagawati, Chakrabarti, & Chakrabarti, 2020; Jaiswal et al., 2017) (Figure 17.3A). Most importantly the incidence of PTHPS was significantly reduced. This might be attributed to increased polarisation from Type-1 macrophage to regulatory and Type-II macrophage in the marrow prior to infusion of donor cells.

Pre-Transplant Immunosuppressive Therapy

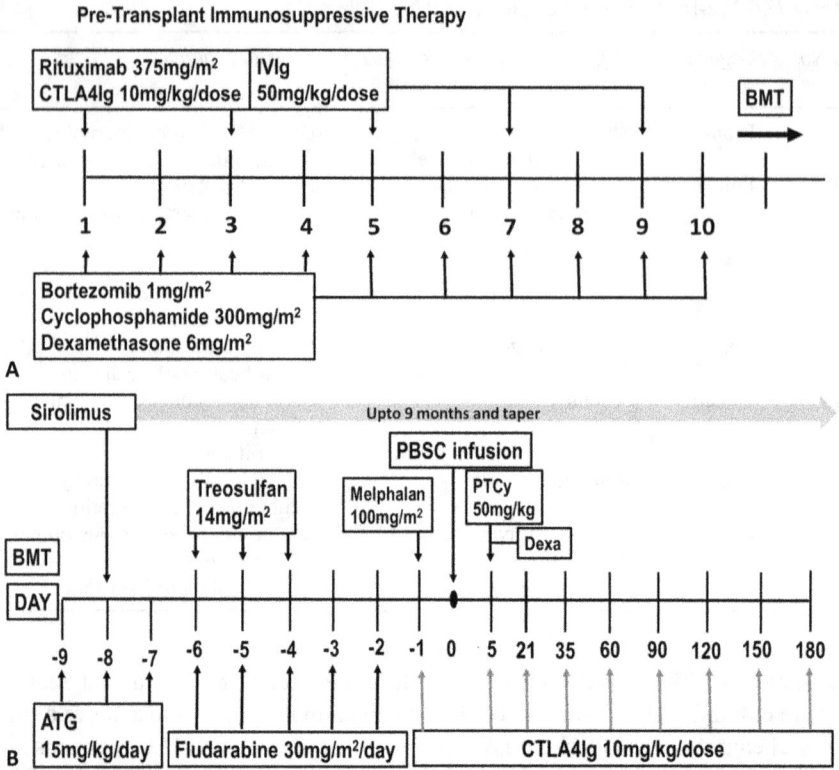

Figure 17.3 Pre- and post-transplant immunosuppression therapy: graphical illustration of (A). Pre-transplant immunosuppressive therapy with abatacept for haploidentical family donor-haematopoietic cell transplantation (HFD-HCT) in patients with SCD. (B) Conditioning and GVHD prophylaxis for HFD-HCT with abatacept in patients with SCD.

Furthermore, this intervention allowed reduction in DSA prior to HCT. Overall, the approach of pTIST as pioneered by Lucarelli and subsequently modified by other groups is an important component of a successful HCT for SCD from HFD or URD by helping the process of tolerance induction and allowing less intense conditioning treatment for HCT (Lucarelli et al., 2012).

HCT Conditioning Regimens

The conditioning regimen used in earlier days was MAC consisting of Bu and Cy. However, subsequently the preclinical studies suggested that even 25% chimerism might be enough to attenuate the process of sickling and that normal erythropoiesis has a survival advantage over sickle erythropoiesis (Kean et al., 2003; Lucarelli et al., 2014). Based on this hypothesis, non-myeloablative (NMC) or reduced Intensity conditioning (RIC) was employed for MSD-HCT in SCD in adults

(Chakrabarti & Bareford, 2004). This has shown a high OS and EFS with the conditioning protocols involving alemtuzumab and low-dose TBI, supplemented with sirolimus as GVHD prophylaxis (Hsieh et al., 2014). Similar results were also observed in the context of haploidentical transplantation when TT-augmented conditioning regimen is used to prevent the graft rejection along with ATG, Flu-Cy-TBI (de la Fuente et al., 2019).

We used a conditioning regimen composed of ATG-Flu-treosulfan-Mel (Figure 17.3B). Busulfan was replaced with treosulfan, which has better immunosuppressive properties, and less hepatic and neurological toxicity in this group of patients, along with reduced dose of Mel (100 mg/m^2) (Jaiswal, Bhakuni, Aiyer et al., 2020; Strocchio et al., 2015) (Figure 17.3B).

However, in TCD-based HCT, a MAC is preferred due to a higher risk of GF. In this context, a CT of Flu-Treo-TT along with rabbit ATG (rATG) has produced excellent outcome in non-malignant disorders (Bertaina et al., 2014).

GVHD Prophylaxis

In the context of MSD HCT, calcineurin inhibitors (CNI), either cyclosporine or tacrolimus with or without methotrexate (Mtx) or mycophenolate mofetil (MMF), have been the gold standard for GVHD prophylaxis. In HCT for SCD, following reports from the French group, ATG or alemtuzumab have been increasingly used for in vivo TCD. This was associated with reduction in both GVHD as well as GF. The same approach has been employed for URD as well. In UCB, in vivo serotherapy is not employed, and a combination of tacrolimus and MMF is the most popular approach.

As discussed earlier, PTCy and TCD are the two approaches to GVHD prophylaxis in HFD-HCT. The choice is clearly dependent on the expertise and experience of the individual centre with no evidence to suggest if one is superior to the other. A novel approach employing T-cell co-stimulatory blockade with abatacept has been pioneered by our group, initially in children with aplastic anemia undergoing HFD-HCT and subsequently in those with haemoglobinopathies as detailed above (Jaiswal et al., 2017). The incidence of GF, aGVHD and cGVHD all have been extremely low with this approach. Following this, a group from the USA has employed abatacept along with tacrolimus and methotrexate in 14 patients each with grafts from MUD and MMUD. The incidence of aGVHD was 28.6% and that of cGVHD was 57%. This was much higher compared to our study, where abatacept was combined with PTCy and sirolimus (Shenoy et al., 2016) (Figure 17.3B).

Graft Source: Mobilised Peripheral Blood Stem Cells (PBSC) or Bone Marrow or Cord Blood

Studies from Europe and North America have reported very similar results after HLA matched sibling transplantation when BM was used as a source of graft. A CIBMTR study on 996 patients did not show any difference between BM, PBSC or

CB as graft sources (Eapen et al., 2019). While BM graft is traditionally associated with less GVHD than PBSC, the latter has certain advantages:

1   PBSC graft is associated with a higher incidence of engraftment in a shorter duration.
2   PBSC contains more of T cells and hence mortality rate due to infections could be less.
3   Graft manipulation can be done easily with PBSC.

Initial results of related cord blood transplantation in children with SCD are extremely encouraging (Locatelli et al., 2003). The Eurocard transplant group reported the outcome of 33 patients with thalassemia and 11 patients with SCD who received matched related cord blood transplantation (median age of all patients, five years; range 1–20 years). At a median follow-up of 24 months, the OS in both disease groups was 100%, with 90% EFS in SCD patients (1/11 SCD patients rejected the graft). The probability of developing aGVHD and cGVHD in all patients was 11% and 6%, respectively. However, this advantage is balanced by higher risk of graft rejection and longer duration of haematological recovery. The results of mismatched unrelated umbilical cord blood (mMUCB) in SCD are less encouraging and only CB units with 7–8/8 match and high cell dose are to be considered within the framework of a clinical trial (Locatelli et al., 2003).

Engraftment and Chimerism

With the current conditioning regimens, the incidence of sustained myeloid engraftment is in excess of 90–95% in MSD-HCT (Krishnamurti et al., 2015), even though this might be a bit lower in alternate donor HCT depending on the following factors:

1   the degree of HLA mismatch,
2   the titre of DSA if present,
3   the intensity of conditioning,
4   the presence of active infection at the time of HCT.

Sequential whole blood chimerism starting at day +30 might give a good idea about graft stability. Assessment of red cell chimerism is challenging, hence split chimerism, sickle haemoglobin percentage (HbS%) and Hb% may provide the additional information regarding red cell chimerism. It has been observed through several earlier studies, where MAC was employed, that unlike malignant disorders, a chimerism of even 10% might sustain the survival advantage of normal erythropoiesis over sickle erythropoiesis (Chakrabarti & Bareford, 2004). In a transgenic mouse model, it was demonstrated that a myeloid engraftment of 40% can result in complete elimination of sickle erythroid clone (Kean et al., 2002). On the other hand, HbS% of greater than 50% suggest likelihood of tending towards autologous recovery. In these situations, more frequent assessment is essential. In this situation, the role of donor lymphocyte infusion in improving the chimerism has been documented but might be at the cost of marrow aplasia. In case of a prolonged cytopenia, CD34+ selected cells may be helpful or a salvage HCT may be required. In a patient with autologous recovery or following the GF, a second HCT may be considered after six months.

Complications Unique to HCT for SCD

Neurological: The incidence of posterior reversible encephalopathy (PRES) syndrome increases during HCT for patients with SCD. Also, the earlier studies have linked the occurrence of PRES to use of CNI as well as decreased serum magnesium (Walters et al., 2010). The management of PRES is conservative and its development is associated with adverse outcome. Hence, it is important to maintain magnesium levels and to avoid the use of CNI in favour of sirolimus as has been demonstrated by our group and others (Hsieh et al., 2014; Jaiswal, Chatterjee, Mukherjee, Ray, & Chakrabarti, 2015).

Renal: Complement-mediated vascular injury is the central phenomenon in patients with SCD. This phenomenon might be aggravated during the process of HCT leading to aggravation of endothelial injury in the end organs, in the form of transplant-associated thrombotic micro angiopathy (TA-TMA). This problem has to be closely monitored, especially control of BP and would be the further reason of not to use CNI during the transplantation for SCD.

Cardiovascular and pulmonary: The individuals with SCD have lower BP compared to age matched peers (Pegelow et al., 1997). Hence base line BP needs to be taken notice of and any alteration should be addressed during the transplantation. A combination of Brain Natriuretic Peptide (BNP) more than 160 pg/ml and echocardiographic TRV more than 3.0 m/s is a strong indicator of mortality and hence it is important to monitor patients both pre- and post-transplantation (Gladwin et al., 2004).

Infections: These patients mostly have auto infarct spleen at a very early age, leading to impairment of splenic function. Hence, they are prone to the opportunistic infection by bacteria, fungus and virus pathogens and are dictated by timeline of immune-deficiency and its re-constitution. Whilst the early post-transplant period is marked by bacterial and fungal infections, the subsequent period may be several months or years depending on the degree of HLA mismatch amongst other things might contributes to recurrent or severe viral infections. However, what is unique in the patients of SCD is splenic dysfunction resulting from recurrent vascular occlusions and auto infarct of spleen. This predisposes them to infection with capsulated organisms' mainly 'Pneumococcus'. This might be aggravated by the appearance of cGVHD. Early pneumococcal vaccination and long-term prophylaxis are the key to prevention of this (Tomblyn et al., 2009).

PTHPS

An allogenic HCT can be complicated by a rare and unexplained phenomenon of haemophagocytosis (HPS) early after HCT. This was initially reported in mismatched unrelated UCB-HCT (Takagi et al., 2009). Our group had reported the increased incidence of the same phenomenon in HFD-HCT (Jaiswal et al., 2016). This was observed predominantly in younger patients who received transplantation for non-malignant disorders. The syndrome itself has been described under several nomenclatures, including macrophage activation syndrome, as no uniform definition existed (Jaiswal et al., 2016).

Several criteria have been used in the past for post-transplant HPS (PTHPS). The original criteria proposed by Henter et al. was modified for haemophagocytic lymphohistiocytosis (HLH-2004) trial (Henter et al., 2007). However, many of these criteria are not applicable in the post-HCT scenario. Takagi et al. had defined PTHPS in the setting of unrelated UCB-HCT (Takagi et al., 2009). However, given the fact that PTHPS in UCB-HCT was strongly related to graft-failure, our group had proposed the following criteria for PTHPS following HFD-HCT. Presence of all five criteria as listed below was essential for diagnosis of PTHPS (Jaiswal et al., 2016):

1   Fever > 38.5°C
2   Cytopenia involving 2/3 cell lineages
3   Serum ferritin >2,000 ng/ml if pre-transplant levels were <1000 ng/ml or a greater than twofold increase from pre-transplant levels if levels were higher pre-transplant
4   Fasting serum triglyceride >1.5 times the upper limit of normal and/or serum fibrinogen values less than 150 mg/dl
5   Demonstration of haemophagocytosis in marrow/lymph node/liver/spleen. Documentation of >5%

Haemophagocytes in BM aspiration cytology was needed to establish histopathological evidence in BM as haemophagocytes are not infrequent findings on marrow specimens after HSCT.

The rationale for the modifications is as follows:

1   The molecular criterion listed in HLH-2004 does not apply to PTHPS.
2   NK-cell activity is usually low or absent early after HSCT depending on the nature of GVHD prophylaxis and hence that was not considered a suitable criterion in this scenario.
3   For similar reasons, soluble IL-2 receptor was also not considered as a criterion.

Since this report, several reports of PTHPS causing increased mortality have been reported after HFD-HCT (Garg et al., 2020; Lima et al., 2018; Yoshihara et al., 2019). It is hypothesised that this arises from marrow resident macrophages which are in a state of activation induced by alloreactive donor T cells and vice versa (Sandler et al., 2020). While PTHPS cause can be triggered by any infection as well, early PTHPS is almost exclusively an alloreactive process (Jaiswal, Bhakuni,

Chakrabarti, & Chakrabarti, 2019; Jaiswal et al., 2016; Yoshihara et al., 2019). One might ponder as to why patients with SCD and thalassemia are more prone to develop PTHPS. Both are haemolytic conditions, resulting in an increased release of heme in the circulation. Heme-iron-loading of macrophages results in phenotypic alteration of macrophages to a proinflammatory state. This has been demonstrated in vitro as well as in mouse models (Vinchi et al., 2016). Heme is sensed by the innate immune cells vis-à-vis macrophages as a danger-associated molecular pattern (DAMP) triggering the toll-like receptor (TLR) and inflammasome pathways (Dutra et al., 2014). In fact, chitotriosidase, a marker of macrophage activation, is markedly elevated in both SCD and thalassemia (Barone, Di Gregorio, Romeo, Schiliro, & Pavone, 1999; Kaddah, Abdel-Salam, Farhan, & Ragab, 2017), which seem to reduce with adequate iron chelation. Thus, macrophages in these conditions of chronic haemolytic state with iron overload are in a heightened state of activation due to the proinflammatory environment induced by release of heme and an iron-overload state. Haemopexin, a heme scavenger, has been shown to reverse this inflammatory phenotype of macrophages in mouse models (Vinchi et al., 2016).

Our group has demonstrated that prolonged use of Abatacept along with Bor-Cy-Dex and rituximab as preconditioning for 8–10 weeks might reduce the incidence of PTHPS (Figure 17.3A) (Jaiswal, Bhakuni, Aiyer et al., 2020). Prolonged exposure to abatacept has been shown to polarise monocytes and macrophages from an inflammatory type 1 phenotype to a regulatory phenotype (Romano et al., 2018).While, further elucidation of this process is ongoing, induction of regulatory phenotype in the monocyte-macrophage axis of both donor and the recipient might prevent this complication.

The treatment of alloreactive PTHPS is extremely unsatisfactory. This is generally refractory to the standard treatment used in HLH. Further research needs to be focussed on the unique complication of HFD-HCT for SCD and escalate it to the next level.

Long-term Outcomes Following HCT

1 The role of donor-derived haematopoiesis on vaso-occlusion: several data confirm that patients neither experience any clinical complication nor require blood transfusion post-HCT. However, their pain may persist for longer durations, especially in older patients. This was more evident in patients with anxiety or prolonged use of pain killers prior to HCT (Darbari et al., 2019). Some restoration of splenic function and osteonecrosis has also been observed (Ferster et al., 1993). There is stabilisation of cerebral vascular disease. Patients who had stable engraftment did not experience any stroke. However, the stroke was not preventable in those who rejected the graft. These effects translated into better Health-Related Quality of Life (HRQoL) with reduced pain and improvement in overall physical functions (Krishnamurti et al., 2019). Neurological complications have occurred in a few patients after HCT, but were mostly self-limiting. One group of investigators showed radiographic progression of or increase in the size of lacunar infarct in five out of nine patients. These possibly reflect the

evolution of cerebro-vascular disease that existed before HCT, as progressive neurocognitive deficit was not observed (Woodard et al., 2005).

2   Pulmonary function had also seen to improve in many patients. This was assessed by per cent change in forced expiratory volume in 1 second (FEV1) and mean predicted forced vital capacity (FVC). In a study by Walters et al., over a median of 3.2 years after HCT, pulmonary function was improved statistically in terms of residual volume (RV) and RV/total lung capacity (TLC), indicating reduced air trapping (Koumbourlis, Lee, & Lee, 2007).

3   Developmental assessment of post-transplant patients:

   a   To understand the effect of HCT on growth and development in paediatric cohorts, patients were enrolled on two trials by Eggleston and his group (CSSCD (co-operative study of SCD) and HUD-KIDS (maximum tolerated dose of hydroxyurea; HU)) and were compared with HCT on 53 children and adolescents. The predicted height velocity in HCT recipient was greater than CSSCD group between 3.6 and 11.6 years of age. However, no growth benefit was seen in HCT group. Similarly, until 12.1 years the linear weight velocity was greater than CSSCD group (Eggleston et al., 2007). Hence this was concluded that no adverse effect on height and weight due to high dose conditioning in the younger children.

   b   The gonadal functions were assessed by Gonadotropin and sex hormone levels. In a large study by Walters et al., the median ages were 21.6 and 21.7 years amongst the males and females, respectively (Walters et al., 2000). Amongst them the endocrine studies with LH and FSH level were available in 14 females and 13 males. However, only 3 of 13 had normal testosterone levels consistent with hypogonadotrophic hypogonadism in most of the pubertal males. In contrast, 8 of 14 females had increased gonadotropin levels and/or below normal estradiol levels, a finding consistent with primary ovarian failure in the majority of post-pubertal females. Only 4 of 14 females had normal oestradiol levels. However, 1 female had a successful pregnancy 13 years after BMT and another female with graft rejection gave birth to a healthy baby following preimplantation genetic diagnosis 14 years after BMT (Eggleston et al., 2007). Study by Bernaudin et al. has shown that post-pubertal female patients (range, 13–22 years) at HCT developed amenorrhea with low serum estradiol and elevated LH and FSH levels during the year following transplantation, necessitating hormone replacement therapy. Most of the girls who were pre-pubertal at transplantation required hormone therapy to develop secondary sexual characteristics when they reached a bone age of 13 years (Bernaudin et al., 2020).

HCT for SCD – A Sub-Saharan Perspective

When over a million people are affected with a chronic illness in a country, it is no longer a matter of personal health but becomes a focal issue for public health (McGann, Hernandez, & Ware, 2017).

The success of MSD-HCT in children with SCD in Europe and the USA suggests that HCT might be a suitable approach to address the burden of SCD in sSA. Optimisation of supportive care in terms of early diagnosis, antibiotics prophylaxis, vaccination and management of SCD-related complications at a national level is essential and would be a stepping stone towards the development of a curative programme (Gladwin et al., 2014; Limerick & Abraham, 2022; Maitra et al., 2017).

The major deterrent to the development of a HCT programme in a resource-constrained country, are the infrastructure cost and lack of trained manpower. With political will and awareness in the population, these bottlenecks can be addressed through global partnerships. Innovations and flexibility would be required to develop HCT programme for patients with SCD at lower costs. A key component for such a programme would be an advanced laboratory and transfusion support. Centralised laboratory and transfusion facilities supporting several centres could be a model worth exploring.

Dedicated training of physicians and pediatricians in the process of HCT along with regular on-site and subsequently online support from global experts' opinions could largely address manpower issues.

Several countries in sSA are making progress in the right direction and HCT for SCD might be a reality in sSA in the next couple of years.

Acknowledgement

We are grateful to Mr. Jaganath Arunachalam, and Mr. Ashraf Saifullah for their secretarial and technical help in formatting the manuscript.

Authorship Contribution: SRJ and SC wrote the manuscript. Both the authors reviewed and approved the manuscript.

Abbreviations

aGVHD	acute graft-versus-host disease
ALEM	Alemtuzumab
ALG	anti-lymphocyte globulin
APCs	antigen-presenting cells
ATG	anti-thymocyte globulin
ATGAM	horse anti-thymocyte globulin
BM	bone marrow
BMT	bone marrow transplant
BNP	brain natriuretic peptide
Bu	busulphan
Campath	CAM PATH
CB	cord blood
cGVHD	chronic graft-versus-host disease
CIBMTR	The Center for International Blood and Marrow Transplant Research
CMV	Cytomegalovirus

CNIs	calcineurin inhibitors
COSBL	T-cell co-stimulation blockade
CR	complete remission
CsA	Cyclosporine
CSSCD	co-operative study of SCD
CT	conditioning treatment
CTLA4Ig	CTLA4 molecule with IgG1
Cy	cyclophosphamide
DAMP	danger-associated molecular pattern
DLI	donor lymphocyte infusions
DSA	donor-specific HLA antibodies
EBMT	The European Group for Blood & Marrow Transplantation
EFS	event-free survival
FEV1	forced expiratory volume in 1 second
Flu	Fludarabine
FVC	forced vital capacity
GVHD	graft-versus-host disease
Gy	gray
GF	graft failure
GFR	Glomerular filtration rate
GVL	graft-versus-leukaemia
GVT	graft-versus-tumour
Hbs	sickle haemoglobin
HCT	haematopoietic cell transplantation
HFD	halfmatched family donor
HLA	human leukocyte antigen
HLH	hemophagocytic lymphohistiocytosis
HPS	haemophagocytosis
HRQoL	health-related quality of life
HSC	haematopoietic stem cells
IL	interleukin
IST	immuno-suppression therapy
kg	kilo gram
MAC	myeloablative conditioning
Mel	Melphalan
mg-	milli gram
MMF	mycophenolate mofetil
mMUCB	mismatched unrelated umbilical cord blood
mMUD	mismatched unrelated donor
MUD	matched unrelated donor
Mtx	methotrexate
MP	Methyl Prednisolone
MRD	matched related donor
MRI	magnetic resonance imaging

MSD	matched sibling donor
N	numbers
NMAC	non-myeloablative conditioning
NRM	non-relapse mortality
OS	overall survival
PB	peripheral blood
PBSC	peripheral blood stem cells
Plt	platelet
Pred	Prednisolone
PRES	encephalopathy syndrome
PTCy	post-transplant cyclophosphamide
PTIS	pre-transplant immunosuppressive therapy
pTIST	pre-transplant conditioning immunosuppressive therapy
PTPHS	post-transplant haemophagocytic syndrome
rATG-	rabbit anti-thymocyte globulin
Qol	quality of life
Ref	refractory
Rel	relapsed
RIC	reduced intensity conditioning
RRT	regimen-related toxicity
RTC	reduced toxicity
rTMac	reduced toxicity MAC
RV	residual volume
SAA	severe aplastic anaemia
SCD	sickle cell disease
Siro-	Sirolimus
sSA	sub-Saharan Africa
TAC	tacrolimus
TA-TMA	transplant associated thrombotic micro angiopathy
TBI	total body irradiation
TCD	T-cell depletion
TCRα	T-cell receptor alpha
TCRβ	T-cell receptor beta
TLC	total lung capacity
TLI	total lymphoid irradiation
TNC	Total Nucleated cell Count
TRV	tricuspid regurgitant velocity
TT	thiotepa
Treo	Treosulfan
UC	umbilical cord
UCB	umbilical cord blood
URD	unrelated donor
VOC	vaso-occlusive crises

References

Angelucci, E., Matthes-Martin, S., Baronciani, D., Bernaudin, F., Bonanomi, S., Cappellini, M. D., … Parties, E. P. W. (2014). Hematopoietic stem cell transplantation in thalassemia major and sickle cell disease: Indications and management recommendations from an international expert panel. *Haematologica, 99*(5), 811–820. https://doi.org/10.3324/haematol.2013.099747

Anurathapan, U., Hongeng, S., Pakakasama, S., Sirachainan, N., Songdej, D., Chuansumrit, A., … Andersson, B. S. (2016). Hematopoietic stem cell transplantation for homozygous beta-thalassemia and beta-thalassemia/hemoglobin E patients from haploidentical donors. *Bone Marrow Transplant, 51*(6), 813–818. https://doi.org/10.1038/bmt.2016.7

Aversa, F., Terenzi, A., Tabilio, A., Falzetti, F., Carotti, A., Ballanti, S., … Martelli, M. F. (2005). Full haplotype-mismatched hematopoietic stem-cell transplantation: A phase II study in patients with acute leukemia at high risk of relapse. *J Clin Oncol, 23*(15), 3447–3454. https://doi.org/10.1200/JCO.2005.09.117

Barone, R., Di Gregorio, F., Romeo, M. A., Schiliro, G., & Pavone, L. (1999). Plasma chitotriosidase activity in patients with beta-thalassemia. *Blood Cells Mol Dis, 25*(1), 1–8. https://doi.org/10.1006/bcmd.1999.0221

Bernaudin, F., Dalle, J. H., Bories, D., de Latour, R. P., Robin, M., Bertrand, Y., … Societe Francaise de Greffe de Moelle et de Therapie, C. (2020). Long-term event-free survival, chimerism and fertility outcomes in 234 patients with sickle-cell anemia younger than 30 years after myeloablative conditioning and matched-sibling transplantation in France. *Haematologica, 105*(1), 91–101. https://doi.org/10.3324/haematol.2018.213207

Bernaudin, F., Socie, G., Kuentz, M., Chevret, S., Duval, M., Bertrand, Y., … Sfgm, T. C. (2007). Long-term results of related myeloablative stem-cell transplantation to cure sickle cell disease. *Blood, 110*(7), 2749–2756. https://doi.org/10.1182/blood-2007-03-079665

Bernaudin, F., Verlhac, S., Arnaud, C., Kamdem, A., Hau, I., Leveille, E., … Pondarre, C. (2016). Long-term treatment follow-up of children with sickle cell disease monitored with abnormal transcranial Doppler velocities. *Blood, 127*(14), 1814–1822. https://doi.org/10.1182/blood-2015-10-675231

Bernaudin, F., Dalle, J. H., Bories, D., de Latour, R. P., Robin, M., Bertrand, Y., … Societe Francaise de Greffe de Moelle et de Therapie, C. (2020). Long-term event-free survival, chimerism and fertility outcomes in 234 patients with sickle-cell anemia younger than 30 years after myeloablative conditioning and matched-sibling transplantation in France. *Haematologica, 105*(1), 91–101. https://doi.org/10.3324/haematol.2018.213207

Bertaina, A., Merli, P., Rutella, S., Pagliara, D., Bernardo, M. E., Masetti, R., … Locatelli, F. (2014). HLA-haploidentical stem cell transplantation after removal of alphabeta+ T and B cells in children with nonmalignant disorders. *Blood, 124*(5), 822–826. https://doi.org/10.1182/blood-2014-03-563817

Bhatia, M., Jin, Z., Baker, C., Geyer, M. B., Radhakrishnan, K., Morris, E., … Cairo, M. S. (2014). Reduced toxicity, myeloablative conditioning with BU, fludarabine, alemtuzumab and SCT from sibling donors in children with sickle cell disease. *Bone Marrow Transplant, 49*(7), 913–920. https://doi.org/10.1038/bmt.2014.84

Blume, K. G., Forman, S. J., & Appelbaum, F. R. (2008). *Thomas' hematopoietic cell transplantation.* John Wiley & Sons.

Bolanos-Meade, J., Cooke, K. R., Gamper, C. J., Ali, S. A., Ambinder, R. F., Borrello, I. M., … Brodsky, R. A. (2019). Effect of increased dose of total body irradiation on graft failure associated with HLA-haploidentical transplantation in patients with severe haemoglobinopathies: A prospective clinical trial. *Lancet Haematol, 6*(4), e183–e193. https://doi.org/10.1016/S2352-3026(19)30031-6

Bolanos-Meade, J., Fuchs, E. J., Luznik, L., Lanzkron, S. M., Gamper, C. J., Jones, R. J., & Brodsky, R. A. (2012). HLA-haploidentical bone marrow transplantation with post-transplant cyclophosphamide expands the donor pool for patients with sickle cell disease. *Blood*, *120*(22), 4285–4291. https://doi.org/10.1182/blood-2012-07-438408

Chakrabarti, S., & Bareford, D. (2004). Will developments in allogeneic transplantation influence treatment of adult patients with sickle cell disease? *Biol Blood Marrow Transplant*, *10*(1), 23–31. https://doi.org/10.1016/j.bbmt.2003.09.004

Chakrabarti, S., & Jaiswal, S. R. (2021). Haploidentical transplantation: Challenges and solutions. *Contemporary Bone Marrow Transplant*, 223–263. https://doi.org/10.1007/978-3-030-36358-1_19.

Chakrabarti, S., Handa, S. K., Bryon, R. J., Griffiths, M. J., & Milligan, D. W. (2001). Will mixed chimerism cure autoimmune diseases after a nonmyeloablative stem cell transplant? *Transplantation*, *72*(2), 340–342. https://doi.org/10.1097/00007890-200107270-00032

Dallas, M. H., Triplett, B., Shook, D. R., Hartford, C., Srinivasan, A., Laver, J., … Leung, W. (2013). Long-term outcome and evaluation of organ function in pediatric patients undergoing haploidentical and matched related hematopoietic cell transplantation for sickle cell disease. *Biol Blood Marrow Transplant*, *19*(5), 820–830. https://doi.org/10.1016/j.bbmt.2013.02.010

Darbari, D. S., Liljencrantz, J., Ikechi, A., Martin, S., Roderick, M. C., Fitzhugh, C. D., … Hsieh, M. (2019). Pain and opioid use after reversal of sickle cell disease following HLA-matched sibling haematopoietic stem cell transplant. *Br J Haematol*, *184*(4), 690–693. https://doi.org/10.1111/bjh.15169

de la Fuente, J., Dhedin, N., Koyama, T., Bernaudin, F., Kuentz, M., Karnik, L., … Kassim, A. A. (2019). Haploidentical bone marrow transplantation with post-transplantation cyclophosphamide plus thiotepa improves donor engraftment in patients with sickle cell Anemia: Results of an international learning collaborative. *Biol Blood Marrow Transplant*, *25*(6), 1197–1209. https://doi.org/10.1016/j.bbmt.2018.11.027

Dedeken, L., Le, P. Q., Azzi, N., Brachet, C., Heijmans, C., Huybrechts, S., … Ferster, A. (2014). Haematopoietic stem cell transplantation for severe sickle cell disease in childhood: A single centre experience of 50 patients. *Br J Haematol*, *165*(3), 402–408. https://doi.org/10.1111/bjh.12737

Drawz, P., Ayyappan, S., Nouraie, M., Saraf, S., Gordeuk, V., Hostetter, T., … Little, J. (2016). Kidney disease among patients with sickle cell disease, hemoglobin SS and SC. *Clin J Am Soc Nephrol*, *11*(2), 207–215. https://doi.org/10.2215/CJN.03940415

Dutra, F. F., Alves, L. S., Rodrigues, D., Fernandez, P. L., de Oliveira, R. B., Golenbock, D. T., … Bozza, M. T. (2014). Hemolysis-induced lethality involves inflammasome activation by heme. *Proc Natl Acad Sci USA*, *111*(39), E4110–4118. https://doi.org/10.1073/pnas.1405023111

Eapen, M., Brazauskas, R., Walters, M. C., Bernaudin, F., Bo-Subait, K., Fitzhugh, C. D., … Tisdale, J. F. (2019). Effect of donor type and conditioning regimen intensity on allogeneic transplantation outcomes in patients with sickle cell disease: A retrospective multicentre, cohort study. *Lancet Haematol*, *6*(11), e585–e596. https://doi.org/10.1016/S2352-3026(19)30154-1

Eggleston, B., Patience, M., Edwards, S., Adamkiewicz, T., Buchanan, G. R., Davies, S. C., … Multicenter Study of HCT for SCA. (2007). Effect of myeloablative bone marrow transplantation on growth in children with sickle cell anaemia: Results of the multicenter study of haematopoietic cell transplantation for sickle cell anaemia. *Br J Haematol*, *136*(4), 673–676. https://doi.org/10.1111/j.1365-2141.2006.06486.x

Ferster, A., Bujan, W., Corazza, F., Devalck, C., Fondu, P., Toppet, M., … Sariban, E. (1993). Bone marrow transplantation corrects the splenic reticuloendothelial dysfunction in sickle cell anemia. *Blood*, *81*(4), 1102–1105. Retrieved from https://www.ncbi.nlm.nih. gov/pubmed/8427992

Foell, J., Kleinschmidt, K., Jakob, M., Troeger, A., & Corbacioglu, S. (2020). Alternative donor: alphass/CD19 T-cell-depleted haploidentical hematopoietic stem cell transplantation for sickle cell disease. *Hematol Oncol Stem Cell Ther*, *13*(2), 98–105. https://doi. org/10.1016/j.hemonc.2019.12.006

Garg, A., Shah, S., Patel, K., Shah, K., Anand, A., Panchal, H., ... Parikh, S. (2020). Posttransplant hemophagocytic lymphohistiocytosis in benign hematological disorders: Experience of 4 cases with review of literature. *Indian J Hematol Blood Transfus*, *36*(4), 674–679. https://doi.org/10.1007/s12288-020-01258-z

Gaziev, J., Isgro, A., Sodani, P., Paciaroni, K., De Angelis, G., Marziali, M., ... Andreani, M. (2018). Haploidentical HSCT for hemoglobinopathies: Improved outcomes with TCRalphabeta(+)/CD19(+)-depleted grafts. *Blood Adv*, *2*(3), 263–270. https://doi.org/10.1182/ bloodadvances.2017012005

Gladwin, M. T., Barst, R. J., Gibbs, J. S., Hildesheim, M., Sachdev, V., Nouraie, M., ... Patients. (2014). Risk factors for death in 632 patients with sickle cell disease in the United States and United Kingdom. *PLoS One*, *9*(7), e99489. https://doi.org/10.1371/journal.pone.0099489

Gladwin, M. T., Sachdev, V., Jison, M. L., Shizukuda, Y., Plehn, J. F., Minter, K., ... Ernst, I. (2004). Pulmonary hypertension as a risk factor for death in patients with sickle cell disease. *N Engl J Med*, *350*(9), 886–895.

Gluckman, E., Cappelli, B., Bernaudin, F., Labopin, M., Volt, F., Carreras, J., ... Marrow Transplant, R. (2017). Sickle cell disease: An international survey of results of HLA-identical sibling hematopoietic stem cell transplantation. *Blood*, *129*(11), 1548–1556. https://doi. org/10.1182/blood-2016-10-745711

Gluckman, E., Fuente, J., Cappelli, B., Scigliuolo, G. M., Volt, F., Tozatto-Maio, K., ... Inborn Errors Working Parties of the, E. (2020). The role of HLA matching in unrelated donor hematopoietic stem cell transplantation for sickle cell disease in Europe. *Bone Marrow Transplant*, *55*(10), 1946–1954. https://doi.org/10.1038/s41409-020-0847-z

Gyurkocza, B., & Sandmaier, B. M. (2014). Conditioning regimens for hematopoietic cell transplantation: One size does not fit all. *Blood*, *124*(3), 344–353. https://doi.org/10.1182/ blood-2014-02-514778

Henter, J. I., Horne, A., Arico, M., Egeler, R. M., Filipovich, A. H., Imashuku, S., ... Janka, G. (2007). HLH-2004: Diagnostic and therapeutic guidelines for hemophagocytic lymphohistiocytosis. *Pediatr Blood Cancer*, *48*(2), 124–131. https://doi.org/10.1002/pbc.21039

Hsieh, M. M., Fitzhugh, C. D., Weitzel, R. P., Link, M. E., Coles, W. A., Zhao, X., ... Tisdale, J. F. (2014). Nonmyeloablative HLA-matched sibling allogeneic hematopoietic stem cell transplantation for severe sickle cell phenotype. *JAMA*, *312*(1), 48–56. https:// doi.org/10.1001/jama.2014.7192

Jaiswal, S. R., Bhakuni, P., Aiyer, H. M., Soni, M., Bansal, S., & Chakrabarti, S. (2020). CTLA4Ig in an extended schedule along with sirolimus improves outcome with a distinct pattern of immune reconstitution following post-transplantation cyclophosphamide-based haploidentical transplantation for hemoglobinopathies. *Biol Blood Marrow Transplant*, *26*(8), 1469–1476. https://doi.org/10.1016/j.bbmt.2020.05.005

Jaiswal, S. R., Bhakuni, P., Bhagawati, G., Aiyer, H. M., Soni, M., Sharma, N., ... Chakrabarti, S. (2021). CTLA4Ig-primed donor lymphocyte infusions following haploidentical transplantation improve outcome with a distinct pattern of early immune reconstitution as compared to conventional donor lymphocyte infusions in advanced hematological malignancies. *Bone Marrow Transplant, 56*(1), 185–194. https://doi.org/10.1038/s41409-020-01002-1

Jaiswal, S. R., Bhakuni, P., Bhagawati, G., Chakrabarti, A., & Chakrabarti, S. (2020). CTLA4Ig-based T-cell costimulation blockade is associated with reduction of adenovirus viremia following post-transplantation cyclophosphamide-based haploidentical transplantation. *Bone Marrow Transplant, 55*(3), 649–652. https://doi.org/10.1038/s41409-019-0549-6

Jaiswal, S. R., Bhakuni, P., Chakrabarti, A., & Chakrabarti, S. (2019). Rotavirus infection following post-transplantation cyclophosphamide based haploidentical hematopoietic cell transplantation in children is associated with hemophagocytic syndrome and high mortality. *Transpl Infect Dis*, e13136. https://doi.org/10.1111/tid.13136

Jaiswal, S. R., Bhakuni, P., Joy, A., Kaushal, S., Chakrabarti, A., & Chakrabarti, S. (2019). CTLA4Ig primed donor lymphocyte infusion: A novel approach to immunotherapy after haploidentical transplantation for advanced leukemia. *Biol Blood Marrow Transplant, 25*(4), 673–682. https://doi.org/10.1016/j.bbmt.2018.12.836

Jaiswal, S. R., Bhakuni, P., Zaman, S., Bansal, S., Bharadwaj, P., Bhargava, S., & Chakrabarti, S. (2017). T cell costimulation blockade promotes transplantation tolerance in combination with sirolimus and post-transplantation cyclophosphamide for haploidentical transplantation in children with severe aplastic anemia. *Transpl Immunol, 43–44*, 54–59. https://doi.org/10.1016/j.trim.2017.07.004

Jaiswal, S. R., Chakrabarti, A., Chatterjee, S., Bhargava, S., Ray, K., & Chakrabarti, S. (2016). Hemophagocytic syndrome following haploidentical peripheral blood stem cell transplantation with post-transplant cyclophosphamide. *Int J Hematol, 103*(2), 234–242. https://doi.org/10.1007/s12185-015-1905-y

Jaiswal, S. R., Chatterjee, S., Mukherjee, S., Ray, K., & Chakrabarti, S. (2015). Pre-transplant sirolimus might improve the outcome of haploidentical peripheral blood stem cell transplantation with post-transplant cyclophosphamide for patients with severe aplastic anemia. *Bone Marrow Transplant, 50*(6), 873–875. https://doi.org/10.1038/bmt.2015.50

Kaddah, A. M., Abdel-Salam, A., Farhan, M. S., & Ragab, R. (2017). Serum hepcidin as a diagnostic marker of severe iron overload in Beta-thalassemia major. *Indian J Pediatr, 84*(10), 745–750. https://doi.org/10.1007/s12098-017-2375-4

Kamani, N. R., Walters, M. C., Carter, S., Aquino, V., Brochstein, J. A., Chaudhury, S., … Shenoy, S. (2012). Unrelated donor cord blood transplantation for children with severe sickle cell disease: Results of one cohort from the phase II study from the blood and marrow transplant clinical trials network (BMT CTN). *Biol Blood Marrow Transplant, 18*(8), 1265–1272. https://doi.org/10.1016/j.bbmt.2012.01.019

Kean, L. S., Durham, M. M., Adams, A. B., Hsu, L. L., Perry, J. R., Dillehay, D., … Archer, D. R. (2002). A cure for murine sickle cell disease through stable mixed chimerism and tolerance induction after nonmyeloablative conditioning and major histocompatibility complex-mismatched bone marrow transplantation. *Blood, 99*(5), 1840–1849. Retrieved from http://www.ncbi.nlm.nih.gov/pubmed/11861303

Kean, L. S., Manci, E. A., Perry, J., Balkan, C., Coley, S., Holtzclaw, D., … Archer, D. R. (2003). Chimerism and cure: Hematologic and pathologic correction of murine sickle cell disease. *Blood, 102*(13), 4582–4593. https://doi.org/10.1182/blood-2003-03-0712

Kharya, G., Bakane, A., Agarwal, S., & Rauthan, A. (2021). Pre-transplant myeloid and immune suppression, upfront plerixafor mobilization and post-transplant cyclophosphamide: Novel strategy for haploidentical transplant in sickle cell disease. *Bone Marrow Transplant, 56*(2), 492–504. https://doi.org/10.1038/s41409-020-01054-3

King, A. A., Kamani, N., Bunin, N., Sahdev, I., Brochstein, J., Hayashi, R. J., … Shenoy, S. (2015). Successful matched sibling donor marrow transplantation following reduced intensity conditioning in children with hemoglobinopathies. *Am J Hematol, 90*(12), 1093–1098. https://doi.org/10.1002/ajh.24183

Koumbourlis, A. C., Lee, D. J., & Lee, A. (2007). Longitudinal changes in lung function and somatic growth in children with sickle cell disease. *Pediatr Pulmonol, 42*(6), 483–488. https://doi.org/10.1002/ppul.20601

Krishnamurti, L., Ross, D., Sinha, C., Leong, T., Bakshi, N., Mittal, N., … Loewenstein, G. (2019). Comparative effectiveness of a web-based patient decision aid for therapeutic options for sickle cell disease: Randomized controlled trial. *J Med Internet Res, 21*(12), e14462. https://doi.org/10.2196/14462

Krishnamurti, L., Sullivan, K. M., Kamani, N. R., Waller, E. K., Abraham, A., Campigotto, F., … Walters, M. C. (2015). Results of a multicenter pilot investigation of bone marrow transplantation in adults with sickle cell disease (STRIDE). *Blood, 126*(23), 543–543. https://doi.org/10.1182/blood.V126.23.543.543

Kuentz, M., Robin, M., Dhedin, N., Hicheri, Y., Peffault de Latour, R., Rohrlich, P., Bordigoni, P., Bruno, B., Socié, G., & Bernaudin, F. (2011). Is there still a place for myeloablative regimen to transplant young adults with sickle cell disease? *Blood, 118*(16), 4491–4492; author reply 4492-3. https://doi.org/10.1182/blood-2011-07-367490. PMID: 22021455.

Leikin, S. L., Gallagher, D., Kinney, T. R., Sloane, D., Klug, P., & Rida, W. (1989). Mortality in children and adolescents with sickle cell disease. Cooperative study of sickle cell disease. *Pediatrics, 84*(3), 500–508. Retrieved from https://www.ncbi.nlm.nih.gov/pubmed/2671914

Lima, V., Gouvea, A. L. F., Menezes, P., Santos, J. D. F., Rochael, M. C., Carvalho, F. R., … Lugon, J. R. (2018). Hemophagocytic lymphohistiocytosis, a rare condition in renal transplant – a case report. *J Bras Nefrol, 40*(4), 423–427. https://doi.org/10.1590/2175-8239-JBN-2018-0012

Limerick, E., & Abraham, A. (2022). Across the myeloablative spectrum: Hematopoietic cell transplant conditioning regimens for pediatric patients with sickle cell disease. *J Clin Med, 11*(13). https://doi.org/10.3390/jcm11133856

Locatelli, F., Rocha, V., Reed, W., Bernaudin, F., Ertem, M., Grafakos, S., … Eurocord Transplant, G. (2003). Related umbilical cord blood transplantation in patients with thalassemia and sickle cell disease. *Blood, 101*(6), 2137–2143. https://doi.org/10.1182/blood-2002-07-2090

Lucarelli, G., Galimberti, M., Giardini, C., Polchi, P., Angelucci, E., Baronciani, D., … Gaziev, D. (1998). Bone marrow transplantation in thalassemia. The experience of Pesaro. *Ann N Y Acad Sci, 850*, 270–275. https://doi.org/10.1111/j.1749-6632.1998.tb10483.x

Lucarelli, G., Isgro, A., Sodani, P., & Gaziev, J. (2012). Hematopoietic stem cell transplantation in thalassemia and sickle cell anemia. *Cold Spring Harb Perspect Med, 2*(5), a011825. https://doi.org/10.1101/cshperspect.a011825

Lucarelli, G., Isgro, A., Sodani, P., Marziali, M., Gaziev, J., Paciaroni, K., … Wakama, T. T. (2014). Hematopoietic SCT for the Black African and non-Black African variants of sickle cell anemia. *Bone Marrow Transplant, 49*(11), 1376–1381. https://doi.org/10.1038/bmt.2014.167

Luznik, L., O'Donnell, P. V., Symons, H. J., Chen, A. R., Leffell, M. S., Zahurak, M., … Fuchs, E. J. (2008). HLA-haploidentical bone marrow transplantation for hematologic malignancies using nonmyeloablative conditioning and high-dose, posttransplantation cyclophosphamide. *Biol Blood Marrow Transplant, 14*(6), 641–650. https://doi.org/10.1016/j.bbmt.2008.03.005

Maitra, P., Caughey, M., Robinson, L., Desai, P. C., Jones, S., Nouraie, M., ... Ataga, K. I. (2017). Risk factors for mortality in adult patients with sickle cell disease: A meta-analysis of studies in North America and Europe. *Haematologica, 102*(4), 626–636. https://doi.org/10.3324/haematol.2016.153791

McGann, P. T., Hernandez, A. G., & Ware, R. E. (2017). Sickle cell anemia in sub-Saharan Africa: Advancing the clinical paradigm through partnerships and research. *Blood, 129*(2), 155–161. https://doi.org/10.1182/blood-2016-09-702324

McPherson, M. E., Hutcherson, D., Olson, E., Haight, A. E., Horan, J., & Chiang, K. Y. (2011). Safety and efficacy of targeted busulfan therapy in children undergoing myeloablative matched sibling donor BMT for sickle cell disease. *Bone Marrow Transplant, 46*(1), 27–33. https://doi.org/10.1038/bmt.2010.60

Nickel, R. S., Seashore, E., Lane, P. A., Alazraki, A. L., Horan, J. T., Bhatia, M., & Haight, A. E. (2016). Improved splenic function after hematopoietic stem cell transplant for sickle cell disease. *Pediatr Blood Cancer, 63*(5), 908–913. https://doi.org/10.1002/pbc.25904

Panepinto, J. A., Walters, M. C., Carreras, J., Marsh, J., Bredeson, C. N., Gale, R. P., ... Marrow Transplant, R. (2007). Matched-related donor transplantation for sickle cell disease: Report from the Center for International Blood and Transplant Research. *Br J Haematol, 137*(5), 479–485. https://doi.org/10.1111/j.1365-2141.2007.06592.x

Pawlowska, A. B., Cheng, J. C., Karras, N. A., Sun, W., Wang, L. D., Bell, A. D., ... Rosenthal, J. (2018). HLA haploidentical stem cell transplant with pretransplant immunosuppression for patients with sickle cell disease. *Biol Blood Marrow Transplant, 24*(1), 185–189. https://doi.org/10.1016/j.bbmt.2017.08.039

Pegelow, C. H., Colangelo, L., Steinberg, M., Wright, E. C., Smith, J., Phillips, G., & Vichinsky, E. (1997). Natural history of blood pressure in sickle cell disease: Risks for stroke and death associated with relative hypertension in sickle cell anemia. *Am J Med, 102*(2), 171–177.

Perronne, V., Roberts-Harewood, M., Bachir, D., Roudot-Thoraval, F., Delord, J. M., Thuret, I., ... Godeau, B. (2002). Patterns of mortality in sickle cell disease in adults in France and England. *Hematol J, 3*(1), 56–60. https://doi.org/10.1038/sj.thj.6200147

Piel, F. B., Patil, A. P., Howes, R. E., Nyangiri, O. A., Gething, P. W., Dewi, M., ... Hay, S. I. (2013). Global epidemiology of sickle haemoglobin in neonates: A contemporary geostatistical model-based map and population estimates. *The Lancet, 381*(9861), 142–151. https://doi.org/10.1016/s0140-6736(12)61229-x

Piel, F. B., Patil, A. P., Howes, R. E., Nyangiri, O. A., Gething, P. W., Williams, T. N., ... Hay, S. I. (2010). Global distribution of the sickle cell gene and geographical confirmation of the malaria hypothesis. *Nat Commun, 1*, 104. https://doi.org/10.1038/ncomms1104

Platt, O. S., Brambilla, D. J., Rosse, W. F., Milner, P. F., Castro, O., Steinberg, M. H., & Klug, P. P. (1994). Mortality in sickle cell disease. Life expectancy and risk factors for early death. *N Engl J Med, 330*(23), 1639–1644. https://doi.org/10.1056/NEJM199406093302303

Rogers, V. E., Marcus, C. L., Jawad, A. F., Smith-Whitley, K., Ohene-Frempong, K., Bowdre, C., ... Mason, T. B. (2011). Periodic limb movements and disrupted sleep in children with sickle cell disease. *Sleep, 34*(7), 899–908. https://doi.org/10.5665/SLEEP.1124

Romano, M., Fanelli, G., Tan, N., Nova-Lamperti, E., McGregor, R., Lechler, R. I., ... Scotta, C. (2018). Expanded regulatory T cells induce alternatively activated monocytes with a reduced capacity to expand T helper-17 cells. *Front Immunol, 9*, 1625. https://doi.org/10.3389/fimmu.2018.01625

Sandler, R. D., Carter, S., Kaur, H., Francis, S., Tattersall, R. S., & Snowden, J. A. (2020). Haemophagocytic lymphohistiocytosis (HLH) following allogeneic haematopoietic stem cell transplantation (HSCT)-time to reappraise with modern diagnostic and treatment strategies? *Bone Marrow Transplant*, *55*(2), 307–316. https://doi.org/10.1038/s41409-019-0637-7

Shah, N., & Krishnamurti, L. (2021). Evidence-based minireview: In young children with severe sickle cell disease, do the benefits of HLA-identical sibling donor HCT outweigh the risks? *Hematology Am Soc Hematol Educ Program*, *2021*(1), 190–195. https://doi.org/10.1182/hematology.2021000322

Shenoy, S. (2011). Hematopoietic stem cell transplantation for sickle cell disease: Current practice and emerging trends. *Hematology Am Soc Hematol Educ Program*, *2011*, 273–279. https://doi.org/10.1182/asheducation-2011.1.273

Shenoy, S., Eapen, M., Panepinto, J. A., Logan, B. R., Wu, J., Abraham, A., ... Kamani, N. (2016). A trial of unrelated donor marrow transplantation for children with severe sickle cell disease. *Blood*, *128*(21), 2561–2567. https://doi.org/10.1182/blood-2016-05-715870

Steinberg, M. H., Barton, F., Castro, O., Pegelow, C. H., Ballas, S. K., Kutlar, A., ... Terrin, M. (2003). Effect of hydroxyurea on mortality and morbidity in adult sickle cell anemia: Risks and benefits up to 9 years of treatment. *JAMA*, *289*(13), 1645–1651. https://doi.org/10.1001/jama.289.13.1645

Strocchio, L., Zecca, M., Comoli, P., Mina, T., Giorgiani, G., Giraldi, E., ... Locatelli, F. (2015). Treosulfan-based conditioning regimen for allogeneic haematopoietic stem cell transplantation in children with sickle cell disease. *Br J Haematol*, *169*(5), 726–736. https://doi.org/10.1111/bjh.13352

Takagi, S., Masuoka, K., Uchida, N., Ishiwata, K., Araoka, H., Tsuji, M., ... Taniguchi, S. (2009). High incidence of haemophagocytic syndrome following umbilical cord blood transplantation for adults. *Br J Haematol*, *147*(4), 543–553. https://doi.org/10.1111/j.1365-2141.2009.07863.x

Tomblyn, M., Chiller, T., Einsele, H., Gress, R., Sepkowitz, K., Storek, J., ... Prevention. (2009). Guidelines for preventing infectious complications among hematopoietic cell transplantation recipients: A global perspective. *Biol Blood Marrow Transplant*, *15*(10), 1143–1238. https://doi.org/10.1016/j.bbmt.2009.06.019

Vermylen, C., Cornu, G., Ferster, A., Brichard, B., Ninane, J., Ferrant, A., ... Sariban, E. (1998). Haematopoietic stem cell transplantation for sickle cell anaemia: The first 50 patients transplanted in Belgium. *Bone Marrow Transplant*, *22*(1), 1–6. https://doi.org/10.1038/sj.bmt.1701291

Vinchi, F., Costa da Silva, M., Ingoglia, G., Petrillo, S., Brinkman, N., Zuercher, A., ... Muckenthaler, M. U. (2016). Hemopexin therapy reverts heme-induced proinflammatory phenotypic switching of macrophages in a mouse model of sickle cell disease. *Blood*, *127*(4), 473–486. https://doi.org/10.1182/blood-2015-08-663245

Walters, M. C., De Castro, L. M., Sullivan, K. M., Krishnamurti, L., Kamani, N., Bredeson, C., ... Petersdorf, E. (2016). Indications and results of HLA-identical sibling hematopoietic cell transplantation for sickle cell disease. *Biol Blood Marrow Transplant*, *22*(2), 207–211. https://doi.org/10.1016/j.bbmt.2015.10.017

Walters, M. C., Hardy, K., Edwards, S., Adamkiewicz, T., Barkovich, J., Bernaudin, F., ... Multi-center Study of Bone Marrow Transplantation for Sickle Cell, D. (2010). Pulmonary, gonadal, and central nervous system status after bone marrow transplantation for sickle cell disease. *Biol Blood Marrow Transplant*, *16*(2), 263–272. https://doi.org/10.1016/j.bbmt.2009.10.005

Walters, M. C., Patience, M., Leisenring, W., Eckman, J. R., Scott, J. P., Mentzer, W. C., ... Sullivan, K. M. (1996). Bone marrow transplantation for sickle cell disease. *N Engl J Med*, *335*(6), 369–376. https://doi.org/10.1056/NEJM199608083350601

Walters, M. C., Storb, R., Patience, M., Leisenring, W., Taylor, T., Sanders, J. E., ... Sullivan, K. M. (2000). Impact of bone marrow transplantation for symptomatic sickle cell disease: An interim report. Multicenter investigation of bone marrow transplantation for sickle cell disease. *Blood, 95*(6), 1918–1924. Retrieved from https://www.ncbi.nlm.nih. gov/pubmed/10706855

Ware, R. E., Rees, R. C., Sarnaik, S. A., Iyer, R. V., Alvarez, O. A., Casella, J. F., ... Investigators, B. H. (2010). Renal function in infants with sickle cell anemia: Baseline data from the BABY HUG trial. *J Pediatr, 156*(1), 66–70 e61. https://doi.org/10.1016/j. jpeds.2009.06.060

Weatherall, D. J. (2010). The inherited diseases of hemoglobin are an emerging global health burden. *Blood, 115*(22), 4331–4336. https://doi.org/10.1182/blood-2010-01-251348

Williams, T. N. (2016). Sickle cell disease in Sub-Saharan Africa. *Hematol Oncol Clin North Am, 30*(2), 343–358. https://doi.org/10.1016/j.hoc.2015.11.005

Woodard, P., Helton, K. J., Khan, R. B., Hale, G. A., Phipps, S., Wang, W., ... Cunningham, J. M. (2005). Brain parenchymal damage after haematopoietic stem cell transplantation for severe sickle cell disease. *Br J Haematol, 129*(4), 550–552. https://doi. org/10.1111/j.1365-2141.2005.05491.x

Yoshihara, S., Li, Y., Xia, J., Danzl, N., Sykes, M., & Yang, Y. G. (2019). Posttransplant hemophagocytic lymphohistiocytosis driven by myeloid cytokines and vicious cycles of T-cell and macrophage activation in humanized mice. *Front Immunol, 10*, 186. https://doi. org/10.3389/fimmu.2019.00186

Zaia, J., Baden, L., Boeckh, M. J., Chakrabarti, S., Einsele, H., Ljungman, P., ... Prevention. (2009). Viral disease prevention after hematopoietic cell transplantation. *Bone Marrow Transplant, 44*(8), 471–482. https://doi.org/10.1038/bmt.2009.258

18 Nursing Care in Sickle Cell Disease

Lessons from East Africa

Eunice Ndirangu-Mugo

Background

Sickle Cell Disease Prevalence and Statistics

Sickle cell disease (SCD) is a global health concern. The disease exerts a significant brunt on healthcare systems, as individuals with SCD require regular medical care, including preventive measures, pain management, and treatment of complications. SCD arises from a disorder of the red blood cells (RBCs), which form a C-shape and become less effective at carrying oxygen to all parts of the body. Such cells have a shorter lifespan, leading to their shortage in the circulatory system (Vacca & Blank, 2017) The c-shape sticks to blood vessels, hence clogging blood flow, which could cause pain, acute chest syndrome, and other serious and fatal conditions such as stroke. SCD is a genetic condition. Thus, children who receive two sickle cell genes, one from each parent, inherit the disorder. Sickle cell is more prevalent among people with African, Indian, and Middle Eastern ancestry with approximately 50–90% of undiagnosed cases in sub-Saharan Africa registering deaths before the fifth birthday (Williams, 2016).

SCD was considered as children's disease because few patients survived past the age of 20 years (Vacca & Blank, 2017). However, SCD patients have increased their life expectancy to between 40 and 60 years, with various disease management techniques, such as vaccination and antibiotics to manage infections, pain medication, high fluid intake, and bone-marrow transplant that can be undertaken to cure the disorder (Lubeck et al., 2019). As cited in Adigwe, Onoja, and Onavbavba (2023), a systematic analysis for the Global Burden of Disease Study 2013 published in Lancet revealed that globally, approximately 43 million people are carriers of the sickle cell trait a genetic condition that can lead to serious complications and even death, despite being initially considered benign (Key & Derebail, 2010; Tantawy, 2014). While approximately 100,000 people have sickle cell in the United States, SCD is more prevalent among African Americans at a rate of 1 in 365 people, followed by Hispanics at 1 in 16, 300, with 1 out of 13 African Americans being sickle cell carriers (Vacca & Blank, 2017). According to the World Health Organization (WHO), approximately 300,000 children born annually suffer from severe hemoglobin disorders (Weatherall & Clegg,

DOI: 10.4324/9781003463931-19

2001), with a prevalence rate of 15–30% in Ghana and Nigeria; and Uganda (45% among the Baamba tribe) registering the highest prevalence rate in East Africa (WHO, 2006). Vos et al. (2015) assert that 4.4 million people around the world had SCD by 2015, with 80% of this figure registered in sub-Saharan Africa. However, studies estimate that SCD cases could be as high as 25 million globally, with disease prevalence spread across the globe due to immigration (Vacca & Blank, 2017).

Within East Africa, the prevalence of the SCD is linked to incidences of subterrain malaria with higher sickle-cell trait cases registered in regions with hyperendemic malaria (Burton, 2019). For instance, a survey of SCD prevalence conducted in Kenya established that 80% of the cases observed were from Western areas, that is, the Lakeside region, where the plasmodium parasite breading sites are high due to proximity to lake Victoria contributing to the high incidence of malaria (Aluoch & Aluoch, 1993). Diallo and Tchernia (2002) estimated that sickle cell cases in some regions in Africa could be as high as 40%, with little medical intervention due to poor access to healthcare. However, a recent study by Williams (2016) found that more than 240,000 children born each year in sub-Saharan Africa have SCD. In East Africa particularly, the prevalence of SCD in Uganda ranges between 13.4% to 17.5%, affecting 0.7% of the population (Ndeezi et al., 2016), while the sickle cell trait prevalence rate may also be relatively high in Burundi and Rwanda. In the Democratic Republic of Congo, Tshilolo et al. (2009) screened 31,204 newborns and established that 16.9% of the sample had the sickle cell trait, while 1.4% were homozygous for hemoglobin S. The prevalence rate holds with increasing incidence in Kenya's malaria prone areas. In Tanzania, the high birth prevalence (11,000 births per year) of SCD in the Northwestern region underscores the need for targeted interventions and management (Ambrose et al., 2018; Tluway & Makani, 2017).

Sickle Cell Disease Burden

The WHO recognized SCD as a major problem of global significance and set goals and targets, which have not been met in most of the countries (Mburu & Odame, 2019). SCD patients suffer from high rates of mortality, morbidity, and low life expectancy. The disease is a proven burden to the patients, communities, and policymakers, as researchers develop practices to aid in nursing care for SCD patients. However, despite the higher prevalence, interventions for care and management of SCD have mostly drawn from research conducted in the United States (Makani et al., 2013). In high resource-settings, various medical interventions have been developed to manage SCD and raise the life expectancy to 40 years. For instance, in 2019, the United States Food and Drug Administration approved new medicines developed by pharmaceutical firm, Novartis AG. The drug, Adakveo, was developed for patients aged 16 and older and required a monthly infusion which would cost between $85,000 and $113,000 annually, depending on dosing (Metzger, Anim, & Johnson, 2021). Such costs are unaffordable, especially for individuals who have no insurance cover.

On the other hand, there has been negligible research progress in sub-Saharan Africa, where the SCD trait is highly prevalent (Makani et al., 2013). SCD burden in East Africa is exacerbated by the prevalence of various other bacterial infections which cause comorbidity among sickle cell patients and lead to high rates of mortality. Bacterial infections caused by encapsulated organisms increase mortality among SCD patients in East Africa (Makani et al., 2013). Apart from invasive bacterial infections, several viral infections, such as Parvovirus B19, can lead to life-threatening anemia among SCD patients (Slavov, Kashima, Pinto, & Covas, 2011, Soltani et al., 2020). Coupled with the brunt of hyperendemic malaria, the East African countries have health systems beset by several challenges which makes it difficult to prioritize research and interventions for SCD (Mburu & Odame, 2019).

Impact of Sickle Cell Disease

Physiological

SCD results from a disorder of the RBCs, whose unusual shapes hinders oxygen flow and require continuous replacement at a faster rate than normal RBCs. The disorder has physiological implications to the human body, including pain, hemolytic anemia and vaso-occlusive crises which could be life threatening. Sickle cells are fragile and normally impacted by mechanical forces in the body during circulation (Iragorri et al., 2018). While normal RBCs have a 120-day lifetime, sickle cells last between 10 and 20 days. Chronic hemolytic anemia and vaso-occlusive crises are characterized by ischemic-reperfusion tissue injury. Acute and chronic vaso-occlusion can also cause painful episodes, acute chest syndrome, organ damage, stroke, and in some cases, death. Pains associated with sickle cell are mostly sudden and always felt at the lower back, joints, and the extremities (Lutz, Meiler, Bekker, & Tao, 2015). Patients described the pain as migratory, continuous, and throbbing, with patients groaning, grunting, crying, twisting, turning and assuming abnormal postures to relieve the pain (Vacca & Blank, 2017).

Furthermore, medical interventions to manage sickle cell, such as blood transfusions, could lead to serious complications. For instance, blood transfusions could increase blood viscosity due to a higher hemoglobin content, which could trigger vaso-occlusive crises (Darbari, Sheehan, & Ballas, 2020). Sickle cell could also cause ischemic stroke, most common in children, which cause substantial morbidity among patients (Guilliams et al., 2019; Kwiatkowski et al., 2015). Adult patients are also exposed to hemorrhagic stroke, which carries a higher risk of death. SCD patients also have asplenia, that is, non-functioning spleen which increases the rate of infection since the spleen is responsible for antibody production and blood filtration.

Osunkwo et al. (2021) established that SCD has severe impact on the daily lives of patients, with the most noticeable symptom being general fatigue. Some of the physiological impacts associated with sickle cell included headaches, bone aches, stiffness in the joints, and breathing difficulties, which hinders patients from being productive and reduces the quality of their lives (Fuggle, Shand, Gill, & Davies,

1996; Palermo, Platt-Houston, Kiska, & Berman, 2005; Rhodes et al., 2020). Other physiological impacts of SCD include insomnia, poor appetite, poor vision, yellow eyes, difficulty adding weight, swelling in body parts, itching, nausea, and numbness or tingling in different parts of the body (Brandow, Zappia, & Stucky, 2017; Elkins, Johnson, & Fisher, 2012). Mental health issues such as anxiety and depression, memory issues, and difficulty in concentrating also present in some SCD cases (Osunkwo et al., 2021).

Sociocultural

In the developed world, the sociocultural impact of SCD is mediated through the experiences of racism among minorities who are mostly impacted by the disease. SCD patients in the United States face stigmatization, which impacts how they are viewed, and the social support received from family and the community (Van der Beek, Bos, Middel, & Wynia, 2013). The National Heart, Lung, and Blood Institute allude that sickle cell patients in the United States often strive to keep their diagnosis secret for fear of stigma and social isolation in the workplace or within their social relationships (Labore, 2012). On the other hand, in sub-Saharan Africa, SCD has been associated with various myths and misconceptions tied within cultural beliefs in various African countries. In Uganda, which has the fifth highest SCD burden in the world, lack of general knowledge regarding the condition has led to social stigma toward SCD patients (Tusuubira, Naggawa, & Nakamoga, 2019). For instance, 68% of the participants assessed did not know that SCD was a genetic disorder and had no comprehension about sickle cell carriers and they underlying mechanism of diseases transmission to their children (Tusuubira et al., 2018). The cultural myths and misconceptions regarding sickle cell in East African countries, such as Uganda, Tanzania, and Kenya are mostly as a result of little awareness regarding the causes, symptoms, treatment, and management of the disease. Some societies associate symptoms such as jaundice with unnatural practices, such as witchery. For instance, most Ugandans believe that patients with SCD should not socialize or interact with other people (Tusuubira et al., 2018). The discrimination, stigma, and little awareness about the disease result in social alienation and isolation of the patients and their families, leading to negative psychosocial effects, and the inability of such patients lead a normal lives in society (Kuerten, 2019; Wonkam et al., 2014). The sociocultural impacts of SCD are also felt by caregivers of SCD patients, with a correlation between SCD and cognitive skills, sleep disorders, poor social relations, and low satisfaction among partners (Madani, Al Raddadi, Al Jaouni, Omer, & Al Awa, 2018).

Economic

SCD results in morbidity and comorbidity in patients, which impacts their productivity in in the society. The body aches and other impacts on well-being hinder daily productive efforts of the patients and their participation in economic and social activities leading to a societal net loss on productivity (Osunkwo et al., 2021).

For instance, an article published in *Blood Advances Journal* estimated the non-elderly lifetime cost of the SCD at $1.7 million with an out of pocket cost of $40,000 (Johnson et al., 2022). In the United States, it is estimated that SCD attribute to an annual loss of $15,000 to individuals, which totals to more than $650, 000 over a lifetime (Holdford, Vendetti, Sop, Johnson, & Smith, 2021). SCD also causes a net national loss of $1.5 billion in the United States (Holdford et al., 2021). Similarly, East African countries bear the economic burden of SCD, as most families struggle to afford the recommended health interventions for SCD management. Parents of children suffering from SCD feel drained of their financial resources when seeking intervention for the treatment of the disease. Wonkam et al. (2014) adduced that the most prevalent financial factors were the cost of drugs, cost of blood, hospital bills, transportation costs, cost of adequate and nutritious food, and the loss of working hours, which inhibits job performance. Furthermore, the high comorbidity rates among SCD patients increase mortality at a young age;, hence, draining the community of its economic productive base. Additionally, Grosse et al. (2011) estimated that sickle cell mortality rates among children in East Africa lies between 50% and 90%, indicating the frequency and the magnitude of the problem, and the economic burden it places on society (Vos et al., 2015, 2016; Wang et al., 2016).

Health Systems

East African countries have registered slow response in the management of SCD due to various challenges related to the health systems of different countries. Aygun and Odame (2012) argue that there has been little progress in the management of SCD due to limited partnerships among the relevant stakeholders, such as the government, professionals, funding agencies, and public health players needed to create awareness regarding the disease. While sickle cell patients need medical interventions to manage pain and other challenges and complications arising from the disease, the health systems among East African countries are not adequately prepared to handle SCD cases. Sickle cell remains a low priority for most governments and policymakers (Vos et al., 2015, 2016; Wang et al., 2016) in sub-Saharan Africa, with most health systems lacking the necessary facilities, knowledge, and empowerment to manage the condition (Grosse et al., 2011). Compared to the developed world which has the necessary facilities to test and diagnose SCD, East African countries still lack the necessities to test for SCD in childhood, leading to high rates of mortality among undiagnosed cases. SCD patients have to contend with poor health systems that lack the facilities and personnel to manage the disease (Aygun & Odame, 2012).

However, lower- and middle-income countries have registered progress due to immunization and improved diet among children in urban regions, which is likely to reflect in SCD management. The increasing number of SCD patients surviving to adulthood in East Africa will confront the health system with the demand for medical procedures and interventions to manage end-organ damage and other critical impacts associated with SCD (Makani, Williams, & Marsh, 2007; Makani et al., 2013). Health systems within sub-Saharan Africa are overstretched and have multiple other priorities limiting their abilities to meet the demand for medical interventions and nursing care required by SCD patients.

Nursing Role in SCD Management

Literature on Nursing Care

Nurse-led interventions are indispensable in raising the health-related quality of life among SCD patients (Pandarakutty et al., 2019). In addition to care strategies, research studies emphasize the importance of nurses in enhancing patients' selfcare and pain managements, as well as educating families about the disease, through both non-pharmacological and pharmacological treatments, especially among children (Freire et al., 2020; Gribbons, Zahr, & Opas, 1995). Despite Africa bearing the heaviest burden of SCD, there has been little intervention to screen newborn babies, diagnose the condition, and implement health interventions to increase the quality of life, with the result being high mortality in infancy (Adewoyin, 2015; Williams, 2016). Additionally, researchers have decried the low rates of screening and the unpreparedness of the health system in the DRC to diagnose and manage SCD in infancy and reduce morbidity and mortality (Tshilolo et al., 2009).While the newborn screening (NBS) working group of the Africa Sickle Cell Research Network (AfroSickleNet) recommended evidence-based interventions in the management of SCD within the African setting, limited research evidence document the practice in sub-Saharan Africa despite the burgeoning SCD burden (Hsu et al., 2018). Although scholars underscores the feasibility and importance of NBS programs (Tshilolo et al., 2009), the sustainability of the process requires an integrated engagement of the community, families, healthcare providers, and health system administrators in developing and implementing reproductive counselling and preventive care to reduce healthcare costs associated with SCD, reduce mortality, and increase the level of the workforce.

Despite the progress made in the developed world in the management of SCD, its treatment and control in sub-Saharan Africa are largely suboptimal (Adewoyin, 2015). Further, there is a need for increased knowledge of SCD phenotypes and the comprehensive care required to manage the disease among healthcare workers to enhance quality of care (Adewoyin, 2015). Overall, the research indicate that East African countries have not made significant progress in SCD management, neither is there an effective government policy, or standards and practice meant to manage SCD (DeBaun, Galadanci, & Vichinsky, 2019; Makani et al., 2007, 2013).

Holistic Care

There are several nursing interventions for SCD patients and among them nurses play critical roles in the care and management of the condition. The nursing interventions for SCD patients include the assessment of the vital signs, grading the amplitude of peripheral pulses, skin color and temperature, skin integrity, and capillary refill (Vacca & Blank, 2017). Equally, nurses need to perform careful pain assessment and evaluate pain relief measures. Other assessments include examining the patients would and initiating wound care, assessing alterations in fluid volume and deficit, assessing for impaired gas exchange, and initiating RBCs transfusion as indicated. Within the developed world, nurse practitioners are critical to the early diagnosis and further management of the condition to reduce morbidity, mortality, and improve the quality of life (Tanyi, 2003). Hydroxyurea treatment is also an effective nursing intervention for the management of SCD (Tshilolo et al., 2019). Scientific observations have shown that hydroxyurea use reduces infections such as malaria, transfusions, vaso-occlusive crises, and death among young SCD patients (Tshilolo et al., 2019). However, sub-Saharan Africa has made little progress in developing medical interventions in the management of SCD, with hydroxyurea treatment limited to few, high-end health facilities.

Various studies have recommended different interventions for the holistic management of the various complications related to SCD (Adewoyin, 2015). A study conducted by Adewoyin (2015) provided treatment guidelines for acute bone pain crisis, including therapeutic interventions that nurses can use effectively. The research further provided guidelines for managing other complications related to SCD such as acute abdominal pain, visceral sequestration crises, aplastic crisis, worsening anemia, cerebrovascular disease, ischemic stroke, acute chest syndrome, priapism, ocular disease, osteomyelitis, as well as chronic morbidities associated with SCD (Adewoyin, 2015). The study author argues that holistic nursing intervention is possible, supported by an effective national policy, increased training and awareness among healthcare workers, and increased involved of physicians in patient care, and understanding the present standards and best practice in SCD management (Adewoyin, 2015). Additionally, a study conducted by Jakubik and Thompson (2000) reported that staff nurses have an indispensable role to provide prompt treatment and institute preventative measures to avoid the adverse outcomes associated with SCD. Indeed, nurses need to understand the pathophysiology of vaso-occlusion, the immune system, the spleen, and hemolysis to manage complications such as bacterial sepsis and cardiovascular issues.

Theoretical and Models of Care

Theories Used in Nursing Care for SCD

Orem's self-care theory has been identified by various researchers as the most effective in nursing care for SCD. Orem's theory of self-care focuses on the practice and performance of the various activities by individuals taken on their behalf to maintaining the normal life functioning, develop oneself, or correct a health condition or deviation (Hartweg, 2015). Prevention of pain crises among SCD patients can only be managed effectively though self-care (Matthie, 2013). Higher SCD self-efficacy, strong social support systems, gainful employment, living with friends and family, high levels of education, high income, and being sex are associated with improved self-care health outcomes (Matthie, 2013). Apparently, the theory of interpersonal relations developed by Hildegard Peplau focusing on strong nurse-patient relationships is also relative in SCD management (Smith, 2019). SCD patients are less aware of their conditions, and effective, appropriate, and frequent communication with nurses could be crucial in improving health outcomes. For instance, a study conducted on the role of self-care management among the SCD patients revealed that individuals who perceived themselves to be better adapted to self-care improved their SCD outcomes and reduced the number of hospital visits (Matthie, 2013). The findings were corroborated by Jenerette and Murdaugh (2008) who argued that self-care management among SCD patients positively alleviates vulnerability factors to improve health outcomes.

Jenerette and Brewer are proponents for patient-centered interventions in SCD management (Jenerette & Brewer, 2011; Jenerette & Murdaugh, 2008). The researchers presented the revised theory of self-care management for SCD as the most effective framework from which health practitioners can derive theory-based interventions to manage SCD. The revised theory of self-care management focuses on creating awareness regarding the four distinct physiologic phases within which SCD crises occur, that is, prodromal, the evolving infarctive phase, the established phase, and the recovery or post-crisis phase. An understanding among patients of the various phases enhances the success of self-care initiatives which improve health outcomes and reduces hospitalizations, and stigma associated with SCD (Jenerette & Brewer, 2011). Patient-centered interventions for SCD also need to consider that patients are unique, hence require specific treatment and health interventions that are unique to their needs, as emphasized in Watson's theory of human caring (Smith, 2019).

Arguably, the theory of self-care is less effective when SCD patients lack accurate knowledge about their condition, which is necessary for primary care (Tavares, do Nascimento, de Luna Neto, Junior, & Christofolini, 2017). In addition, it perhaps does not consider the transitional phase which is the hallmark of individuals living with the SCD. For East Africa, nursing care for SCD should focus on patient education to enhance their understanding and improve self-care outcomes with respect to the multiple points of transition. As a result, the nursing process theory, which focuses on professionalism and increased relationship between nurses and patients, can be effective in evaluating patient progress and creating awareness to supplement self-care initiatives (Smith, 2019).

Transitions Theory

Transitions theory is a conceptual framework that focuses on human experiences, responses, and the consequences of transitions on people's well-being. This framework is designed to aid people go through healthy transitions including the mastery of behavior, sentiments, cues, symbols, and behaviors associated with new identities and roles to enhance health outcomes (Meleis, 2010). The objective of the transitions theory is to prepare individuals for developmental, situational, and health illness transitions, as well as care for patients during transitions to enhance quality and well-being. The theory acknowledges that individuals' priorities evolve based on the points of transition. The role of nursing therefore becomes one of providing support, treatment, and health promotion during the health and illness experience during life changes. The theory seeks to describe, explain, and predict human beings' experiences in various types of transitions including health/illness transitions, situational transitions, developmental transitions, and organizational transitions (Liehr & Smith, 2017). Further, the theory takes into account the increased risk to vulnerability during the points of social, physical, health/illness, and developmental transitions (Meleis, Sawyer, Im, Messias, & Schumacher, 2000). This makes the transitions theory very apt for contexts with marked complexities and diversities such as the East African region.

The transitions theory applies in the management of SCD as patients transit from the original onset of SCD symptoms, movement between wellness and illness, as well from childhood to adulthood. According to Molter and Abrahamson (2015) the transition point between pediatric and adult care is characterized by particular vulnerabilities for patients, which increase the risk of poor pain management and poor health outcomes. The author notes self-efficacy as significant for patient outcomes during transition from pediatric to adult care, hence the need to identify individuals with low self-efficacy at transitory periods and develop proper interventions (Molter & Abrahamson, 2015).

Transitions theory goes hand in hand with self-care management theory, as young people learn to become more responsible for their health at the point when the management of their conditions is passed to adult healthcare providers. Labore, Mawn, Dixon, & Andemariam (2017) opine that transition finds meaning in lived time, space, body, and human relationships, which effectively aid SCD patients to be more prepared for self-care management. Medical advances have changed SCD from a childhood disease to a chronic lifelong disease, hence the need to prioritize transition of young adults from pediatric care. There is a need for proper communication, access to adult healthcare providers and insurance coverage and reimbursement, and the financial independence as among critical factors managing transition for SCD patients (Treadwell et al., 2011). Medical interventions in the management of SCD have been suboptimal in East Africa, which has recorded high rates of infant mortality due to undiagnosed SCD (Matthie, 2013; Tluway & Makani, 2017). As health systems improve their capacity for SCD management, East African countries will need to manage the transition from pediatric care to adult care and enhance the self-efficacy among patients to improve the outcomes of their self-care management (Faremi, 2020).

Challenges and Opportunities of Nursing Care

SCD is a significant public health challenge in East African countries where the disease has high prevalence. There has been little progress in infant screening and identification of SCD cases in childhood, leading to lower health-related quality of life among SCD infant patients. Despite scientific advancements and medical interventions for management of SCD, nursing interventions are suboptimal in East Africa, which is among the regions impacted by the SCD burden (Makani et al., 2007; Matthie, 2013). Apart from poor health systems, little awareness of SCD,

stigma, and cultural beliefs, East African countries have not made SCD management a health priority, despite its high prevalence in the region. Makani et al. (2013)
estimated that infant SCD patients have the highest mortality rates before age three,
with most cases undiagnosed. There are few medical facilities to identify, diagnose,
and manage the disease, leading to high rates of mortality (DeBaun et al., 2019).

Increasing knowledge and awareness regarding sickle cell will help in managing sociocultural aspects of the disease that cause stigma and social isolation
in patients and their families. Medical advances in SCD management will also
enhance nursing interventions toward SCD care. There is an opportunity for East
African countries to practice NBS for all infants for identification and intervention
for SCD. Medical advances and increasing knowledge and awareness among practitioners will also lead to more evidence-based interventions, such as hydroxyurea
treatments to manage vaso-occlusion, reduce pain, and manage other crises associated with SCD, hence increasing the rate of transition from childhood to adulthood
(DeBaun et al., 2019). East African health systems should be improved to enhance
capacity to screen, diagnose, and manage SCD, hence reduce comorbidities and the
high rates of mortality associated with the disease.

Recommendations for Practice, Research, and Policy

East African countries need to show commitment to SCD management by integrating SCD management in national health policies and plans. Various stakeholders
should be encouraged to collaborate in research on patient-centered interventions
for SCD care, while taking into considerations the socio-economic and cultural
contexts of various groups within East Africa. Aside from public health policy to
manage SCD, East African countries also need to improve health facilities to be
better equipped to screen, diagnose, and manage SCD in infancy. Governments
need to allocate funding and hire more healthcare workers with SCD management
as priority. Additionally, government policies should reduce the costs of SCD care
and include SCD treatment as part of the national health insurance coverage, hence
reduce healthcare cost burdens to families and communities affected by SCD.

East African countries also need to collaborate with national and international
stakeholders such as the WHO to enhance their capacity for SCD management. Part-
nering with the WHO should assist to increase awareness, train medical personnel,
develop treatment protocols, provide patient support and genetic counselling, undertake screening for all newborns, and provide clinical, laboratory, diagnostic and
imaging facilities at different levels of the health system in line with global best
practice. Increased public awareness campaigns are also needed to reduce stigma associated with SCD and support families or communities bearing the burden of SCD.

Furthermore, countries in East Africa should partner with the developed world
for research and best practice for SCD management. Various stakeholders should
be encouraged to collaborate in research on patient-centered interventions for SCD
care, while taking into consideration the socio-economic and cultural contexts of
various groups within East Africa. There is a need for funding on quality improvement in clinical care for SCD as well as the role of nurses in SCD management

(Smith et al., 2006). Makani et al. (2011) also recommend further research on the etiology, pathophysiology, and appropriate and effective care management strategies for SCD. However, there is a dearth of research on awareness regarding SCD and the appropriate intervention strategies required to reduce the disease burden within communities. Nursing interventions such as hydroxyurea therapy have been applied in developed countries with much success and could be effective in treating the disease and its adverse effects, hence improving the quality of life and lengthening the life expectancy of patients. Research is needed to assess the effectiveness of hydroxyurea and the potential side effects of hydroxyurea therapy on SCD patients.

Emphasis on self-care as an effective SCD management approach should also consider the psychosocial well-being of SCD patients and its impact on healthcare outcomes. With the higher incidences of SCD patients as children, adolescents, and young adults, there is a need for emphasis on mental health and psychological factors necessary for effective care from childhood, teenage to adulthood. An understanding of the pathophysiology of SCD needs to be accompanied by a thorough understanding of the psychosocial influences related to the disease (Edwards et al., 2005). SCD, like many conditions with chronic pain, has psychosocial components whose understanding is critical for healthcare outcomes. Cognitive, behavioral, coping capacity and style, among other psychosocial factors, are necessary for SCD care. Indeed, SCD and its associated stigmas cause alienation, isolation, and loneliness, which expose the patients to mental health challenges such as depression, and suicide ideation, which could lead to suicides. Psychosocial issues are critical in SCD care, considering that chronically ill patients in most conditions are likely to attempt suicide out of despair. Among the psychosocial factors that SCD interventions require include resilience building among patients, and the improvement of self-efficacy (Edwards et al., 2009). Resilience, defined as the ability to bounce back or recover quickly from difficulty, is required among SCD patients to cope and recover from SCD crises and pain episodes. Self-efficacy will emphasize the patient's ability to bear the adverse consequences of the condition. Higher SCD self-efficacy, strong social support systems, gainful employment, living with friends and family, high levels of education, high income, and being male are associated with better self-care health outcomes (Matthie, 2013).

Overall, the last two decades have seen an increasing number of SCD patients transition to adulthood. However, although the self-care and transitions theory have been discussed in this study, there is a need for the application of life-course approach, which will require building support among patients from their childhood as they transition toward adulthood. The life-course approach is designed to increase the effectiveness of interventions throughout a person's life (Rowlands et al., 2019). The life-course approach will be crucial in identifying and utilizing evidence-based positive factors to enhance health and wellness of SCD patients, such as positive social relationships, and networks, healthy balanced diet, quality housing and environment, among other factors. SCD interventions will also create awareness among patients regarding negative experiences, behaviors, and actions that worsen their quality of life, such as drug and substance abuse, crime, and violence, among others.

References

Adewoyin, A. S. (2015). Management of sickle cell disease: A review for physician education in Nigeria (sub-Ssaharan Africa). *Anemia*, 791498.

Adigwe, O. P., Onoja, S. O., & Onavbavba, G. (2023). A critical review of sickle cell disease burden and challenges in Sub-Saharan Africa. *Journal of Blood Medicine, 14*, 367–376.

Aluoch, J., & Aluoch, L. (1993). Survey of sickle disease in Kenya. *Tropical and Geographical Medicine, 45*(1), 18–21.

Ambrose, E. E., Makani, J., Chami, N., Masoza, T., Kabyemera, R., Peck, R. N., Kamugisha, E., Manjurano, A., Kayange, N., & Smart, L. R. (2018). High birth prevalence of sickle cell disease in Northwestern Tanzania. *Pediatric Blood & Cancer, 65*(1), e26735.

Aygun, B., & Odame, I. (2012). A global perspective on sickle cell disease. *Pediatric Blood & Cancer, 59*(2), 386–390.

Brandow, A. M., Zappia, K. J., & Stucky, C. L. (2017). Sickle cell disease: A natural model of acute and chronic pain. *Pain, 158*(Suppl 1), S79.

Burton, E. K. (2019). Red crescents: Race, genetics, and sickle cell disease in the middle east. *Isis, 110*(2), 250–269.

Darbari, D. S., Sheehan, V. A., & Ballas, S. K. (2020). The vaso-occlusive pain crisis in sickle cell disease: Definition, pathophysiology, and management. *European Journal of Haematology, 105*(3), 237–246.

da Silva Freire, A. K., de Mendonça Belmont, T. F., Palmeira do Ó, K., da Silva, A. S., Farias, I. C. C., de Fátima Alves Aguiar Carvalho, M., …, de Mendonça Cavalcanti, M. d. S (2020). Nursing care in pain management in children with sickle cell anemia: Na integrative review. *Research, Society and Development, 9*, e182953353.

DeBaun, M. R., Galadanci, N. A., & Vichinsky, E. P. (2019). Sickle cell disease in sub-Saharan Africa. Alphen aan den Rijn: Wolters Kluwer UpToDate.

Diallo, D., & Tchernia, G. (2002). Sickle cell disease in Africa. *Current Opinion in Hematology, 9*(2), 111–116.

Edwards, C. L., Green, M., Wellington, C. C., Muhammad, M., Wood, M., Feliu, M., … Barksdale, C. (2009). Depression, suicidal ideation, and attempts in black patients with sickle cell disease. *Journal of the National Medical Association, 101*(11), 1090–1095.

Edwards, C. L., Scales, M. T., Loughlin, C., Bennett, G. G., Harris-Peterson, S., Castro, L. M. D., … Johnson, S. (2005). A brief review of the pathophysiology, associated pain, and psychosocial issues in sickle cell disease. *International Journal of Behavioral Medicine, 12*(3), 171–179.

Elkins, G., Johnson, A., & Fisher, W. (2012). Cognitive hypnotherapy for pain management. *American Journal of Clinical Hypnosis, 54*(4), 294–310.

Faremi, F. A. (2020). *Outcome of nursing intervention on self-care ability and quality of life of adolescents living with sickle cell disease in Oyo and Ekiti States* (Doctoral dissertation)

Fuggle, P., Shand, P., Gill, L., & Davies, S. (1996). Pain, quality of life, and coping in sickle cell disease. *Archives of Disease in Childhood, 75*(3), 199–203.

Gribbons, D., Zahr, L. K., & Opas, S. R. (1995). Nursing management of children with sickle cell disease: An update. *Journal of Pediatric Nursing, 10*(4), 232–242.

Grosse, S. D., Odame, I., Atrash, H. K., Amendah, D. D., Piel, F. B., & Williams, T. N. (2011). Sickle cell disease in Africa: A neglected cause of early childhood mortality. *American Journal of Preventive Medicine, 41*(6), S398–S405.

Guilliams, K. P., Kirkham, F. J., Holzhauer, S., Pavlakis, S., Philbrook, B., Amlie-Lefond, C., … Carpenter, J. L. (2019). Arteriopathy influences pediatric ischemic stroke presentation, but sickle cell disease influences stroke management. *Stroke, 50*(5), 1089–1094.

Hartweg, D. L. (2015). Dorothea Orem's self-care deficit nursing theory. *Nursing Theories and Nursing Practice, 35*(1), 105–132.

Holdford, D., Vendetti, N., Sop, D. M., Johnson, S., & Smith, W. R. (2021). Indirect economic burden of sickle cell disease. *Value in Health*, *24*(8), 1095–1101.

Hsu, L., Nnodu, O. E., Brown, B. J., Tluway, F., King, S., Dogara, L. G., … Cooper, R. S. (2018). White paper: Pathways to progress in newborn screening for sickle cell disease in sub-Saharan Africa. *Journal of Tropical Diseases & Public Health*, *6*(2), 260.

Iragorri, M. A. L., El Hoss, S., Brousse, V., Lefevre, S. D., Dussiot, M., Xu, T., … Kashima, S. (2018). A microfluidic approach to study the effect of mechanical stress on erythrocytes in sickle cell disease. *Lab on a Chip*, *18*(19), 2975–2984.

Jakubik, L. D., & Thompson, M. (2000). Care of the child with sickle cell disease: Acute complications. *Pediatric Nursing*, *26*(4), 373–373.

Jenerette, C., & Brewer, C. (2011). Situation, background, assessment, and recommendation (SBAR) may benefit individuals who frequent emergency departments: Adults with sickle cell disease. *Journal of Emergency Nursing*, *37*(6), 559–561.

Jenerette, C. M., & Murdaugh, C. (2008). Testing the theory of self-care management for sickle cell disease. *Research in Nursing & Health*, *31*(4), 355–369.

Johnson, K. M., Jiao, B., Ramsey, S. D., Bender, M., Devine, B., & Basu, A. (2022). Lifetime medical costs attributable to sickle cell disease among nonelderly individuals with commercial insurance. *Blood Advances*, *7*(3), 365–374.

Key, N. S., & Derebail, V. K. (2010). Sickle-cell trait: Novel clinical significance. *Hematology/the Education Program of the American Society of Hematology*, *2010*(1), 418–422.

Kuerten, B. G. (2019). Psychosocial burden of childhood sickle cell disease on family members and caregivers, Homa Bay, Kenya. *Journal of Pediatric Psychology*, *45*(5), 561–572.

Kwiatkowski, J. L., Kanter, J., Fullerton, H. J., Voeks, J., Debenham, E., Brown, D. G., … Adams, R. J. (2015). Ischemic stroke in children and young adults with sickle cell disease (SCD) in the post-stop era. *Blood*, *126*(23), 68.

Labore, N. (2012). *Transition to self-management: The lived experience of 21-25 year olds with sickle cell disease*. Massachusetts: University of Massachusetts Lowell.

Labore, N., Mawn, B., Dixon, J., & Andemariam, B. (2017). Exploring transition to self-management within the culture of sickle cell disease. *Journal of Transcultural Nursing*, *28*(1), 70–78.

Liehr, P., & Smith, M. J. (2017). Middle range theory: A perspective on development and use. *Advances in Nursing Science*, *40*(1), 51–63.

Lubeck, D., Agodoa, I., Bhakta, N., Danese, M., Pappu, K., Howard, R., … Lanzkron, S. (2019). ("Sickle Cell Anemia (Nursing) – StatPearls – NCBI Bookshelf") estimated life expectancy and income of patients with sickle cell disease compared with those without sickle cell disease. *JAMA Network Open*, *2*(11), e1915374.

Lutz, B., Meiler, S. E., Bekker, A., & Tao, Y.-X. (2015). Updated mechanisms of sickle cell disease-associated chronic pain. *Translational Perioperative and Pain Medicine*, *2*(2), 8.

Madani, B. M., Al Raddadi, R., Al Jaouni, S., Omer, M., & Al Awa, M.-I. (2018). Quality of life among caregivers of sickle cell disease patients: A cross sectional study. *Health and Quality of Life Outcomes*, *16*(1), 1–9.

Makani, J., Cox, S. E., Soka, D., Komba, A. N., Oruo, J., Mwamtemi, H., … Mgaya, J. (2011). ("Sickle Cell Disease – Medicine bibliographies – Cite This For Me") mortality in sickle cell anemia in Africa: A prospective cohort study in Tanzania. *PLoS One*, *6*(2), e14699.

Makani, J., Ofori-Acquah, S., Nnodu, O., Wonkam, A., & Ohene-Frempong, K. (2013). Sickle cell disease: New opportunities and challenges in Africa. *The Scientific World Journal*, *2013*, 193252.

Makani, J., Williams, T., & Marsh, K. (2007). Sickle cell disease in Africa: Burden and research priorities. *Annals of Tropical Medicine & Parasitology*, *101*(1), 3–14.

Matthie, N. (2013). Sickle cell disease: The role of self-care management. *Pain Management Nursing*, *16*(3), 257–266.

Mburu, J., & Odame, I. (2019). Sickle cell disease: Reducing the global disease burden. *International Journal of Laboratory Hematology, 41*, 82–88.

Meleis, A. I. (2010). *Transitions theory: Middle range and situation specific theories in nursing research and practice.* New York: Springer.

Meleis, A., Sawyer, L., Im, E., Messias, D. K. H., & Schumacher, K.(2000). Experiencing transitions: An emerging middle-range theory. *Advances in Nursing Science, 23*(1), 12–28.

Metzger, A. H., Anim, M., & Johnson, C. (2021). Outcomes and barriers to use of novel sickle cell therapeutic agents in a Community Health Center. *Journal of Hematology Research, 8*(1), 1–5.

Molter, B. L., & Abrahamson, K. (2015). Self-efficacy, transition, and patient outcomes in the sickle cell disease population. *Pain Management Nursing, 16*(3), 418–424.

Ndeezi, G., Kiyaga, C., Hernandez, A. G., Munube, D., Howard, T. A., Ssewanyana, I., ..., Aceng, J. R. (2016). Burden of sickle cell trait and disease in the Uganda Sickle Surveillance Study (US3): A cross-sectional study. *The Lancet Global Health, 4*(3), e195–e200.

Osunkwo, I., Andemariam, B., Minniti, C. P., Inusa, B. P., El Rassi, F., Francis-Gibson, B., ... Arlet, J. B. (2021). Impact of sickle cell disease on patients' daily lives, symptoms reported, and disease management strategies: Results from the international Sickle Cell World Assessment Survey (SWAY). *American Journal of Hematology, 96*(4), 404–417.

Palermo, T. M., Platt-Houston, C., Kiska, R. E., & Berman, B. (2005). Headache symptoms in pediatric sickle cell patients. *Journal of Pediatric Hematology/Oncology, 27*(8), 420.

Pandarakutty, S., Murali, K., Arulappan, J., & Thomas, D. S. (2019). Effectiveness of nurse led intervention on health related quality of life among children with sickle cell disease in Oman: A pilot study. *Advances in Hematology, 2019*, 6045214

Rhodes, A., Martin, S., Wolters, P., Rodriguez, Y., Toledo-Tamula, M. A., Struemph, K., ... Tisdale, J. (2020). Sleep disturbance in adults with sickle cell disease: Relationships with executive and psychological functioning. *Annals of Hematology, 99*(9), 2057–2064.

Rowlands, G., Protheroe, P., Saboga-Nunes, L., Van den Broucke, S., Levin-Zamir, D., & Okan, O. (2019). Health literacy and chronic conditions: A life course perspective. *International Handbook of Health Literacy, 183.*

Slavov, S. N., Kashima, S., Pinto, A. C. S., & Covas, D. T. (2011). Human parvovirus B19: General considerations and impact on patients with sickle-cell disease and thalassemia and on blood transfusions. *FEMS Immunology & Medical Microbiology, 62*(3), 247–262.

Smith, M. C. (2019). *Nursing theories and nursing practice.* Philiadelphia: FA Davis.

Smith, L. A., Oyeku, S. O., Homer, C., & Zuckerman, B. (2006). Sickle cell disease: A question of equity and quality. *Pediatrics, 117*(5), 1763–1770.

Soltani, S., Zakeri, A., Tabibzadeh, A., Zandi, M., Ershadi, E., Akhavan Rezayat, S., ... Farahani, A. (2020). A literature review on the parvovirus B19 infection in sickle cell anemia and β-thalassemia patients. *Tropical Medicine and Health, 48*(1), 1–8.

Tantawy, A. (2014). The scope of clinical morbidity in sickle cell trait. *Egyptian Journal of Medical Human Genetics, 15*(4), 319–326.

Tanyi, R. A. (2003). Sickle cell disease: Health promotion and maintenance and the role of primary care nurse practitioners. *Journal of the American Academy of Nurse Practitioners, 15*(9), 389–397.

Tavares, N. B. F., do Nascimento, N. M. A., de Luna Neto, R. T., Junior, J. G., & Christofolini, D. M. (2017). Self-care practice in people with sickle cell anemia. *Revista Brasileira em Promoção da Saúde, 30*(4), 1–7.

Tluway, F., & Makani, J. (2017). Sickle cell disease in Africa: An overview of the integrated approach to health, research, education and advocacy in Tanzania, 2004–2016. *British Journal of Haematology, 177*(6), 919–929.

Treadwell, M., Telfair, J., Gibson, R. W., Johnson, S., & Osunkwo, I. (2011). Transition from pediatric to adult care in sickle cell disease: Establishing evidence-based practice and directions for research. *American Journal of Hematology, 86*(1), 116.

Tshilolo, L., Aissi, L., Lukusa, D., Kinsiama, C., Wembonyama, S., Gulbis, B., & Vertongen, F. (2009). Neonatal screening for sickle cell anaemia in the Democratic Republic of the Congo: Experience from a pioneer project on 31 204 newborns. *Journal of Clinical Pathology, 62*(1), 35–38.

Tshilolo, L., Tomlinson, G., Williams, T. N., Santos, B., Olupot-Olupot, P., Lane, A., ... McGann, P. T. (2019). Hydroxyurea for children with sickle cell anemia in sub-Saharan Africa. *New England Journal of Medicine, 380*(2), 121–131.

Tusuubira, S. K., Naggawa, T., & Nakamoga, V. (2019). To join or not to join? A case of sickle cell clubs, stigma and discrimination in secondary schools in Butambala district, Uganda. *Adolescent Health, Medicine and Therapeutics, 10*, 145.

Tusuubira, S. K., Nakayinga, R., Mwambi, B., Odda, J., Kiconco, S., & Komuhangi, A. (2018). Knowledge, perception and practices towards sickle cell disease: A community survey among adults in Lubaga division, Kampala Uganda. *BMC Public Health, 18*(1), 1–5.

Vacca Jr, V. M., & Blank, L. (2017). Sickle cell disease: Where are we now? *Nursing, 47*(4), 26–34.

van der Beek, K. M., Bos, I., Middel, B., & Wynia, K. (2013). Experienced stigmatization reduced quality of life of patients with a neuromuscular disease: A cross-sectional study. *Clinical Rehabilitation, 27*(11), 1029–1038.

Vos, T., Allen, C., Arora, M., Barber, R. M., Bhutta, Z. A., Brown, A., ... Chen, A. Z. (2016). Global, regional, and national incidence, prevalence, and years lived with disability for 310 diseases and injuries, 1990–2015: A systematic analysis for the Global Burden of Disease Study 2015. *The Lancet, 388*(10053), 1545–1602.

Vos, T., Barber, R. M., Bell, B., Bertozzi-Villa, A., Biryukov, S., Bolliger, I., ... Dicker, D. (2015). Global, regional, and national incidence, prevalence, and years lived with disability for 301 acute and chronic diseases and injuries in 188 countries, 1990–2013: A systematic analysis for the Global Burden of Disease Study 2013. *The Lancet, 386*(9995), 743–800.

Wang, H., Naghavi, M., Allen, C., Barber, R., Carter, A., Casey, D., ... Coggeshall, M. (2016). Global, regional, and national life expectancy, all-cause mortality, and cause-specific mortality for 249 causes of death, 1980–2015: A systematic analysis for the Global Burden of Disease Study 2015. *The Lancet, 388*(10053), 1459–1544.

Weatherall, D., & Clegg, J. B. (2001). Inherited haemoglobin disorders: An increasing global health problem. *Bulletin of the World Health Organization, 79*, 704–712.

WHO. (2006). Sickle-Cell Anaemia. Retrieved from https://apps.who.int/gb/ebwha/pdf_files/WHA59/A59_9-en.pdf

Williams, T. N. (2016). Sickle cell disease in sub-Saharan Africa. *Hematology/Oncology Clinics, 30*(2), 343–358.

Wonkam, A., Mba, C. Z., Mbanya, D., Ngogang, J., Ramesar, R., & Angwafo, F. F. (2014). Psychosocial burden of sickle cell disease on parents with an affected child in Cameroon. *Journal of Genetic Counseling, 23*(2), 192–201.

19 Access to Blood Products for Sickle Cell Disease Warriors in Nigeria

Challenges and Opportunities

Adaeze Oreh

Introduction

Sickle cell disease (SCD) is the most common genetic disorder amongst Black people and one of the major chronic non-communicable diseases (NCDs) affecting children. With regard to the global burden of the disease, Nigeria ranks the highest in the world for the number of cases of sickle cell disease. Each year, approximately 150,000 babies are born in the country with SCD, and between 70% and 90% of them die before they reach the age of five (Fraiwan et al., 2019). The disease is a source of significant psycho-socio-economic burden, not only to those who suffer from this disease, but also on their families and caregivers (Adegoke & Kuteyi, 2012; Edwards et al., 2005). The impact on the family is worse in developing countries such as Nigeria because of inadequate healthcare and social welfare services (Adegoke & Kuteyi, 2012).

Clinical research evidence continues to validate the role of safe, quality blood transfusion as a critical intervention in the management of SCD patients (Howard, 2016). This therapy is often necessary to effectively address the acute vaso-occlusive complications of SCD which frequently arise, namely acute chest syndrome, acute anemia, acute ischemic stroke, acute pain, acute priapism, multiorgan failure, acute sickle hepatopathy, severe sepsis, and other painful events which require that the oxygen-carrying capacity of the patient's blood is bolstered (Table 19.1) (Diaku-Akinwumi et al., 2016; Howard & Telfer, 2015; National Heart Lung and Blood Institute [NHLBI], 2014).

Therefore, up to 40–60% of patients with sickle cell anemia (SCA) require frequent blood transfusions, even from as early as childhood, to address their complications and ensure a good quality of health and well-being (Diaku-Akinwunmi et al., 2016; Howard, 2016). Additionally, there is a documented increase in the rate of maternal and foetal morbidity and mortality in women with SCD. In a prospective research study conducted in the United Kingdom, 26 out of 109 women (24%) were transfused during pregnancy, and transfusion was even more frequent in women with HbSS (45%) than in those with HbSC (5%) (Oteng-Ntim et al., 20154).

There are vast differences between how blood is utilized in high-income settings compared to low income. In high-income countries, blood transfusions are most

DOI: 10.4324/9781003463931-20

Table 19.1 Summary of emergency indications for blood transfusion in SCD (Howard, 2016; Howard & Telfer, 2015; Martone et al., 2021; NHLBI, 2014; Wang & Dwan, 2013).

Indication	Comment
Acute anemia	Simple transfusion to baseline hemoglobin
Acute ischemic stroke	Prophylactic transfusions to prevent severe vaso-occlusion and stroke, or therapeutic exchange transfusion
Acute pain	Not currently indicated unless additional complication is present
Acute chest syndrome	No transfusion, simple or exchange transfusion depending on severity
Acute priapism	Consider simple or exchange transfusion if no response to initial treatment
Multiorgan failure, acute sickle hepatopathy, severe sepsis	Simple top-up transfusion or exchange transfusion

Source: Adapted from Howard (2016).

frequently indicated following heart and transplant surgeries, in the management of massive trauma or during cancer treatment. In such scenarios, nearly 80% of transfusions are administered to patients above 60 years (Tancred & Bates, 2019). The picture however differs greatly in low- and middle-income countries (LMICs), where two-thirds of blood transfusions are given to children with anemia under the age of five, followed by the transfusion of women during complications in pregnancy and childbirth (World Health Organization [WHO], 2022).

Also, in high-income countries, the blood usage rate reported is approximately 32 units of blood per 1,000 persons, 12.5 units in upper middle-income countries, 5.38 units in lower middle-income countries and 3.41 units in low-income countries (Bonnar, 2000; Rath, 2011). The huge differences in these data across country income levels point at a massive under-utilisation of blood in LMICs (WHO, 2022). According to WHO guidelines of ten units for each 1,000 population, approximately 13 million units of blood are required to meet the blood transfusion demand of over 1.37 billion people in Africa (WHO, 2009). However, each year, an estimated 4.4 million units of blood are collected, thereby addressing less than 35% of the estimated need (Loua et al., 2018). Of course, under-reporting of blood collection data is also an important consideration on the continent. Several factors drive the demand for blood, and in sub-Saharan Africa, these include but are not limited to obstetric bleeding, road traffic accidents, armed conflict, SCD and childhood anaemia, malnutrition, HIV, malaria, and parasitic infections (Bloch et al., 2012). This highlights the fact that a lack of access to safe blood and blood products disproportionately affects the young in whom most transfusions are required, thus exacting a severe economic toll on a region that is already considerably economically challenged (Bloch et al., 2012).

Certain factors place a significant amount of strain on the blood supply in sub-Saharan Africa, and some of these include the weak health and transfusion services infrastructure, dearth of skilled workforce, high prevalence of anemia, and high malaria burden (Lund et al., 2013).

A cross-sectional study conducted across 31 public and secondary hospitals in Nigeria revealed that more than 78% of clinicians were unable to transfuse an SCD patient because of unavailability of blood between once a month and three or more times monthly (Diaku-Akinwunmi et al., 2016). Challenges which were regularly reported by up to 80% of patients while engaging with blood establishments included financial constraints, inadequate blood availability, and delays in accessing blood (Diaku-Akinwunmi et al., 2016).

Following the 2006 survey conducted by World Health Organization (WHO) on the *Status of Blood Safety in the WHO African Region*, the United Nations agency projected that by the year 2012, safe and sustainable blood transfusion services would have been actualized in sub-Saharan Africa (WHO, 2009). Unfortunately, the current reality is that despite the development of policies aimed at providing safe, affordable, and readily available blood units to patients in need, the implementation of these policies and the impact on the people have fallen quite short (Lund et al., 2013; Tagny et al, 2008). Globally, it is recognized that a robust supply of safe blood units is critical to the effective delivery of healthcare services to save lives in various clinical settings (Aneke & Okocha, 2017). Therefore, for numerous African countries, the failure to have achieved this goal has translated to a perpetuation of negative health indices especially for maternal health, malaria, anemias, trauma, cancers, and of course SCD.

Challenges of Access to Blood and Blood Products in Nigeria

Management of Blood Transfusion Services

An overview of blood transfusion services in the African region presented by WHO reports the presence of a national blood transfusion service in 42 countries – Nigeria being one of such countries. National coordination of the service by government was reported in 36 (78%) of the 46 countries, and national blood policies were either fully or partially developed in 44 (96%) out of 46 countries. However, only 38 (83%) countries had developed plans to operationalize their policies while such policies were only being implemented in 23 (50%) of the countries (WHO, 2009).

Regarding enabling legislature, only 33 (72%) countries had enacted or were in the process of enacting legislation for their National Blood Services at the time of the survey (WHO, 2009). Although a significant number of the African countries surveyed by WHO reported a functioning transfusion service with legislation and national policies in place, eight countries had no national blood transfusion service, the majority lacked a legal framework for blood transfusion policy nationally, and most were reliant on external financial and technical assistance from international agencies such as WHO, the United Nations AIDS program, the United States President's Emergency Fund for AIDS Relief, and the Global Fund for AIDS, Tuberculosis and Malaria (Bloch et al., 2012; WHO, 2009). In fact, Nigeria's National Blood Service was only recently provided full legislative backing under the provisions of the National Blood Service Commission Act of 2021 (Federal Republic of Nigeria [FRN], 2021).

Nigeria's National Blood Service commenced operations in 2005 following a bilateral partnership between the Federal Government of Nigeria (FGN) and the United States government (USG) through the United States (US) President's Emergency Fund for AIDS Relief (PEPFAR) as the National Blood Transfusion Service [NBTS] (2020). The organization currently has a nationwide presence with a national headquarters, and 17 blood collection, screening, and distribution centres across the 6 geopolitical zones of Nigeria, including the Federal Capital Territory (FCT) Abuja (Figure 19.1) (Oreh et al., 2022). Through a pool of regular donations by voluntary, unpaid blood donors, NBSC collects, screens, stores, and distributes approximately 50,000 safe blood units each year, making them available to patients following requests from partner hospitals across the country.

Although approximately 3.2 million units of blood are transfused annually in secondary and tertiary hospitals across Nigeria, majority of these donations are sourced from paid commercial blood donors (NBTS, 2020). Only recently, with the passage of the NBSC Act of 2021, does the National Blood Service have the requisite legislative powers to regulate, coordinate, and ensure the safe provision of blood services nationwide. Whereas the National Health Act of 2014 recognized the role of the National Blood Service, clear legislative backing for the Service to regulate blood establishments nationwide with regard to safety and quality was only provided in 2021 (FRN, 2014, 2021). The NBSC's presence in 17 of Nigeria's

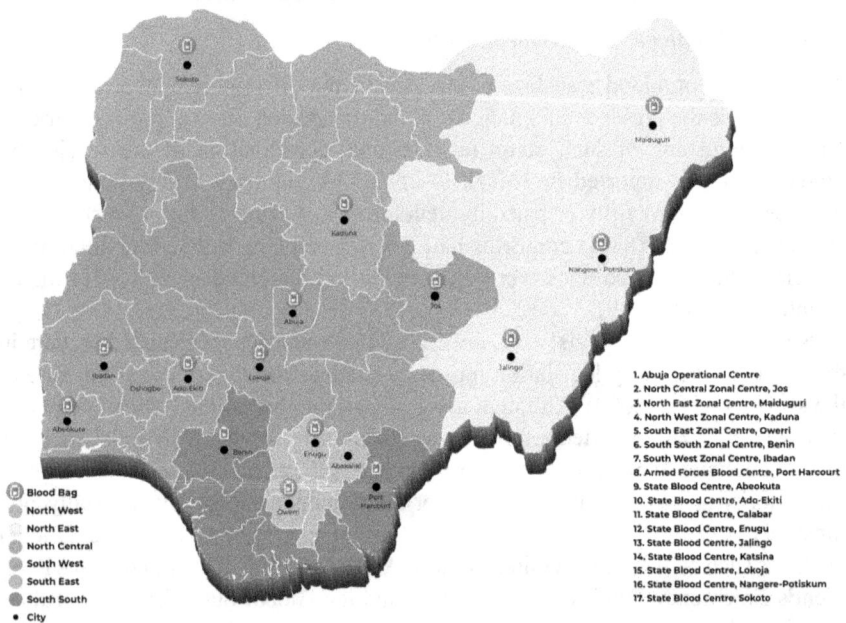

1. Abuja Operational Centre
2. North Central Zonal Centre, Jos
3. North East Zonal Centre, Maiduguri
4. North West Zonal Centre, Kaduna
5. South East Zonal Centre, Owerri
6. South South Zonal Centre, Benin
7. South West Zonal Centre, Ibadan
8. Armed Forces Blood Centre, Port Harcourt
9. State Blood Centre, Abeokuta
10. State Blood Centre, Ado-Ekiti
11. State Blood Centre, Calabar
12. State Blood Centre, Enugu
13. State Blood Centre, Jalingo
14. State Blood Centre, Katsina
15. State Blood Centre, Lokoja
16. State Blood Centre, Nangere-Potiskum
17. State Blood Centre, Sokoto

Figure 19.1 Distribution of National Blood Service Commission (NBSC) centres across Nigeria.

Source: Oreh et al. (2022).

36 states and the federal capital territory, and the Lagos State Blood Transfusion Service leaves 18 other states that need to establish State Blood Transfusion Services (SBTS) with NBSC providing technical support. Given Nigeria's vast land mass and population size, this state coverage gap in blood service provision is relevant to the gaps experienced by patients in critical need of safe blood country wide.

Blood Donor Mobilisation

Approximately 118.4 million blood donations are collected globally – 40% of these are collected in high-income countries, which are home to a mere 16% of the world's population, while donors from LMICs which make up about 48% of the world's population contribute only 24% of the global blood supply (WHO, 2021, 2022).

These wide disparities in blood donation signal the marked difference in the level of access to blood between low- and high-income countries, as the whole blood donation rate is an indicator for the general availability of blood in a country (Tancred & Bates, 2019). For every 1,000 people in high-income countries, there are 33.1 donations and 4.6 donations in low-income countries (WHO, 2022). Globally, differences have been noted in people's perceptions regarding blood donation, and in LMICs, despite considerable levels of altruistic motivations, these perceptions are driven by significant myths and misconceptions about the purpose and safety of blood donation (Asamoah-Akuoko et al., 2017; Zanin et al., 2016).

Some of these beliefs include fears of finding out their HIV status, fear that unsterile needles will be used, thereby transmitting infections such as HIV and hepatitis, beliefs that blood lost in a donation is not replenished, and fear that one's blood once collected could be used for witchcraft (Muthivhi et al., 2015; Shenga, Pal & Sengupta, 2018). Other fears observed as deterrents to would-be donors include fear of side effects such as weight loss, sudden death, sexual disorders, high blood pressure, and convulsions (Aneke & Okocha, 2017). Researchers have also found that in many developing countries challenged by a dearth of voluntary blood donors, there is often a wide gap between awareness of voluntary blood donation and the actual commitment to donating blood amongst young populations (Ciepiela et al., 2017; Ossai et al., 2018; Ugwu et al., 2019). Other reasons for low voluntary unpaid donations in low-resource settings include deferred donations in prospective blood donors due to low hemoglobin counts from anemia, malaria, and poor nutrition. Ironically, the environments which desperately need safe blood supplies are lacking sufficiently large numbers of healthy blood donors (Oreh, 2020).

In Nigeria, like in many other LMICs, transfusion services are predominantly hospital-led. For anyone seeking blood, it is often the responsibility of the family to find a replacement donor whose blood is used to replace the blood unit transfused to the patient. Most often, these donors are actually paid or commercial blood donors, and not family replacement donors. Additionally, these donations are screened for transfusion-transmissible infections (TTIs) and also undergo grouping and compatibility testing at the hospital laboratory. Unfortunately, this system is prone to significant delays, inconvenience, and untold distress for most patients and their families (Bates, Manyasi & Lara, 2007).

Screening of Blood and Transfusion-Transmissible Infections

The major TTIs such as human immunodeficiency virus (HIV), hepatitis B (HBV), hepatitis C (HCV), and syphilis are a global concern. Furthermore, other infestations including malaria and filariasis could be transmitted via blood transfusion (Choudhury et al., 2003; Kitchen & Chiodini, 2006). The prevalence of TTIs however varies significantly between geographical location and population of study, but the relatively high prevalence in LMICs coupled with poor screening equipment and documentation in numerous blood establishments are quite concerning (Bloch et al., 2012).

In sub-Saharan Africa, 1.3% of blood units were estimated to be reactive to HIV, 4.2% to hepatitis B virus, 1.0% to hepatitis C virus, and 0.8% to syphilis (Loua et al., 2018; WHO, 2022). Stockouts of testing kits for TTIs are quite common in LMICs, and Nigeria is no exception. With exponentially rising inflation rates, difficulties in foreign-exchange transactions, and supply chain disruptions in the wake of COVID-19, these shortages have heightened. Globally, HIV testing rates for blood for transfusion range from 91.5% to 99.7%, hepatitis B virus testing from 26.8% to 98.5%, hepatitis C virus from 17.5% to 99%, and syphilis from 66% to 98.4% (WHO, 2022).

Over the years, due to financial constraints, rapid test kits (RTKs) were promoted, especially in LMICs as a cost-efficient means of screening blood donated for transfusion. However, these rapid test kits are of variable sensitivity and need validation before use (Garraud et al., 2016; Pruett et al., 2015). Thus, the screening results are often unreliable with a significant number of false negative results and subsequent transfusion with TTI-infected blood. Ideally, screening tests for the most prevalent transfusion-transmittable infections, such as HIV, hepatitis B virus, and hepatitis C virus, should be highly sensitive to reduce the risk of transmitting infection to blood recipients (Pirozzolo & LeMay, 2007). As the largest recipients of blood donations, pregnant women and children below the age of five are at the greatest risk of acquiring such infections (Roberts et al., 2017). During the public hearing for the bill to establish Nigeria's National Blood Service Commission, a member of the House of Representatives who sponsored the bill shared a family experience of hepatitis B transmission following blood transfusion to his daughter, a young SCD survivor (Nda-Isaiah, 2020). Although maximum sensitivity is provided by nucleic acid testing, this method is prohibitively expensive for LMICs (Jani & Peter, 2022; Roberts et al., 2017; Tancred & Bates, 2019).

Appropriate Clinical Use of Blood and Regulation of Blood Donor and Recipient Safety

Blood transfusions are life-saving, however, due to the risks, they must only be used when necessary. Health facilities in Africa record post-transfusion case fatality rates of 6–20% (Hassall et al., 2020; Tancred & Bates, 2019). Furthermore, blood transfusions are expensive. In Nigeria, the cost of one unit of whole blood transfused can exceed 25 USD, and 500 USD for platelet concentrate. And for certain clinical conditions or surgical procedures, patients can be asked to get three or four units of blood, and in most cases the blood is eventually not transfused. Given that the average expenditure per capita on health in LMICs is 30 USD, these expenses and wastages can be catastrophic for patients and their families (WHO, 2014).

Until the establishment of NBSC in late 2021, there was no legal framework enabling any government entity to register blood establishments nationwide, probe their processes, and require facility mandatory reporting of adverse transfusion events (Ciepiela et al., 2017;, FRN, 2021; NBTS, 2020). This means that a comprehensive national database of recognized, regulated, and registered blood establishments is yet unavailable. The previous status quo therefore enabled all manner of unscrupulous and profiteering practices in blood services nationwide with dire consequences for the safety of Nigeria's blood donors and recipients.

Opportunities to Improve Access to and Availability of Safe Blood and Blood Products

Governance and Financing

A coordinated national blood transfusion service that can provide in a timely manner adequate supplies of safe blood and blood products for all patients who require it has been recommended by the WHO as a key to achieving blood safety in any country (WHO, 2011). To facilitate this, given Nigeria's political structure, with health being a sector on the concurrent legislative list (FRN, 1999), it is paramount that all state governments establish and operate their own SBTS with technical support and guidance from NBSC.

In 2016, at the 58th meeting of Nigeria's highest decision-making body for health, the National Council on Health (NCH) which held in Sokoto State, it was agreed that all state governments should be encouraged to establish SBTS and take over management of those states which already had (then) NBTS centres located in their states (NBTS, 2020).

By encouraging the establishment of SBTSs, more adequate funding will be available for regulation, coordination of blood services, public awareness, blood donor mobilization and engagement, staff training, quality equipment for highly sensitive laboratory screening of blood for transfusion, transportation and cold chain maintenance, waste disposal management, and other operations. At the hospital facility level, adequate governance includes the establishment and operationalization of Hospital Transfusion Committee. The key role of these committees is to ensure that blood and blood products are used appropriately, local policies governing transfusion processes are developed, clinicians are educated, and blood use within the hospital is audited regularly (Haynes & Torella, 2004).

Adequate financing is also vitally important for recruiting and retaining voluntary blood donors. Research conducted in West Africa revealed that media and communication strategies such as regular newsletters, group meetings, social media engagement, mobile telephone communication, radio and television dramas about blood donations in various local languages; and media celebration of donor milestones were critical to blood donor motivation (Appiah et al., 2013). These activities however do not come cheap.

Health Workforce and Service Delivery

The process of recruiting voluntary blood donors from the community can be quite complex and expensive (Bates et al., 2007). This relies heavily on blood drives held in various communities, some of which in LMICs can be quite remote. Certain useful community groups include faith-based groups, women groups, youth clubs, higher institutions of learning, and even schools where the message of blood donation can be shared for students to act upon when they reach the age of donation (18 years) (National Blood Service Commission [NBSC], 2022).

Earlier in this chapter, reference was made to the myths and misconceptions that trail blood donation in sub-Saharan Africa. These cultural beliefs and misconceptions especially those surrounding blood's relationship with personal health and kinship for individuals and societies are not so different from those that were held in England close to a century ago before blood donation became an acceptable practice there (Starr, 2002).

Therefore, well-trained staff and volunteers who can engage in community mobilization, public enlightenment, advocacy, client-centered care, donor motivation, recruitment, retention, and appreciation are required to promote blood donations, address these myths and misconceptions, and increase Nigeria's pool of safe blood. Additionally, expertise is required to counsel donors professionally, collect blood safely, and ensure appropriate storage and issuance of blood to hospitals.

Medical Technologies, Information, and Research

Presently, no comprehensive data platform exists which captures all blood transfusion data from across the NBSC zonal and state centers, and all the secondary level and tertiary health institutions in Nigeria. There is therefore significant potential for disruptive digital technologies to optimize the operations of blood services and blood establishments.

First, through donor management software platforms, coded and confidentially stored data could shorten the length of donor recruitment. The age range for blood donation in Nigeria is 18–65 years (NBSC, 2022). This is an economically productive age group, who would rather not spend an undue amount of time filling forms before donating blood. These time delays discourage many potential voluntary donors. Therefore, technology could shorten the process of blood donation, aid the recruitment of new blood donors, and keep returning donors motivated.

Secondly, using technology and artificial intelligence, specific blood donor groups can be matched with the groups of patients in need, enhancing speed of access to safe blood, and minimizing adverse transfusion reactions. Jela's Development Initiatives (JDI) is a non-governmental organization (NGO) which developed and launched *J Blood Match*, an Artificial Intelligence (AI) service in Nigeria aimed at directly connect willing blood donors and recipients at no cost (Abubakar, 2019; Simon, 2023). Third, drone-delivery of blood using unmanned aerial vehicles has made it possible to speedily deliver safe blood to remote locations, and according to Zipline, a medical logistics company, "reducing delivery time from four hours by road to 20 minutes, using drones that travel up to 100 km per hour at a time" (Onukwue, 2021, p. 1). While operational in Rwanda and Ghana, this technology has only fairly recently become available in Nigeria. Also, tech-forward companies such as Life Bank through partnerships with Google Nigeria map out locations, connecting facilities where blood needs to be transfused with blood banks and dispatch riders (Salaudeen, 2019).

Fourth, data on blood donation and transfusion is critical to haemovigilance, a vital aspect of blood regulation and involves collecting and evaluating all information on adverse events during blood donation and transfusion to improve donor and patient safety (Samukange et al., 2021). Finally, distilling information through research across the blood supply chain is necessary for evidence-based policy to enhance access and availability of safe blood.

Conclusion

Despite the numerous challenges surrounding the availability and access to safe and quality blood products for SCD warriors, opportunities exist to surmount them. Using the WHO health system framework to highlight these opportunities underlines the role of political willingness, and mobilizing people and communities towards enhancing access to life-saving blood and blood products equitably and sustainably. This will ensure that for Nigerians living with SCD and other conditions requiring safe blood, no one is left behind.

References

Abubakar, B. (2019). Meet your Match: J Blood Artificial Intelligence connects blood donors to receivers in the FCT. Retrieved March 7, 2022, from Nigeria Health Watch website: https://nigeriahealthwatch.com/meet-your-match-jblood-artificial-intelligence-connects-blood-donors-to-receivers-in-the-fct/

Adegoke, S. A., & Kuteyi, E. A. (2012). Psychosocial burden of sickle cell disease on the family, Nigeria. *African Journal of Primary Health Care & Family Medicine, 4*(1), 1–6. Retrieved from https://phcfm.org/index.php/phcfm/article/view/380/376

Aneke, J., & Okocha, C. (2017). Blood transfusion safety; current status and challenges in Nigeria. *Asian Journal of Transfusion Science, 11*(1), 1–5. https://doi.org/10.4103/0973-6247.200781

Appiah, B., Bates, I., Owusu-Ofori, S., & Dunn, A. (2013). Culturally relevant communication interventions to promote voluntary blood donations in Ghana: An observational, interview-based study. *The Lancet, 382*(Supplement 1), 8. https://doi.org/10.1016/s0140-6736(13)62169-8

Asamoah-Akuoko, L., Hassall, O. W., Bates, I., & Ullum, H. (2017). Blood donors' perceptions, motivators and deterrents in Sub-Saharan Africa – a scoping review of evidence. *British Journal of Haematology, 177*(6), 864–877. https://doi.org/10.1111/bjh.14588

Bates, I., Manyasi, G., & Lara, A. M. (2007). Reducing replacement donors in Sub-Saharan Africa: Challenges and affordability. *Transfusion Medicine, 17*(6), 434–442. https://doi.org/10.1111/j.1365-3148.2007.00798.x

Bloch, E. M., Vermeulen, M., & Murphy, E. (2012). Blood transfusion safety in Africa: A literature review of infectious disease and organizational challenges. *Transfusion Medicine Reviews, 26*(2), 164–180. https://doi.org/10.1016/j.tmrv.2011.07.006

Bonnar, J. (2000). Massive obstetric haemorrhage. *Best Practice & Research Clinical Obstetrics & Gynaecology*, *14*(1), 1–18. https://doi.org/10.1053/beog.1999.0060

Choudhury, N., Murthy, P. K., Chatterjee, R. K., Khan, M. A., & Ayyagari, A. (2003). Transmission of filarial infection through blood transfusion. *Indian Journal of Pathology & Microbiology*, *46*(3), 367–370.

Ciepiela, O., Jaworska, A., Łacheta, D., Falkowska, N., Popko, K., & Demkow, U. (2017). Awareness of blood group and blood donation among medical students. *Transfusion and Apheresis Science*, *56*(6), 858–864. https://doi.org/10.1016/j.transci.2017.10.002

Diaku-Akinwumi, I. N., Abubakar, S. B., Adegoke, S. A., Adeleke, S., Adewoye, O., Adeyemo, T., ... Kangiwa, G. U. (2016). Blood transfusion services for patients with sickle cell disease in Nigeria. *International Health*, *8*(5), 330–335. https://doi.org/10.1093/inthealth/ihw014

Edwards, C. L., Scales, M. T., Loughlin, C., Bennett, G. G., Harris-Peterson, S., Castro, L. M. D., ... Killough, A. (2005). A brief review of the pathophysiology, associated pain, and psychosocial issues in sickle cell disease. *International Journal of Behavioral Medicine*, *12*(3), 171–179. https://doi.org/10.1207/s15327558ijbm1203_6

Estcourt, L. J., Kohli, R., Hopewell, S., Trivella, M., & Wang, W. C. (2020). Blood transfusion for preventing primary and secondary stroke in people with sickle cell disease. *Cochrane Database of Systematic Reviews*, *7*(7), CD003146. https://doi.org/10.1002/14651858.cd003146.pub4

Federal Republic of Nigeria. (2014). National Health Act. Official Gazette Government Notice No. 208 2014; Lagos: Federal Government of Nigeria FGP 156/122015/1.200. Retrieved February 28, 2022, from National Blood Service Commission website: https://nbsc.gov.ng/wp-content/uploads/2022/05/National-Health-Act-FGN-2014.pdf

Federal Republic of Nigeria. (2021). National Blood Service Commission Act. Official Gazette Government Notice No. 186 2021; Lagos: Federal Government of Nigeria FGP 153/092021/250. Retrieved February 28, 2022, from National Blood Service Commission website: https://nbsc.gov.ng/wp-content/uploads/2022/05/National-Blood-Service-Commission-Act-2021.pdf

Federal Republic of Nigeria. (1999). Constitution of the Federal Republic of Nigeria. Retrieved February 28, 2022, from National Human Rights Commission website: https://nigeriarights.gov.ng/files/constitution.pdf

Fraiwan, A., Hasan, M. N., An, R., Rezac, A. J., Kocmich, N. J., Oginni, T., ... Gurkan, U. A. (2019). Advancing healthcare outcomes for sickle cell disease in Nigeria using Mobile health tools. *Blood*, *134*(Supplement_1), 2173. https://doi.org/10.1182/blood-2019-131344

Garraud, O., Filho, L. A., Laperche, S., Tayou-Tagny, C., & Pozzetto, B. (2016). The infectious risks in blood transfusion as of today – A no black and white situation. *La Presse Médicale*, *45*(7–8), e303–e311. https://doi.org/10.1016/j.lpm.2016.06.022

Hassall, O., Bates, I., & M'baya, B. (2020). 19 - Blood transfusion in resource-limited settings. In E. T. Ryan, D. R. Hill, T. Solomon, N. E. Aronson, & T. P. Endy (Eds.), *Hunters tropical medicine and emerging infectious diseases* (10th edition, pp. 153–158). Elsevier.

Haynes, S. L., & Torella, F. (2004). The role of hospital transfusion committees in blood product conservation. *Transfusion Medicine Reviews*, *18*(2), 93–104. https://doi.org/10.1016/j.tmrv.2003.12.005

Howard, J. (2016). Sickle cell disease: When and how to transfuse. *Hematology*, *2016*(1), 625–631. https://doi.org/10.1182/asheducation-2016.1.625

Howard, J., & Telfer, P. (2015). *Sickle cell disease in clinical practice*. Springer. https://doi.org/10.1007/978-1-4471-2473-3

Jani, I. V., & Peter, T. F. (2022). Nucleic acid point-of-care testing to improve diagnostic preparedness. *Clinical Infectious Diseases*, *75*(4), 723–728. https://doi.org/10.1093/cid/ciac013

Kitchen, A. D., & Chiodini, P. L. (2006). Malaria and blood transfusion. *Vox Sanguinis*, *90*(2), 77–84. https://doi.org/10.1111/j.1423-0410.2006.00733.x

Loua, A., Nikiema, J., Kasilo, O., & Tagny, C. T. (2018). Blood safety and availability in the WHO African region. *Global Surgery*, *4*(4), 1–7. https://doi.org/10.15761/gos.1000189

Lund, T. C., Hume, H., Allain, J. P., McCullough, J., & Dzik, W. (2013). The blood supply in Sub-Saharan Africa: Needs, challenges, and solutions. *Transfusion and Apheresis Science*, *49*(3), 416–421. https://doi.org/10.1016/j.transci.2013.06.014

Martone, G. M., Nanjireddy, P. M., Craig, R. A., Prout, A. J., Higman, M. A., Kelly, K. M., & Ambrusko, S. J. (2021). Acute hepatic encephalopathy and multiorgan failure in sickle cell disease and COVID-19. *Pediatric Blood and Cancer*, *68*(5), e28874. https://doi.org/10.1002/pbc.28874

Muthivhi, T. N., Olmsted, M. G., Park, H., Sha, M., Raju, V., Mokoena, T., ... Reddy, R. (2015). Motivators and deterrents to blood donation among Black South Africans: A qualitative analysis of focus group data. *Transfusion Medicine*, *25*(4), 249–258. https://doi.org/10.1111/tme.12218

National Blood Service Commission. (2022). *Operational guidelines for blood transfusion practice in Nigeria* (2nd edition). Retrieved March 7, 2022, from National Blood Service Commission website: https://nbsc.gov.ng/wp-content/uploads/2022/05/OPERATIONAL%20GUIDELINES%20FOR%20BLOOD%20TRANSFUSION%20PRACTICE%20IN%20NIGERIA.pdf

National Blood Transfusion Service (NBTS). (2020). Ten-Year Strategic Plan Planning a future for a Safe, Quality, Regulated, Coordinated and Accessible Blood System in Nigeria 2021–2030. Retrieved February 28, 2022, from National Blood Service Commission website: https://nbsc.gov.ng/wp-content/uploads/2022/05/NBTS-10-YEAR-STRATEGIC-PLAN-2021-2030.pdf

National Heart Lung and Blood Institute. U.S Department of Health and Human Services. (2014). *Evidence Report Quick Guide Evidence-Based Management of Sickle Cell Disease Expert Panel Report, 2014: Guide to Recommendations*. Retrieved from https://www.nhlbi.nih.gov/sites/default/files/media/docs/Evd-Bsd_SickleCellDis_Rep2014.pdf

Nda-Isaiah, J. (2020). Need for Blood Safety Crisis regulation, quality, and innovation in Nigeria. Retrieved March 4, 2022, from Leadership NG website: https://leadership.ng/need-for-blood-safety-crisis-regulation-quality-innovation/

Onukwue, A. (2021). Zipline needs Nigeria to support its drone delivery medical service – as Rwanda and Ghana did. Retrieved March 7, 2022, from Quartz website: https://qz.com/africa/2086752/what-zipline-brings-to-nigeria-after-5-years-in-rwanda-and-ghana/

Oreh, A. C. (2020). Is COVID-19 convalescent plasma an option for Africa? *Africa Sanguine*, *22*(2), 1–2. https://doi.org/10.4314/asan.v22i2.1

Oreh, A. C., Irechukwu, C., Biyama, F., Nnabuihe, A., Ihimekpen, A., Oshiame, D., ... Amedu, O. J. (2022). COVID-19 impact on Nigeria's national blood service commission – lessons for low- and middle-income countries (LMICs). *The Nigerian Postgraduate Medical Journal*, *29*(1), 6–12. https://doi.org/10.4103/npmj.npmj_720_21

Ossai, E. N., Eze, N. C., Chukwu, O., Uguru, U. A., Ukpai, E. C., & Ihere, E. (2018). Determinants of practice of blood donation among undergraduate students of Ebonyi State University Abakaliki, Southeast Nigeria. *Archives of Community Medicine and Public Health*, *4*(1), 001–007.

Oteng-Ntim, E., Ayensah, B., Knight, M., & Howard, J. (2015). Pregnancy outcome in patients with sickle cell disease in the UK – a national cohort study comparing sickle cell anaemia (HbSS) with HbSC disease. *British Journal of Haematology, 169*(1), 129–137. https://doi.org/10.1111/bjh.13270

Pirozzolo, J. J., & LeMay, D. C. (2007). Blood-borne infections. *Clinics in Sports Medicine, 26*(3), 425–431. https://doi.org/10.1016/j.csm.2007.04.010

Pruett, C. R., Vermeulen, M., Zacharias, P., Ingram, C., Tayou Tagny, C., & Bloch, E. M. (2015). The use of rapid diagnostic tests for transfusion infectious screening in Africa: A literature review. *Transfusion Medicine Reviews, 29*(1), 35–44. https://doi.org/10.1016/j.tmrv.2014.09.003

Rath, W. H. (2011). Postpartum hemorrhage – update on problems of definitions and diagnosis. *Acta Obstetricia et Gynecologica Scandinavica, 90*(5), 421–428. https://doi.org/10.1111/j.1600-0412.2011.01107.x

Roberts, D., Kitchen, A., Field, S., Bates, I., Allain, J., & Delaney, M. (2017). Blood transfusion in a global context. In M. Murphy, D. Roberts, & M. Yazer (Eds.), *Practical transfusion medicine* (5th edition, pp. 254–263). Wiley-Blackwell.

Salaudeen, A. (2019). This company is powering blood donations in Nigeria through Google maps. Retrieved March 8, 2022, from CNN website: https://edition.cnn.com/2019/08/23/africa/lifebank-nigeria-intl/index.html

Samukange, W. T., Kluempers, V., Porwal, M., Mudyiwenyama, L., Mutoti, K., Aineplan, N., … Nuebling, C. M. (2021). Implementation and performance of haemovigilance systems in 10 sub-Saharan African countries is sub-optimal. *BMC Health Services Research, 21*(1), 1258. https://doi.org/10.1186/s12913-021-07235-0

Shenga, N., Pal, R., & Sengupta, S. (2008). Behavior disparities towards blood donation in Sikkim, India. *Asian Journal of Transfusion Science, 2*(2), 56–60. https://doi.org/10.4103/0973-6247.42692

Simon, S. (2023). Nigerian organization launches software to address unpaid blood donations. Retrieved May 23, 2023, from Voice of Nigeria website: https://von.gov.ng/nigerian-organization-launches-software-to-address-unpaid-blood-donations/#:~:text=Nigerian%20organization%20launches%20software%20to%20address%20unpaid%20blood

Starr, D. (2002). *Blood: An epic history of medicine and commerce* (1st edition, pp. 1–310). Harper Collins.

Tagny, C. T., Mbanya, D., Tapko, J.-B., & Lefrère, J.-J. (2008). Blood safety in sub-Saharan Africa: A multi-factorial problem. *Transfusion, 48*(6), 1256–1261. https://doi.org/10.1111/j.1537-2995.2008.01697.x

Tancred, T., & Bates, I. (2019). Improving blood transfusion services. *Best Practice & Research Clinical Obstetrics & Gynaecology, 61*. https://doi.org/10.1016/j.bpobgyn.2019.05.007

Ugwu, N., Oti, W., Ugwu, C., & Uneke, C. (2019). Voluntary non-remunerated blood donation: Awareness, perception, and attitude among potential blood donors in Abakaliki, Nigeria. *Nigerian Journal of Clinical Practice, 22*(11), 1509–1515. https://doi.org/10.4103/njcp.njcp_159_19

Wang, W. C., & Dwan, K. (2013). Blood transfusion for preventing primary and secondary stroke in people with sickle cell disease. *The Cochrane Database of Systematic Reviews,* (11), CD003146. https://doi.org/10.1002/14651858.CD003146.pub2

World Health Organization. (2011). Aide-mémoire for ministries of health: developing a national blood system. Retrieved March 7, 2022, from www.who.int website: https://www.who.int/publications/i/item/WHO-EHT-11.01

World Health Organization. (2021). Global status report on blood safety and availability 2021. Retrieved from www.who.int website: https://www.who.int/publications-detail-redirect/9789240051683

World Health Organization. (2022). Blood safety and availability. Retrieved May 22, 2022, from WHO.int website: https://www.who.int/news-room/fact-sheets/detail/blood-safety-and-availability

World Health Organization. Regional Office for Africa, Tapko, J. B., Mainuka, P., & Diarra-Nama, A. J. (2009). Status of blood safety in the WHO African Region: Report of the 2006 Survey. In *apps.who.int*. World Health Organization. Regional Office for Africa. Retrieved from https://apps.who.int/iris/handle/10665/364673

World Health Organization. Regional Office for Africa. (2014). WHO African Region Expenditure Atlas, November 2014. In *apps.who.int*. World Health Organization. Retrieved from https://apps.who.int/iris/handle/10665/145197

Zanin, T. Z., Hersey, D. P., Cone, D. C., & Agrawal, P. (2016). Tapping into a vital resource: Understanding the motivators and barriers to blood donation in Sub-Saharan Africa. *African Journal of Emergency Medicine*, 6(2), 70–79. https://doi.org/10.1016/j.afjem.2016.02.003

Index

For Product Safety Concerns and Information please contact our EU
representative GPSR@taylorandfrancis.com
Taylor & Francis Verlag GmbH, Kaufingerstraße 24, 80331 München, Germany

www.ingramcontent.com/pod-product-compliance
Lightning Source LLC
Chambersburg PA
CBHW052118230326
41598CB00080B/3817

9 7 8 1 0 3 2 7 3 3 8 5 2